Volume 29, Number 1 — 1999

JOURNAL OF

DRUG
EDUCATION

CONTENTS

Executive Editor:

SEYMOUR EISEMAN, DR.P

Baywood Publishing Company, Inc.

ISSN 0047-2379

Journal of DRUG EDUCATION

EXECUTIVE EDITOR
SEYMOUR EISEMAN, DR. P.H.
Department of Health Sciences
California State University, Northridge

The *Journal of Drug Education* is a peer-refereed journal.

Journal of Drug Education is noted in: *Abstracts on Criminology and Penology; Academic Abstracts; Adolescent Mental Health Abstracts AGRICOLA; ALCONARC: ASSIA: All-Russian Institute of Scientific and Technical Information; Applied Social Sciences Index & Abstracts; Cambridge Scientific Abstracts; Cancer Prevention and Control Database; Counseling and Personnel Services Information Center; Criminal Justice Abstracts; Criminology, Penology and Police Service Abstracts; Current Contents; Current Index to Journals in Education; Cumulative Index to Nursing & Allied Health Literature (CINAHL); Dokumentation Gefahrdung durch Alkohol, Rauchen, Drogen, Arzneimittel; Drug Abuse and Alcoholism Review; EMBASE/Excerpta Medica; Health Promotion and Education Database; International Bibliography of Periodical Literature; International Bibliography of Book Reviews; International Pharmaceutical Abstracts; Kindex Medicus; MEDLINE; NCJRS Catalog; National Institute on Alcohol Abuse and Alcoholism's Alcohol and Alcohol Problems Science Database, ETOH; Psychological Abstracts; Smoking and Health Database; Safety and Health at Work ILO-CIS Bulletin;* and *Sociological Abstracts, Inc.*

The *Journal of Drug Education* is published by the Baywood Publishing Company, Inc., 26 Austin Ave., P.O. Box 337, Amityville, NY 11701. Subscription rate per Volume (four issues): Institutional—$160.00 Individual—$45.00 (prepaid by personal check or credit card). Add $6.50 per volume for postage inside the U.S. and Canada and $11.75 elsewhere. Back list volumes are available at $149.60. Subscription is on a volume basis only and must be prepaid. Copies of single issues are not available. No part of this journal may be reproduced in any form without written permission from the publisher.

J. DRUG EDUCATION, Vol. 29(1) 1-3, 1999

EDITORIAL: CONSENSUS STATEMENT, 14th JULY 1997 OF THE FARMINGTON CONFERENCES

The purpose of *this* statement is to define the basis for shared identity, commitment, and purpose among journals publishing in the field of psychoactive substance use and associated problems. Our aim has enhanced the quality of our endeavors in this multidisciplinary field. We share common concerns and believe that we do well to join together in their solution. To that end we accede to this document as a statement of our consensus and as basis for future collaboration.

1. Commitment to the peer review process

1.1 We are committed to peer review and would expect research reports and scientific reviews to go through this process. As regards the extent to which other material will be so reviewed, we see that as a matter for editorial discretion, but policies should be declared.

1.2 Referees *should be told* that their access to the article on which they have been requested to commit is in strict confidence. Confidentiality should not be broken by pre-publication statements on the content of the submission. Manuscripts sent to reviewers should be returned to the editor or destroyed.

1.3 Referees *should be asked* to declare to the editor if they have a conflict of interest in relation to the material which they are invited to review, and if in doubt they should consult the editor. We define "conflict of interest" as a situation in which professional, personal, or financial considerations could be seen by a fair-minded person as potentially in conflict with independence of judgement. Conflict of interest is not in itself wrong-doing.

2. Expectations of authors

2.1 **Authorship:** All listed authors on an article should have been personally and substantially involved in the work leading to the article.

1

2.2 Avoidance of double publication: Authors are *expected to ensure* that no significant part of the submitted material has been published previously and that it is not concurrently being considered by another journal. An exception to this general position may be made when previous publication has been limited to another language, to local publication in report, or publication of a conference abstract. All such instances, we would expect authors should consult the editor. Editors are encouraged to develop policies concerning electronic publication. Authors are asked to provide the editor at the time of submission with copies of published or submitted reports that *are related to that submission.*

2.3 Sources of funding for the submitted paper must be declared *and will be published.*

2.4 Conflicts of interest experienced by authors: *Authors should* declare to the editor if their relationship with any type of funding source might fairly be construed as exposing them to potential conflict of interest.

2.5 Protection of human and animal rights: *Where applicable* authors *should* give an assurance that ethical safeguards have been met.

2.6 Technical preparation of articles: We will publish guidance for authors on the technical preparation of articles with the form of instruction at the discretion of individual journals.

3. Formal response to breach of expectations by an author

3.1 Working in collaboration with our authors, we have a responsibility to support the expectations of good scientific publishing practice. To that end each journal will have defined policies for response to attempted or actual instances of *duplicate* publicatplagiarismarism, or scientific fraud.

4. Maintaining editorial independence

4.1 *We are committed to independence in the editorial process. To the extent the owner or another body may influence the editorial process, this should be declared, and in that case any sources of support from the alcohol, tobacco, pharmaceutical, or other relevant interests should be published in the journal.*

4.2 *We will publish declarations on any sources of support received by a journal, and will maintain openness in regard to connections which a journal or its editorial staff may have established which could reasonably be construed as conflict of interest.*

4.3 Funding for journal supplements: when we publish journal supplements, an indication will be given of any sources of support for their production.

4.4 **Refereeing journal supplements:** An editorial note will be published to indicate whether it has or has not been peer reviewed.

4.5 **Advertising:** Acceptance of advertising will be determined by, or in consultation with, the editor of each journal.

Seymour Eiseman

FOCUS ON ALCOHOL

Edited by SEYMOUR EISEMAN

PRIMARY ORIENTATION: **prevention of drug misuse**
A must for the drug educator

To adequately address and deal with the detrimental effects of alcohol, attempts must be made to learn and understand the motivations and attitudes which contribute to its use and misuse.

This essential collection represents a psychosocial perspective of the effects of alcohol while providing relatively unknown—but central research needed for a comprehensive understanding of the behaviors associated with alcohol use.

Table of Contents

Format: 6' × 9", 272 pages, Paper, ISBN: 0-89503-083-7

Price: $35.95 + $4.00 postage and handling

Baywood Publishing Company, Inc.
26 Austin Avenue, Amityville, NY 11701
call (516) 691-1270 **fax** (516) 691-1770 **orderline** (800) 638-7819
e-mail: baywood@baywood.com ● **web site:** http://baywood.com

J. DRUG EDUCATION, Vol. 29(1) 5-24, 1999

IS THERE EVIDENCE TO SHOW THAT FETAL ALCOHOL SYNDROME CAN BE PREVENTED?*

MAJELLA G. MURPHY-BRENNAN, B.A. (HONS.)

TIAN P. S. OEI, PH.D.

The University of Queensland, Australia

ABSTRACT

Fetal Alcohol Syndrome (FAS) is currently the major cause of mental retardation in the Western world. Since FAS is not a natural phenomenon and is created by mixing alcohol and pregnancy, the solution to decreasing the incidence of all alcohol-related birth defects is therefore entirely preventable. To date, little is known about the effectiveness of prevention programs in reducing the incidence of FAS. Therefore, it is the intention of this article to review the effectiveness of prevention programs in lowering the incidence of FAS. The present review revealed that prevention programs, to date, have been successful in raising awareness of FAS levels across the groups examined. However, this awareness has not been translated into behavioral changes in "high risk" drinkers as consumption levels in this group have decreased only marginally, indicating prevention programs have had minimal or no impact in lowering the incidence of FAS. Urgent steps must now be taken to fully test prevention programs, and find new strategies involving both sexes, to reduce and ultimately eliminate the incidence of FAS.

Since the recognition of Fetal Alcohol Syndrome (FAS) in the late 1960s, research has focused mainly on the characteristics and problems associated with FAS. There is no doubt now that maternal alcohol consumption during the conceptual period, and throughout pregnancy, has serious effects on the health of the

*This article was partially supported by grants from NH + MRC and ARC to Dr. Oei.

developing embryo and fetus [1-6]. It is also known that the damage to a child born with alcohol-related birth defects, such as FAS and Fetal Alcohol Effects (FAE), is irreversible and permanent. Since FAS and FAE are not natural phenomena and totally created by human beings by mixing alcohol and pregnancy, the solution to decreasing the incidence of all alcohol-related birth defects is entirely preventable. In fact, it is argued that prevention is the only solution to FAS and FAE.

Despite being totally preventable FAS still remains the major cause of mental retardation with a known aetiology in the developed world, surpassing Down's syndrome, cerebral palsy, and spina bifida [7]. In addition, FAS is the third most common cause of congenital defects in newborns [8, 9]. In Australia, a nation with one of the highest alcohol consumption rates in the Western world [10], health authorities acknowledge alcohol consumption as the casual factor in the development of FAS [11].

While there has been sufficient literature examining the characteristics and problems of FAS and FAE, research now needs to expand beyond the interventionist approach and focus more on appropriate preventable measures. To date, little is known about the effectiveness of educative prevention programs in lowering the incidence of FAS and FAE. Therefore, it is the aim of this article to examine the efficacy of prevention programs in FAS and FAE. The present review is divided into two major parts. Part one consists of prevalence and general information on clinical factors of FAS and FAE. This sets the stage for part two which reviews the empirical evidence of prevention programs.

Several criteria were established to select empirically-based studies for inclusion in this review. Only those studies that specifically investigated prevention programs about alcohol use during pregnancy, as opposed to drug use in general, were included. In addition, secondary prevention programs aimed at educating pregnant women of the dangers of alcohol use during pregnancy, were also included. Those studies that related to consumption patterns and reduction of alcohol intake only with pregnant women, were not included as empirical evidence for this had been addressed by other authors [12, 13]

CLINICAL FEATURES OF FAS AND FAE

Children exposed to alcohol consumption in-utero exhibit characteristics which range along a continuum from extremely severe symptoms to milder manifestations. Extensive research findings have established FAS in its most severe form causes lifetime disabilities [4, 5, 8]. The most widely used classification system, the *International Classification of Diseases, Tenth Revision, Clinical Modification* (ICD-10-CM), used for identifying the major characteristics associated with FAS, clusters symptoms into five main areas. These are central nervous system

(CNS) deficits, growth retardation, facial and skeletal abnormalities, behavioral problems, and miscellaneous abnormalities [14, 15]. When children display symptoms in each of these categories a diagnosis of FAS is made.

Mental retardation is the most debilitating and frequently occurring CNS abnormality found in approximately 44 percent of children with FAS [4]. The degree of mental retardation has been linked to the severity of physical abnormalities. In particular, microcephaly (i.e., small head circumference below the third percentile) is related to deficient brain growth [4]. Sensory hypersensitivity in the form of exaggerated responses to the environment also contributes to learning and behavioral problems, eating and sleeping irregularities, and hyperactivity [2].

Growth deficiencies, in both height and weight, are observed in FAS children with many remaining small in size with no significant catch-up growth throughout childhood [15]. Facial anomalies also differentiate infants with FAS from normal children. Narrow forehead, lowset ears, short eye slits, epicanthal folds, short upturned nose, cleft palate, and thin upper lip are the most commonly noted facial malformations. Skeletal deformities affecting fingers, toes, and feet are not uncommon [1].

Miscellaneous abnormalities, such as speech and language deficits, and motor dysfunction demonstrate the variability associated with the diagnosis of FAS. Furthermore, behavioral problems (e.g., attention deficit disorder) are evident throughout childhood with adolescents displaying deviant behaviors uncharacteristic of children with other types of mental retardation (e.g., Down's syndrome) [16].

Children affected by FAE experience some of, but not all, the characteristics associated with FAS. FAE is the single most prevalent cause of cognitive dysfunction [15]. Children with FAE usually display deficits encompassing learning disabilities, hyperactivity with attention deficit, impulsivity, short attention span, and are developmentally delayed in comparison to other children. Despite these problems most children with FAE exhibit intellectual functioning within the normal range [14]. Kleinfeld [17] has noted, undiagnosed children are often labelled as being wilful, difficult, and disruptive in behavior [14]. In addition, a proportion of children with FAE have some of the physical and facial abnormalities characteristic of FAS.

The weight of literature clearly shows that the clinical factors of FAS and FAE are directly related to alcohol consumption [18, 19].

PREVALENCE OF FAS AND FAE

The exact prevalence of FAS is difficult to determine due to the use of different diagnostic criteria by professionals, difficulty in identifying the constellation of features at birth, case finding methodologies, professional under reporting, and prevalence rates between different population subgroups [20]. A review of medical records, which assessed the usefulness of the ICD-9-CM classification code 760.71 in identifying FAS, found American statistics do not reflect full FAS. Instead, figures tend to only reflect developmental and behavioral problems in children associated with in-utero exposure to alcohol.

Recent conservative estimates based on prospectively collected data (i.e., examining births that occurred while the study was in progress) suggest the overall rate for FAS in the Western world is .29 per 1000 for Caucasians and .48 per 1000 for African Americans [21].

Widespread research collating data from different countries (e.g., United States, Canada, United Kingdom, Sweden, New Zealand, and Australia) supports general population estimates of between one and three per 1000 live births for full diagnosis of FAS [21, 22]. These incidence rates have been confirmed by reports from Australian obstetric hospitals [23].

Official statistics are not available in Australia as many authorities do not consider FAS and FAE notifiable disorders. Possibly, clinically recognizable FAS represents only the tip of the iceberg with many cases remaining undiagnosed at birth. Instead, alcohol-related birth defects are classified into the ICD-9-CM code 655.4 category, which includes suspected damage to the fetus from other diseases in the mother. This classification is ambiguous as a number of other maternal conditions affecting the fetus are assigned to this code [11]. As a result, health authorities, despite acknowledging FAS, have concluded there is insufficient evidence to support birth defects are caused by alcohol consumption during pregnancy [11]. However, in the absence of local data, American figures of 1.9 per 1000 live births have been applied to Australian Bureau of Statistics birth data [24]. This figure suggests approximately 500 children are born annually in Australia with a full diagnosis of FAS.

It has been estimated FAS births average twenty-five per 1000 in women who are chronic sufferers of alcoholism, with 17 percent of children dying in the first week of life from heart failure, upper respiratory tract infections, or convulsions [1]. High estimates have also been associated with indigenous populations in Australia, who comprise the highest recorded percentage of problem drinkers worldwide [23]. In addition, an increased prevalence of FAS has been linked to indigenous groups in the United States and Canada [7].

Far more widespread is FAE which affects a greater number of families, many of whom are not identified as having an alcohol consumption problem [16]. Current statistics estimate the incidence of FAE to occur in approximately five to six per 1000 live births [22]. In terms of Australian figures, this reflects a conservative estimate of approximately 1600 births diagnosed per annum based on recent census date [24].

THE IDENTIFICATION OF "AT RISK" GROUPS

An important step in implementing prevention programs is to identify and target *at risk* populations. The targeting of these groups with specialized prevention programs will help in decreasing the incidence of FAS in the future. At the extreme end of the continuum, all fertile sexually-active women who consume alcohol could be identified as being *at risk*. It must also be noted, birth rates for teenagers and women between the age of thirty and forty-four years are on the increase [24].

Research has shown that heavy drinkers are significantly more likely to be African America, poorly educated, and multiparous, in comparison to moderate and light drinkers [25]. However, extensive clinical research by Mills and Graubard has identified women at most risk for alcohol consumption during pregnancy are of European descent, highly educated, twenty to thirty-four year olds [26]. Therefore, women who are not alcohol abusers/dependent, but for whom alcohol plays a role in social interaction, need to be targeted [27]. Research shows women most commonly quote social reasons for drinking alcohol, as opposed to drinking to experience the intoxicating effects of alcohol [28].

Female population subgroups at most risk in Australia are sexually-active teenagers, younger adults, career women, and female aboriginals. However, recent statistics indicate consumption levels in ethnic groups is low [10] minimizing the need for targeting specific cultural groups. The 1993 National Drug Strategy household survey found 50 percent of women drink alcohol at least one day per week [29]. In addition, 50 percent of teenage girls consume alcohol prior to fifteen years of age with two-thirds of young female drinkers classified as heavy drinkers, which represents the highest rate of any population group [29]. Also of concern is knowledge that younger adults (20 to 24 years) drink more heavily when they drink (i.e., binge drink), even though they drink less often than older groups [29].

Furthermore, American and Australian studies have confirmed between 55 and 88 percent of women drink at least once during pregnancy, while approximately 20 to 35 percent drink regularly throughout the gestational period [14, 25, 30]. Generally, consumption rates tend to be highest at conception with marked decreases in drinking patterns occurring on confirmation of pregnancy in the first trimester. Unfortunately, these drinking patterns are known to overlap with embryonic development [31].

Recent large-scale longitudinal studies by Bruce, Adams, and Shulman report percentage rates for American women drinking alcohol throughout pregnancy decreased from 53.8 percent for light drinking (defined in the present study as 1 to 6 drinks per week), in the three months prior to pregnancy to 15.1 percent in the final trimester of pregnancy [32]. Moderate consumption (i.e., 7 to 13 drinks per week) decreased from 3 percent to .30 percent while heavy drinking rates (i.e., 14 or more drinks per week) decreased from 1.3 percent to .13 percent.

These results, which in overall terms are in accordance with the Australian National Drug Strategy [33] statistics for women, show drinking levels in the conceptual period are excessive. This highlights the importance of targeting all sexually-active women of child-bearing age to reduce the incidence of alcohol-related birth defects.

O'Connor has revealed in remote regions 26 percent of pregnant Aboriginal women consume alcohol regularly throughout pregnancy, while 8 percent were reported highly intoxicated at least every week [34]. Furthermore, 25 percent of babies born to these women experienced growth retardation and poor nutrition. However, intervening with such "at risk" populations is a complex task which must account for the individual and cultural needs of each target group.

Reports comprised for Australian health authorities acknowledging alcohol consumption among pregnant Australian women is uncommon at harmful and hazardous levels [11] need to be treated cautiously. Meta-analytical studies by English et al., assessing alcohol intake in pregnant women, have been based on Tasmanian hospital surveys which may not reflect consumption levels on mainland Australia [11]. According to the Australian Bureau of Statistics, the state of Tasmania has the lowest overall alcohol consumption rates in Australia [10]. Such conclusions can be harmful to women, as by denying the true extent of maternal alcohol consumption in Australia these reports hamper the implementation of prevention programs.

REVIEW OF PREVENTION STRATEGIES—
AN OVERVIEW

The importance of prevention programs has been widely acknowledged. To date, two main approaches have been adopted in implementing FAS and FAE prevention programs. Primary prevention programs have targeted the wider community including children and adults of all ages. School-based programs have aimed to increase the level of awareness in children and adolescents. Community groups have also worked to support educational programs at all levels. In addition, media and industry-based programs have targeted the general population through advertising campaigns and warning labels on alcohol beverages.

Secondary prevention procedures have been aimed at pregnant women in the clinic to raise awareness of FAS and dangers associated with maternal alcohol consumption. Information disseminated through clinic-based programs has targeted "at risk" women to decrease or cease alcohol consumption. Culturally-oriented clinical programs have also targeted indigenous groups in America.

School-Based Programs

Despite an emphasis in scientific literature on the importance of targeting schools for implementing primary prevention programs, there remains a paucity of empirically-based research examining the effects of programs undertaken in the classroom. Parental consent, confidentiality issues, and the nature of the topic—pregnancy and alcohol—have conceivably imposed limitations on this research. The limited literature available on classroom-based programs has revealed that the dissemination of information to students about pregnancy and alcohol has been combined with general drug and alcohol educational programs [35, 36]. These programs have focused on drug abuse, unplanned pregnancy, and sexually transmitted diseases, with an emphasis on abstinence as opposed to addressing pregnancy and alcohol directly. Educational programs aimed at adolescents, in particular, need to be taken a step further. In developing specific programs for adolescents on pregnancy and alcohol, emphasis needs to be placed on pre-conception care; unplanned pregnancy; FAS and FAE; the teratogenic effects of alcohol; and problems confronted by parents of children with FAS and FAE.

Community-Based Programs

The role of community organizations has been important in educating at risk groups. Specialist programs on FAS have focused on high risk teenage groups exposed to substance abuse in the home, economically disadvantaged children, and those populations with high teenage pregnancy rates [37, 38]. Such programs have received strong community support despite a lack of direct parental involvement. Peer support programs aimed at teenagers can also be an important component of community-based programs [39, 40]. Research by Perry found peer-led drug abuse prevention programs focusing on life skills help teenagers with respect to drug related behavior [40]. Significant changes in attitudes and behavior were noted when compared with teacher-led programs [40]. Adolescents learning to support one another can offer assistance when encountering "high risk" situations.

Media Campaigns

Large-scale media campaigns have targeted the general population. Only newspapers, magazines, radio, and television advertising adopting a non-moralistic approach have been successful in changing attitudes toward the use of alcohol in pregnancy [41, 42]. Messages that have been linked to fear and lack information on how to affect behavioral change have been ineffective in changing drinking patterns and raising awareness of FAS and FAE [43]. In addition, public service announcements directed at women of child-bearing age recommending abstinence, or a decrease in drinking patterns, have had only a limited impact [3]. A major disadvantage of media campaigns is that high risk women are least responsive to the broad approach associated with this form of advertising.

Industry's Response to Prevention

The legislation of the Beverage Labelling Act in 1988 in the United States of America forced the alcohol industry to adopt responsibility for informing pregnant women of the risk of birth defects associated with alcohol consumption. As noted by Hankin, Sloan, Firestone, Ager et al. [44, 45], the labeling law is a social intervention designed to reduce the prevalence of all alcohol-related birth defects. Even prior to implementation the warning label concept received overwhelming support from all population subgroups surveyed, including heavy drinkers [46].

Within four months of the industry responding to this law a significant increase in awareness about the warning label occurred in young women [44] who comprise a high risk group. An overall decline in drinking patterns amongst lighter drinkers was also noted [42, 45]. However, despite these U.S. findings, the 1988 recommendation by the Australian College of Paediatrics that all alcoholic beverages should be labeled *Alcohol consumption during pregnancy is not recommended* is yet to be implemented in Australia.

Clinical Programs

A variety of clinically-based prevention programs have targeted both pregnant and nonpregnant women. At the individual level self-help programs, cognitive therapies, and behavioral management programs have been effective in helping the problem drinker. In particular, counseling has been effective in reducing alcohol consumption in alcohol abuse/dependence.

However, at a global level clinics have also been effective in educating pregnant women about the dangers of drinking, encouraging a reduction in consumption during pregnancy, and promoting abstinence in subsequent pregnancies. The distribution of pamphlets in antenatal clinics, combined with verbal instruction from medical professionals, has been effective in raising awareness of FAS and FAE [13]. However, written material in the form of well presented booklets has proven to be more popular among clinical clients. Knowledge also increased in pregnant adolescents when targeted by a clinically-based substance abuse educational program and 47.6 percent of subjects decreased or ceased substance abuse [47].

Culture-Specific Prevention Programs

A great deal of care has been taken in developing community based programs for indigenous North Americans which reflect cultural ways. Tribal health centers have had a positive impact in raising awareness of FAS and FAE in the local communities. The distribution of prenatal packages and implementation of school-based programs have raised awareness, with 50 percent of women able to describe some of the features of FAS [48] compared with 21 percent in the general population [49]. In addition, when pregnancy is diagnosed a drinking history is taken for each woman receiving prenatal care. Those who positively respond to alcohol consumption, regardless of amount, are referred to the "Fetal Alcohol Program" [50]. Over 90 percent of clients attending this program ceased drinking after undertaking education programs, viewing pictures and video tapes of children with FAS, and undergoing counseling.

A DESCRIPTION OF EMPIRICAL STUDIES

Table 1 displays a description of five studies chosen for analysis based on the selection criteria previously mentioned. The limited availability of empirically-based studies determined the type of prevention program to be reviewed. Studies addressed prevention across a range of populations including the general public, pregnant women, community samples, school children, and indigenous groups. Of the five studies reviewed, three focused on the effects of warning labels on alcoholic beverages as a means of raising awareness. One study addressed the combined effect of educational programs delivered by trained personnel dispensing print and video material. The final study adopted an innovative method of educating low-income women by using an interactive computer-based multimedia package.

Limitations occurred with two of the studies analyzed in Table 1 as non-randomized groups were used for date collection [see 38, 51]. The May et al. [38] study focused on indigenous people while Kinzie et al. [51] recruited low income women with low literacy levels as participants. Furthermore, three studies (refer to Table 1) focused on clinical populations with results indicative of awareness levels in pregnant women, but not representative when applied to the general population. Only the Hilton et al. [46] study utilized random sampling. In addition, control groups were not used for comparative studies. This can be justified in terms of clinical research as it would be unethical to identify pregnant women who consumed alcohol and withhold education and assistance. Large sample sizes were used with three of the five studies. Only one study, Kinzie et al., relied on a small sample set. Baseline data was not collected in any of the studies reviewed [51]. Despite the methodological flaws in the above studies all revealed an increase in awareness of FAS and the detriments associated with maternal alcohol consumption among the populations targeted. The large-scale study by Hankin and colleagues [44, 45], in terms of sample size and duration of the study, added weight to the interpretation of this research when all studies were compared. However, despite an increase in awareness of FAS and FAE, this knowledge was not reflected in a reduction in drinking patterns of high risk drinkers [45]. These results must be interpreted cautiously, as to reveal the true effectiveness of prevention programs well designed longitudinal studies are required. This research would need to monitor the reduction in alcohol consumption levels in women and decreased incidence of FAS, in conjunction with the use of prevention programs.

Table 1. Results of the Five Empirical Studies Reviewed on
Alcohol and Pregnancy

Study	n	Sample Demographics	Design
Hilton et al. (1991)	2006	General Population Males and Females (18-60+)	Telephone survey
Hankin et al. (1993a)	5169	Pregnant Women Mean age = 23.9 years	Antenatal screening questionnaire
Hankin et al. (1993b)	12026	Pregnant Women Mean age = 23.7 years	Antenatal screening questionnaire
May et al. (1989)	473	Schoolchildren ($n = 215$) Indigenous Community sample ($n = 258$)	Survey
Kinzie et al. (1993)	99	Pregnant women Time 1 $n = 40$ Time 2 $n = 59$	Antenatal clinic: Computer administered questions

Many advantages associated with prevention programs have been identified in the five studies reviewed. All studies reported increases in knowledge levels and/or support for public prevention campaigns (e.g., labeling, printed material). Warning labels on beverages have a place in prevention as they increase awareness of FAS and FAE in younger women and the nonrisk drinker [45]. Labeling alcoholic beverages has not been entirely effective as a decrease in alcohol consumption in heavier drinkers has not been found, which is consistent with the low response by this group to media campaigns [42, 45]. Pregnant at risk drinkers continue to consume alcohol despite warning labels. Hankin found prior success in pregnancy outcome, when combined with maternal alcohol consumption, accounted for continued alcohol consumption in ongoing pregnancies of those studied [42].

The macro-level FAS prevention program targeting indigenous Americans was successful in targeting all age groups from children in Grade 5 onward, as well as community and prenatal groups [38]. Pamphlets and fact sheets were distributed by trained personnel throughout the entire community with posters placed in strategic positions. Slides were also used in delivering the program to participants. Retention of knowledge evaluated in follow-up sessions showed

Type of Prevention Program	Duration	Results
Public support for warning labels on alcoholic beverages	2mths*	87 percent supported warning labels
Knowledge obtained from warning labels	3 years	Time series analysis showed awareness increased from 31 percent to 75 percent in three years
Reduction in consumption levels due to labeling	5 years	No decrease in drinking levels for risk drinkers
Awareness based on information presented by trained personnel, video, posters, leaflets, fact sheets	Not stated, 2-3 month follow-up	50 percent increase in knowledge gained in children and 71 percent increase in community sample, *84 percent of all groups retained knowledge on retest
Interactive computer-based alcohol education programs	Not stated	*75 percent to 81 percent of subjects increased knowledge levels

significant information retention with 84 percent of subjects still aware of FAS. The enthusiasm, motivation, and positivity generated by the trained personnel also contributed to the success of the program [38].

The innovative method of using an interactive computer-based multimedia package trialed by Kinzie et al., has taken advantage of technological advances [51]. Low-income poorly educated women in a rural region were targeted with this method. Of the two groups surveyed, 75 to 81 percent of subjects increased knowledge levels of FAS and FAE. Additionally, interest was expressed in other educational packages based on this system. Advantages of computer-based learning programs are that less demand is placed on staff, thus allowing health-care workers to become involved with clinical tasks, as well as reducing running costs. The disadvantage associated with using computer-based prevention programs is the initial installation costs.

Limitations are evident in the direction prevention strategies have adopted to date. Despite the increased awareness of the dangers associated with alcohol consumption and pregnancy, this knowledge has not necessarily resulted in behavioral change. The prevention programs reviewed identified the characteristics associated with FAS, and detriments of maternal alcohol consumption in pregnancy, but failed to offer strategies for behavioral modification. This possibly accounts for the failure of high risk drinkers to reduce alcohol consumption during pregnancy. Future programs need to be more specific and not only address the characteristics of FAS but detail the teratogenic effects of alcohol. Greater awareness of alcohol's effect on physiological processes in males and females, combined with effective psychological strategies for adopting behavior change, are essential. The continuation of specialist clinical intervention programs, and outreach, provided at an individual level must be maintained for high risk drinkers in addition to prevention programs.

IDENTIFYING EFFECTIVE APPROACHES IN PREVENTION

Effective preventative measures which are influential in adopting change are threefold. The importance of school-based and clinical programs provided in conjunction with support from community organizations, as adopted by indigenous groups in America, cannot be overemphasized. Due to the increasing changes in family structure, schools will continue to play an important role in prevention. The teenage population represents the most important group to target when implementing prevention programs for long-term success.

As noted by Amatetti, effective school-based prevention programs must move beyond the classroom and target the family, community, and society as a whole [35]. Adolescents can play a role in disseminating information to these groups through the distribution of leaflets provided in school programs [e.g., 52]. In addition, the alcohol industry can work with the community by sponsoring speakers to target women's groups, mothers at child care centers and preschools, as well as parent bodies attached to schools.

The successful components of culture-specific programs on FAS and FAE (i.e., outreach within the community, community-based workshops delivered by trained personnel, and distribution of printed material) can be adopted in raising the awareness of Aboriginal women in Australia. These programs could also be applied to the general population. Modeling the approach taken with North American Indian groups [e.g., 50] will be a positive step in adopting FAS prevention programs for Aboriginal women in Australia.

FUTURE DIRECTION FOR PREVENTION PROGRAMS

To date, access to prevention programs has been minimal despite the Australian College of Paediatrics recommendation supporting education of the general public about the risks associated with combining alcohol and pregnancy [53]. Overseas prevention programs have played a particularly important role in raising awareness of FAS as nations strive toward the World Health Organizations goal of reducing the incidence of FAS to 0.12 per 1000 by the year 2000 [49].

Generally speaking, prevention programs overseas have been successful in raising public awareness [54]. To achieve a successful outcome in implementing prevention programs in Australia, a multi-faceted approach needs to be adopted to significantly decrease the incidence of all alcohol-related birth defects, in particular, FAS and FAE.

First, acknowledgment of all alcohol-related birth defects by health authorities is essential. Training schemes need to target established medical professionals, as well as trainee students in health-related disciplines, in raising awareness of alcohol-related birth defects and care of clients. Health care providers need to play an active role in decreasing FAS and FAE by identifying and assisting women at risk. The compilation of a drinking history for all pregnant women should become a routine part of antenatal care. Also as part of routine clinical care a personal approach by health professionals, combined with the provision of printed material, is recommended for informing all pregnant women about the dangers associated with alcohol and pregnancy [55]. Pre-conception care courses are an ideal medium for informing women of dangers associated with alcohol consumption [56]. The provision of written material combined with verbal instruction has been found to decrease alcohol consumption levels in pregnant women [19, 52]. The inclusion of information on the effects of alcohol in planning pregnancy in these courses is warranted.

Second, schools need to be targeted as a primary source of disseminating information by increasing priority in human relations courses of the importance of health care prior to and during pregnancy. Moreover, an emphasis needs to be placed on the teratogenic effects of alcohol and detriments associated with binge drinking, by increasing awareness about the dangers associated with pregnancy and alcohol consumption. In addition, the focus needs to address relationship issues which encompass the importance of safe sex and planned pregnancy, as it has been suggested that a tripartite link exists between unprotected sex, unplanned pregnancy, and alcohol consumption [36].

Third, awareness in the general community can be increased through media exposure. Women need to be encouraged to modify social drinking habits as many remain unaware of their pregnancy in the important early stages. In addition, the alcohol and beverage industry needs to accept responsibility and acknowledge to consumers there are dangers associated with mixing alcohol and pregnancy. Labeling in America has been effective in educating younger women who, in Australia, comprise the highest risk group for alcohol consumption and unplanned pregnancy. However, a viable alternative in targeting all "at risk" women exists. The funding of prevention programs by the alcohol and beverage industry as a tax incentive could lessen the financial burden of implementing such programs.

Fourth, due to Australia's high alcohol consumption levels educational programs on pregnancy and alcohol need to address paternal drinking patterns as well. Recent research indicates alcohol affects the condition of the sperm, leading to behavioral problems and intellectual impairment in the offspring [57]. Furthermore, males can play an important role as a supportive person in helping to reduce alcohol consumption in pregnant partners, or those planning a pregnancy [3].

Finally, for Australia's indigenous people, specialist culture-specific programs that account for cultural values, traditions, and taboos need to be developed to target Aboriginal women [34]. Success will only be achieved when programs such as these are sanctioned by elders and delivered by indigenous women.

Prevention needs to be multifaceted to be effective, and this costs money. However, the lifetime care for one child with FAS costs the community approximately US$596,000 [58]. The cost of prevention cannot be argued, only the means of implementation. Furthermore, costs associated with the more prevalent FAE will also decrease, therefore, money channeled into prevention is dollars saved in long-term care.

ETHICAL CONCERNS RELATED TO PREVENTION ISSUES

The identification and targeting of women for the implementation of prevention programs is not without its problems. Civil liberties dictate that everyone has the right to drink alcohol by choice. Recent statements made by the Australian Medical Association, from an inquiry into fetal welfare and the law [59], support the rights of the mother ahead of those of the fetus [60]. Pregnant women in Australia have the legal right to consume alcohol during pregnancy, despite the well-documented damages associated with fetal development and in-utero alcohol exposure resulting in conditions such as FAS. However, in moral terms, one must question if women are ethically obliged to protect the health of the unborn child. To make such a choice, women first need to be informed of the dangers associated with maternal alcohol consumption.

The issue of fetal dependence upon the mother needs to be considered [61]. Extensive empirical evidence has chronicled the dangers to the fetus associated with alcohol consumption. Therefore, in terms of implementing prevention programs a shift in government policy and attitudes among professional bodies is warranted. Legislation needs to adopt a supportive approach, as laws that criminalize drinking women only exacerbate the problem [62]. More importantly, legislation which promotes just and balanced laws, with a positive outcome for both the mother and unborn child [63], will strengthen preventative efforts in targeting "at risk" women.

The role of health-care professionals also needs to be addressed. Reports by Lelong, Kaminski, Chwalow, Bean, and Subtil indicate those best able to assist women abstaining or at least decreasing alcohol consumption during pregnancy are partners, doctors, and midwives [64]. This study also highlighted 70 percent of heavy smokers who were advised to reduce their intake by the medical profession during pregnancy, while only 20 percent of heavy drinkers were advised to reduce alcohol consumption. An additional survey of American practitioners found only 53 percent questioned clients routinely about maternal drinking patterns [65]. With such widespread evidence documenting fetal deficits associated with alcohol consumption, the lack of information provision and support to clients from health-care professionals is disappointing, as women have the right to be informed. Health-care professionals have an important role to play in the detection, education, and, where necessary, referral of at risk pregnant clients [66].

In addition, the alcohol industry's failure to respond to the Australian College of Pediatricians recommendation should be addressed. Consumer groups need to target the marketing, availability, and labeling of alcoholic beverages aimed at women [67]. The introduction of health warnings on alcoholic beverages will raise awareness among women, even at a minimal level, and protect the alcohol industry from future litigation.

SUMMARY AND CONCLUSION

This article has reviewed the role of prevention in decreasing the incidence of FAS and FAE by raising awareness of "at risk" groups. The characteristics, mechanisms, and prevalence of FAS and FAE were addressed to increase knowledge of this identifiable syndrome and its partial effects. An analysis of prevention programs has drawn attention to successful strategies which can be modified and adapted for targeting "at risk" women worldwide. The identification of "at risk" women has found a number of groups—adolescents, binge drinkers, the social consumer, and indigenous women—need to be targeted for education. Most importantly, government health authorities and professional bodies need to be made more aware of the ethical issues concerning alcohol and pregnancy.

From the above research it can be concluded FAS is a disorder which, in time, can be reduced in prevalence with the implementation of effective prevention programs. Alcohol will continue to be a part of the social fabric of society, therefore, prevention programs to decrease alcohol-related birth defects are essential. Despite the ongoing need for prevention, programs so far have not been entirely successful in lowering the overall incidence of FAS. If the reduced prevalence rates obtained from clinical studies published by Abel and Sokol reflect population-based figures, FAS has decreased in America since the introduction of prevention strategies [21]. However, this finding needs to be replicated in population and community-based studies. An additional flaw in prevention programs has been reflected in alcohol consumption patterns in heavy drinkers, those at greatest risk. Only moderate success has been achieved in reducing consumption patterns in 'high risk' pregnant women as noted by the Hankin et al. [45] study.

Prevention strategies used to date have been effective in raising awareness levels, as the five studies reviewed found increased awareness levels across all groups. The challenge now becomes one of extending this so changes are reflected in behavior of both males and females. Prevention strategies need to take a new direction and focus on teaching strategies for behavioral change as a priority. Furthermore, there is sufficient evidence to support the implementation of prevention programs in Australia. However, to be successful prevention programs need to target specific "at risk" groups. The outcome of prevention programs for specialist groups has shown prevention strategies do work if tailored to the needs of the specific group [38].

Finally, the importance of implementing prevention programs to build awareness cannot be overemphasized as an early solution in targeting all "at risk" groups. Ongoing research is required to improve the present approaches in prevention so that maternal alcohol consumption continues to decrease across all groups. There is no safe level, or time, for consuming alcohol when pregnant or planning a pregnancy. Prevention is the only solution in decreasing the overall incidence of all alcohol-related birth defects.

REFERENCES

1. B. F. Williams, V. F. Howard, and T. F. McLaughlin, Fetal Alcohol Syndrome: Developmental Characteristics and Directions for Further Research, *Education and Treatment of Children, 17:*1, pp. 86-97, 1994.
2. L. Weiner and B. A. Morse, Intervention and the Child with FAS, *Alcohol Health & Research World, 18:*1, pp. 67-72, 1994.
3. E. J. Waterson and I. M. Murray-Lyon, Preventing Alcohol Related Birth Damage: A Review, *Social Science Medicine, 30:*3, pp. 349-364, 1990.
4. J. C. Overholser, Fetal Alcohol Syndrome: A Review of the Disorder, *Journal of Contemporary Psychotherapy, 20:*3, pp. 163-176, 1990.
5. L. Burd and J. T. Martsolf, Fetal Alcohol Syndrome: Diagnosis and Syndromal Variability, *Physiology & Behavior, 46,* pp. 39-43, 1989.
6. M. H. Kaufman, An Hypothesis Regarding the Origin of Aneuploidy in Man: Indirect Evidence from an Experimental Model, *Journal of Medical Genetics, 22,* pp. 171-178, 1985.
7. L. Phelps and J. Grabowski, Fetal Alcohol Syndrome: Diagnostic Features and Psychoeducational Risk Factors, *School Psychology Quarterly, 7:*2, pp. 112-128, 1992.
8. J. M. Aase, Clinical Recognition of FAS: Difficulties of Detection and Diagnosis, *Alcohol Health & Research World, 18:*1, pp. 5-9, 1994.
9. R. L. Bratton, Fetal Alcohol Syndrome: How You Can Help Prevent It, *Postgraduate Medicine, 98:*5, pp. 197-200, 1995.
10. Australian Bureau of Statistics, *1989-1990 National Health Survey: Alcohol Consumption, Australia* (Catalogue No. 4381.0), Australian Government Publishing Service, Canberra, 1992

11. D. R. English, C. D. J. Holman, E. Milne, M. G. Winter, G. K. Hulse, J. P. Codde, C. I. Bower, B. Corti, N. de Klerk, M. W. Knuiman, J. J. Kurinczuk, G. F. Lewin, and G. A. Ryan, *The Quantification of Drug Caused Morbidity and Mortality in Australia*, Commonwealth Department of Human Services and Health, Canberra, 1995.
12. J. B. Schorling, The Prevention of Prenatal Alcohol Use: A Critical Analysis of Intervention Studies, *Journal of Studies on Alcohol, 54:*3, pp. 261-267, 1992.
13. E. J. Waterson and I. M. Murray-Lyon, Preventing Fetal Alcohol Effects; A Trial of Three Methods of Giving Information in the Antenatal Clinic, *Health Education Research, 5:*1, pp. 53-61, 1990.
14. R. H. Short and G. C. Hess, Fetal Alcohol Syndrome: Characteristics and Remedial Implications, *Developmental Disabilities Bulletin,, 23:*1, pp. 12-29, 1995.
15. W. D. Ugent, M. H. Graf, and A. S. Ugent, Fetal Alcohol Syndrome: A Problem that School Psychologists Can Help Recognize, Treat, and Prevent, *School Psychology International, 7,* pp. 55-60, 1986.
16. A. P. Streissguth, A Long-Term Perspective of FAS, *Alcohol Health & Research World, 18:*1, pp. 74-81, 1994.
17. J. Kleinfeld, Fetal Alcohol Syndrome in Alaska: What the Schools Can Do, cited in *Fetal Alcohol Syndrome: Characteristics and Remedial Implications,* R. H. Short and G. C. Hess (eds.), *Developmental Disabilities Bulletin, 23:*1, pp. 12-29, 1995.
18. E. K. Michaelis and M. L. Michaelis, Cellular and Molecular Bases of Alcohol's Teratogenic Effects, *Alcohol Health & Research World, 18:*1, pp. 17-21, 1994.
19. G. A. Niccols, Fetal Alcohol Syndrome: Implications for Psychologists, *Clinical Psychology Review, 14:*2, pp. 91-111, 1994.
20. Morbidity Mortality Weekly Report, *Use of International Classification of Diseases Coding to Identify Fetal Alcohol Syndrome—Indian Health Service Facilities: 1981-1992, 44:*13, pp. 253-261, 1995.
21. E. L. Abel and R. J. Sokol, A Revised Conservative Estimate of the Incidence of FAS and its Economic Impact, *Alcoholism: Clinical Experimental Research, 15,* pp. 514-524, 1991.
22. E. L. Abel and R. J. Sokol, Incidence of Fetal Alcohol Syndrome and Economic Impact of FAS-Related Anomalies, *Drug and Alcohol Dependence, 19,* pp. 51-70, 1987.
23. T. Lipson, The Fetal Alcohol Syndrome in Australia, *The Medical Journal of Australia, 161,* pp. 461-462, 1994.
24. Australian Bureau of Statistics, *Births, Australia 1993* (Catalogue No. 3301.0), Australian Government Publishing Service, Canberra, 1994.
25. M. Behnke and F. D. Eyler, The Consequences of Prenatal Substance Use for the Developing Fetus, Newborn, and the Young Child, *The International Journal of the Addictions, 28:*13, pp. 1341-1391, 1993.
26. J. L. Mills and B. I. Graubard, Is Moderate Drinking during Pregnancy Associated with an Increased Risk for Malformations? *Pediatrics, 80,* pp. 309-314, 1987.
27. T. Remkes, Saying No—Completely, *Canadian Nurse, 89:*6, pp. 25-28, 1993.
28. E. J. Waterson and I. M. Murray-Lyon, Drinking and Smoking Patterns Amongst Women Attending an Antenatal Clinic—1: Before Pregnancy, *Alcohol & Alcoholism, 24:*2, pp. 153-162, 1989.

29. Department of Human Services and Health, *Statistics on Drug Abuse in Australia,* Australian Government Publishing Service, Canberra, 1994.
30. G. Kesby, G. Parker, and E. Barrett, Personality and Coping Sytle as Influences on Alcohol Intake and Cigarette Smoking During Pregnancy, *The Medical Journal of Australia, 155,* pp. 229-233, 1991.
31. M. Russell and J. B. Skinner, Early Measures of Maternal Alcohol Misuse as Predictors of Adverse Pregnancy Outcome, *Alcoholism, 12,* pp. 824-830, 1988.
32. F. C. Bruce, M. M. Adams, and H. B. Shulman, Alcohol Use Before and During Pregnancy, *American Journal of Preventative Medicine, 9:5,* pp. 267-273, 1993.
33. Department of Human Services and Health, *Statistics on Drug Abuse in Australia,* Commonwealth of Australia, Canberra, 1994.
34. M. C. O'Connor, Women's Business: An Introduction to the Cultural Aspects of Aboriginal Obstetric and Gynecological Care, *Perinatal Newsletter, 21,* pp. 3-6, 1993.
35. S. L. Amatetti, A Prevention Primer: Putting Theory to Work in the Classroom, *Alcohol Health & Research World, Summer Issue,* pp. 38-43, 1987.
36. L. Strunin and R. Hingson, Alcohol, Drugs and Adolescent Sexual Behaviour, *The International Journal of the Addictions, 27:2,* pp. 129-146, 1992.
37. F. R. Walton, V. D. Ackiss, and S. N. Smith, Education versus Schooling— Project LEAD: High Expectations! *Journal of Negro Education, 60:3,* pp. 441-453, 1991.
38. P. A. May and K. H. Hymbaugh, A Macro-Level Fetal Alcohol Syndrome Prevention Program for Native Americans and Alaska Natives: Description and Evaluation, *Journal of Studies on Alcohol, 50:6,* pp. 508-518, 1989.
39. K. L. Corn and D. D. Moore, Reach for the S.T.A.R.S.—Students Teaching and Reaching Students: A Two-Faceted Peer Facilitating Program at Greenfield-Central High School, *The School Counsellor, 40,* pp. 68-73, 1992.
40. C. L. Perry, Results of Prevention Programs with Adolescents, *Drug and Alcohol Dependence, 20,* pp. 13-19, 1987.
41. B. M. Ihlen, A. Amundsen, and L. Tronnes, Reduced Alcohol Use in Pregnancy and Changed Attitudes in the Population, *Addiction, 88,* pp. 389-394, 1993.
42. J. R. Hankin, FAS Prevention Strategies: Passive and Active Measures, *Alcohol Health & Research World, 18:*1, pp. 62-66, 1994.
43. L. Weiner, B. A. Morse, and P. Garrido, FAS/FAE: Focusing Prevention on Women at Risk, *The International Journal of the Addictions, 24:5,* pp. 385-395, 1989.
44. J. R. Hankin, J. J. Sloan, I. J. Firestone, J. W. Ager, R. J. Sokol, S. S. Martier, and J. Townsend, The Alcohol Beverage Warning Label: When Did Knowledge Increase? *Alcoholism: Clinical and Experimental Research, 17:2,* pp. 428-430, 1993a.
45. J. R. Hankin, J. J. Sloan, I. J. Firestone, J. W. Ager, R. J. Sokol, and S. S. Martier, A Time Series Analysis of the Impact of the Alcohol Warning Label on Antenatal Drinking. *Alcoholism: Clinical and Experimental Research, 17:2,* pp. 284-289, 1993b.
46. M. E. Hilton and L. Kaskutas, Public Support for Warning Labels on Alcoholic Beverage Containers, *British Journal of Addiction, 86,* pp. 1323-1333, 1991.

47. P. D. Sarvela and T. D. Ford, An Evaluation of a Substance Abuse Education Program for Mississippi Delta Pregnant Adolescents, *Journal of School Health, 63:*3, pp. 147-152, 1993.

48. K. Plaisier, Fetal Alcohol Syndrome Prevention in American Indian Communities of Michigan's Upper Michigan, *American Indian and Alaska Native Mental Health Research, 3:*1, pp. 16-33, 1989.

49. M. C. Dufour, G. D. Williams, K. E. Campbell, and S. S. Aitken, Knowledge of FAS and the Risk of Heavy Drinking during Pregnancy, 1985-1990, *Alcohol Health & Research World, 18:*1, pp. 86-92, 1994.

50. E. B. Harvey, Mental Health Promotion Among American Indian Children, *Arctic Medical Research, 54:*1, pp. 101-106, 1995.

51. M. B. Kinzie, J. B. Shorling, and M. Siegel, Prenatal Alcohol Education for Low-Income Women with Interactive Multimedia, *Patient Education and Counselling, 21,* pp. 51-60, 1993.

52. T. P. S. Oei and A. Baldwin, Smoking Prevention and Education Program: A Developmental Model, *Journal of Drug Education, 22,* pp. 155-188, 1991.

53. E. Tindle, A Can of Worms in a Hornet's Nest: Controversial Issues on Alcohol in Pregnancy, *Drugs in Society, 4,* pp. 32-36, 1991.

54. A. M Vener, L. R. Krupka, and M. D. Engelmann, Drugs in the Womb: College Student Perceptions of Maternal v. Fetal Rights, *Journal of Drug Education, 22:*1, pp. 15-24, 1992.

55. T. P. S. Oei, L. Anderson, and J. Wilks, Public Attitudes To and Awareness of Fetal Alcohol Syndrome in Young Adults, *Journal of Drug Education, 16:*2, pp. 135-147, 1986.

56. B. W. Jack and L. Culpepper, Preconception Care, *The Journal of Family Practice, 32:*3, pp. 306-315, 1991.

57. T. J. Cicero, Effects of Paternal Exposure to Alcohol on Offspring Development, *Alcohol Health & Research World, 18:*1, pp. 37-41, 1994.

58. G. Bloss, The Economic Cost of FAS, *Alcohol Health & Research World, 18:*1, pp. 53-54, 1994.

59. J. Seymour, Inquiry into Fetal Welfare and the Law, *Australian Health Law Bulletin, 2:*5, pp. 53-56, 1994.

60. G. Schloss, Foetal Rights "Second to Mum," *The Courier Mail,* April 22, 1995.

61. P. J. Perez, Navigating Ethical Dilemmas at the Disclosure of Fetal Alcohol Exposure: A Family Therapist's Search for Effective Treatment, *Journal of Family Psychotherapy, 4:*4, pp. 53-68, 1993.

62. B. Bennett, Pregnant Women and the Duty to Rescue: A Feminist Response to the Foetal Rights Debate, *Law in Context, 9:*1, pp. 70-91, 1991.

63. S. A. Garcia, Maternal Drug Abuse: Laws and Ethics as Agents of Just Balances and Therapeutic Interventions, *The International Journal of the Addictions, 28:*13, pp. 1311-1339, 1993.

64. N. Lelong, M. Kaminiski, J. Chwalow, K. Bean, and D. Subtil, Attitudes and Behaviour of Pregnant Women and Health Professionals towards Alcohol and Tobacco Consumption, *Patient Education and Counselling, 25,* pp. 39-49, 1995.

65. B. A. Morse, R. K. Idelson, W. H. Sachs, L. Weiner, and L. C. Kaplan, Pediatricians' Perspectives on Fetal Alcohol Syndrome, *Journal of Substance Abuse, 4,* pp. 187-195, 1992.
66. S. LaFlash, R. A. Aronson, and S. Uttech, Alcohol Use During Pregnancy: Implications for Physicians, *Wisconsin Medical Journal, 92:9,* pp. 501-506, 1993.
67. S. B. Blume, Women and Alcohol: A Review, *Journal of the American Medical Association, 256:11,* pp. 1467-1470, 1986.

Direct reprint requests to:

Professor Tian Oei
School of Psychology
The University of Queensland
Brisbane, Qld. 4072
Australia

J. DRUG EDUCATION, Vol. 29(1) 25-39, 1999

PSYCHOSOCIAL MODERATORS OF SUBSTANCE USE AMONG MIDDLE SCHOOL-AGED ADOLESCENTS

GORDON MACNEIL, PH.D.

ALLAN V. KAUFMAN, PH.D.

WILLIAM W. DRESSLER, PH.D.

The University of Alabama

CRAIG WINSTON LECROY, PH.D.
Arizona State University

ABSTRACT

Recent statistics show a decrease in the overall use of drugs and alcohol in the general population [1]. In sharp contrast to this trend is the indication that adolescents' use of drugs and alcohol is increasing [2]. Because the use of drugs and alcohol can have serious implications for adolescents' physical, emotional, and social development, it is important that human service practitioners working with them understand those factors that influence their substance use, in order to develop effective interventions to deal with this growing problem. This article reports the findings of a study of drug and alcohol use among a sample of 779 adolescents who attended middle schools in a large urban city in the southwest United States. The study examines the relationships between substance use, social support, and a variety of other psychosocial factors. The implications of those relationships for human service practice and research are discussed.

ADOLESCENT SUBSTANCE USE

The United States, of all industrialized nations in the world, has the highest rate of drug use among adolescents [2, 3]. In response to national prevention programs, adolescent drug use decreased in the 1980s and early 1990s. However, recent reports indicate that drug and alcohol use is currently increasing among

25

our nation's youth [4]. Johnson, O'Malley, and Bachman, found that 67 percent of eighth grade students reported that they had used alcohol, with 26 percent of those reporting that they had been drunk at least once. [2]. In this same study, nearly 13 percent of the eighth grade respondents reported that they had tried marijuana. These drugs are commonly referred to as gateway drugs, since continued experimentation with them often leads to use of other more powerful drugs such as hallucinogens, amphetamines, and heroin [5].

Dryfoos estimates that almost nine million (32%) of the nation's twenty-eight million ten- to seventeen-year-olds drink regularly, about three million (11%) use marijuana, and more than 800,000 (3%) have tried cocaine [1]. She further estimates that between 25 percent and 50 percent of the youths who are using these substances, are at moderate or high risk of experiencing serious consequences of their substance use. The most significant negative consequences associated with adolescent substance use are health problems, poor school or work performance, impaired emotional functioning, and lowered social competence [6]. Kandel has found correlations between adolescent substance use and the experience of future problems with marital stability and parenting [7].

A rich and extensive body of research literature on adolescent alcohol and drug use has been compiled over the past thirty years. Two excellent reviews of this literature by Dryfoos [1] and Jensen [4] identify a number of risk factors that are associated with the likelihood that adolescents will use or abuse drugs, and a number of protective factors that have been found to mediate the effects of certain risk factors.

One set of risk and protective factors encompasses an adolescent's environment, and includes such variables as family income level, neighborhood substance use patterns, local availability of drugs and alcohol, prevailing cultural norms regarding substance use, and degree of neighborhood crime and disorganization. A second identified group of risk and protective factors includes individual biological and psychosocial characteristics such as an adolescent's degree of impulse control, the age at which an adolescent first experiments with drugs or alcohol, an adolescent's family history regarding alcoholism, and the degree to which an adolescent is subject to attention deficit problems or is oriented toward sensation-seeking experiences.

A third set of risk and protective factors have been found to relate to the social world of the adolescent and the nature of his or her interpersonal relationships. This set of factors includes such variables as the characteristics of the adolescent's social relationships, the nature of parental supervision and disciplinary practices, the degree of drug and alcohol use by peers and family members, the adolescent's orientation to school and education, and the level of the adolescent's academic performance. It is this set of risk and protective factors that appear to have the most crucial influence upon adolescent drug and alcohol use.

SOCIAL SUPPORT

In view of the critically important influences that social environments and interpersonal relationships can have upon the physical, social, and emotional development and well-being of children and adolescents [8, 9], the apparent influence of these factors upon adolescent substance use is not surprising. What is surprising, however, is the lack of attention given by researchers to the potential relationships between adolescent substance use and those products of social environments and interpersonal relationships often referred to as social support.

Social support as both a construct and a process is multidimensional. No single definition adequately captures the nature, quality, or range of behaviors and activities that have been associated with social support [10]. Epidemiological studies have suggested links between social support and a variety of health conditions and emotional states. Other studies have demonstrated that social support may have important implications for a variety of complex human behaviors such as the manner in which individuals enact their social roles [10].

A particularly intriguing aspect of social support research has involved examinations of the direct effect and the stress-buffer hypotheses [10, 11]. These hypotheses suggest that social support may enhance health and well-being in two different ways. In the direct or main effect model, individuals' positive perceptions regarding their social network relationships, and certain types of supportive behaviors engaged in by members of those networks, are seen as providing positive direct contributions to their health and well-being, regardless of the individuals' stress levels. In this model, people may directly benefit from the receipt of social support in a variety of ways. For example, they engage in more healthy behaviors (reducing their smoking or the use of alcohol) or avoid the stress that would otherwise be associated with certain life situations (loneliness or isolation, job loss, birth of a child) that could have harmful consequences for their physical or psychological health. Thus, simply having social support networks, and using them, can lead to positive health outcomes for individuals.

The buffering model suggests that social support can moderate the amount of stress individuals experience. In this model, certain attributes of individuals' social networks and certain qualities of social support received from members of those networks, under certain circumstances, can lessen peoples' experience of stress. This, in turn, may have an ameliorative influence on certain stress related phenomena such as disease states, emotional conditions or problematic behaviors [11].

Researchers examining the phenomenon of social support have usually focused their attention on factors or variables that generally fall into one of three broad categories. The first contains variables that are related to the structural characteristics of social support networks, including network size, composition, and density. The second category encompasses factors that reflect the nature and type of social support transactions that take place between individuals and members of their social networks. Research in this area has examined such phenomena as the types of supportive behaviors engaged in by social network members and the quality and reciprocity of social network relationships. A third area of focus for researchers has been on those psychological and cognitive factors that are presumed to influence the provision and utilization of social support. Included here are studies that have looked at how factors such as individuals' subjective assessments of their social network relationships, and their attitudes and values regarding seeking or accepting help from others, influence the nature of supportive relationships [10, 12, 13].

Vaux has indicated that, while relatively few studies have focused on social support and adolescence, the research that does exist suggests that a variety of processes, challenges, and issues affecting growth and development during the adolescent years are strongly influenced by the nature and quality of the social support adolescents receive from members of their social networks [10]. Citing the results of a study that he did on social support among high school students, Vaux reported relationships between the youths' use of tobacco, marijuana, and alcohol, and their reports of family and peer support.

One focus of the study reported in this article was to gain a better understanding of the influence of social networks and social support on adolescent substance use. More specifically, we were interested in examining the degree to which adolescent substance use is related to the supportive behaviors of adolescents' social networks, to adolescents' assessments of the nature and quality of their social network relationships, and to adolescents' attitudes regarding the use of those relationships as sources of help and guidance.

We were also interested in examining the impact of several other psychosocial factors on the substance use of early adolescents. Since our sample contained a fairly high percentage of Hispanic and Native American middle school students, we were interested in looking at whether ethnicity had any relationship to the substance use behavior of our subject sample. Also, in view of the strong influence, suggested by previous studies, that peer and family member substance use seems to have on the use of alcohol and drugs by members of this age group [4, 14], we were curious to see how these variables were related to the substance use of our sample. Finally, we wanted to look at how the attitudes and beliefs that the early adolescents in our sample had about their own futures were associated with their use of alcohol and drugs.

METHODS

Sample

Data for this research come from the Youth Plus Survey, which was a component of a larger longitudinal study funded by the federal Center of Substance Abuse Prevention [15]. The goal of the Youth Plus Survey was to identify factors related to early adolescent substance use that would assist in the development of substance abuse prevention programs targeting middle school aged children. Data for the Youth Plus Survey were collected from four cohorts. Data for the study reported here were collected from the 1995 cohort.

Survey data were collected from an initial sample of 809 students who attended two middle schools in a large southwestern city. The schools were located in lower-income neighborhoods and served predominately minority populations. Thirty students not belonging to one of the three main ethnic groups in the sample (Anglos, Hispanics, or Native Americans) were excluded from the data analysis, resulting in a final sample of 779 subjects.

Fourteen percent of the students were Anglo, 13 percent were Native American, and 73 percent were Hispanic. Fifty percent of the subjects were male, and the students ranged in age from eleven to fifteen (mean = 12.81). Forty-five percent of the students were in the seventh grade, and 55 percent were in the eighth grade.

Of students who knew their parents' education level, most reported that their parents had a high school degree or less. However, 26 percent of the sample did not know their mother's level of education, and 37 percent did not know their father's. Most subjects reported that their mothers were either unemployed (35%) or held unskilled jobs (48%). Their fathers tended to hold unskilled (28%) or skilled (36%) jobs. Only 9 percent of the subjects reported that their fathers were unemployed. Fifty-five percent of the adolescents reported that their families were receiving some form of government assistance.

Ninety-four percent of the subjects were living with at least one natural parent, while over half of them (52%) reported living with both natural parents. Additionally, 13 percent reported that extended family members were living in their homes.

Procedure for Data Collection

On the day data were collected, two-person teams of graduate student research assistants met with individual classes during their regular fifty-minute class periods. The research assistants distributed the instruments and monitored the students as they completed the self-administered questionnaires. A Spanish version of the questionnaire and Spanish-speaking assistants were available for those students with limited English language skills. All students attending school on the day of administration were included in the overall sample.

Measures—Family, Peer, and Subject Substance Use

The instrument developed for the Youth Plus Survey was multidimensional and was designed to identify factors in family, peer, school, and substance use domains that would serve as predictor and outcome measures of early adolescent substance use. Brooks, Stuewig, and LeCroy used factor analysis to formulate the predictor and outcome scales from questionnaire items [15]. Items were grouped according to domain (i.e., peers, family, substance use) and subjected to a factor analysis using a promax rotation within each domain. The factor patterns were used as starting points in determining the composition of the scales. Reliability analyses were then conducted on each scale to insure face and construct validity. Cronbach's alpha was computed for each scale. For a more detailed discussion of the development of this instrument see Brooks, Stuewig, and LeCroy [15].

Two sets of variables in the Youth Plus Survey instrument addressed the measurement of substance use: one targeted lifetime substance use, the other targeted substances the respondent had used during the past month. The respondents' scale scores for each of these two aspects of substance use had a Pearson correlation coefficient of .81, suggesting that the two scales were measuring the same phenomenon. We chose to focus our attention on whether our subjects had ever used drugs or alcohol, rather than examining their current patterns of substance use. Therefore, we used the Lifetime Substance Use scale from the Youth Plus Survey as our dependent variable. This scale, as originally developed, was composed of six items that asked students to identify any of the following substances that they had ever used: tobacco, marijuana, cocaine/crack, inhalants, alcohol, or other drugs (e.g., uppers, speed, tranquilizers, hallucinogens, heroin). The number of the substances that students reported they had ever used were summed to create a substance use score ($\alpha = .76$, as reported by Brooks et al.). In the current study we excluded tobacco from our analyses, resulting in a five-item substance use scale with a Cronbach's alpha of .60. Our initial review of the frequency distribution for this scale indicated that our sample was skewed, with nearly 50 percent of the respondents reporting that they had never tried any of the substances listed. Because of this, we discotomized the scale into "never" and "ever" use categories.

The following predictor variables for this study were taken directly from the Youth Plus Survey: ethnicity, socio-economic status, family substance use, friend substance use, and the student's expectations about the future. Family substance use was computed by summing three items that measured the student's report of family members' use of alcohol, marijuana, and other drugs such as cocaine, inhalants, or heroin ($\alpha = .52$). Friend substance use was computed by summing four items that measured the student's report of how many of their friends use alcohol, marijuana, inhalants, or other drugs such as cocaine/crack or pills ($\alpha = .78$). All items on both of these scales used 5-point Likert type response categories ranging from "none" to "all."

Expectations students had about their future (Future Beliefs) was measured by a seven-item scale created by Brooks, Stuewig, and LeCroy [15]. The scale included such items as: the highest level of education that the student would like to achieve, the likelihood of the student achieving that level of education, the student's excitement about his/her chances of getting a good job, his/her expectation of getting "the good things in life," his/her expectations of living a long life, and the student's general optimism about the future ($\alpha = .79$).

Measures—Social Support

We developed additional predictor variables that focused on social support. In our study we used a multidimensional approach to the measurement of social support, based on the work of Vaux [10, 16]. Based on this approach, social support is viewed as a metaconstruct composed of four domains: social support resources, social support behaviors, social support appraisals, and social network orientation. Social support resources encompasses the structural attributes of an individual's social support networks, and includes such factors as network size, composition, and density. Social support behaviors refers to the modes of support exchanged by members of social networks, and includes the provision of material and emotional assistance, advice, guidance, and socialization. Social support appraisals encompasses an individual's assessments about the degree to which the person feels accepted and valued by his or her network members based on the network's supportive activities. Network orientation refers to an individual's attitudes and values regarding social networks as appropriate sources of assistance, and the individual's willingness to request or utilize help from his or her network members.

We used items from the Youth Plus Survey to create three indexes that corresponded with three of the above domains. (There were insufficient data available from this survey to generate a measure of social support resources.) The first index, Appraisals of Support (AOS), was composed of fourteen items and measured the extent to which the students felt accepted, valued, and cared for by parents, school personnel, and friends. The index included items such as: "When we talk about things, my parents listen to what I have to say." "My friends care about what happens with me." "Teachers and staff at this school care about me." A 5-point Likert-type scale was used to score responses with choices that ranged from "not true" to "always true." Scores for the individual items were summed to create an AOS score. Cronbach's alpha for this scale was .80.

A fourteen-item Support Behaviors (SB) index measured the degree to which students used parents or friends as sources of advice, guidance, and emotional support. Included in this index were items such as: "How often do you talk with your parents about problems you have?" "How often do you talk with your friends about things you have done that you are worried or feel guilty about?" Responses were scored using a 5-point Likert-type scale with possible response choices that ranged from "never" to "very often." Scores for the individual items were summed to create an SB score. This index also had a Cronbach's alpha of .80.

A Support Orientation (SO) index contained eight items, and measured the student's attitudes and willingness to use parents, friends, or teachers as sources of help. This index included such items as: "I can count on my parents to help me if I need it." "Being with my friends makes me feel better when I feel angry or sad." "If you had a problem at school or with a friend, how easy would it be to talk to your parents about it?" As with the above indexes, 5-point Likert-type response scales were used. Scores for the individual items were summed to create an SO score. Cronbach's alpha for this index was .61. Although this was somewhat lower than the other two measures, it still indicated an acceptable level of reliability.

RESULTS

Table 1 shows descriptive statistics for the entire sample, and broken down by ethnic group. There are no significant differences among the three ethnic groups in overall level of substance use (about half the students in each group report substance use). Similarly, there is no gender difference among the three groups.

With respect to several potential predictors of substance use, however, there are substantial differences among the three groups. Anglos tend to have higher parental socioeconomic status than either Hispanics or Native Americans. Substance use by both family and friends tends to be higher for Native Americans, followed by Hispanics and Anglos. With respect to the social support variables and beliefs about the future, there are no significant differences (although the differences for beliefs about the future approaches statistical significance, $p = .058$).

Next, the bivariate and multivariate associations between the independent variables and substance use were examined. Due to the distribution of substance use

Table 1. Descriptive Statistics for the Total Sample and for Each Ethnic Group

Variables	Total Sample ($n = 779$)	Anglos ($n = 113$)	Hispanics ($n = 567$)	Native Americans ($n = 99$)
Total drug use (%)	50.2	47.8	51.0	49.5
Gender (% male)	50.0	51.3	52.4	40.4
Socioeconomic status**	0.00 (± 0.57)	0.34 (± 0.60)	0.00 (± 0.55)	0.01 (± 0.57)
Family substance abuse**	4.53 (± 1.62)	4.05 (± 1.35)	4.56 (± 1.62)	4.88 (± 1.79)
Friend substance use*	6.28 (± 2.77)	5.80 (± 2.31)	6.29 (± 2.79)	6.75 (± 3.04)
Support Orientation	29.6 (± 5.67)	29.6 (± 5.88)	29.7 (± 5.63)	28.7 (± 5.66)
Appraisals of Support	54.8 (± 9.33)	54.7 (± 9.47)	54.9 (± 9.41)	54.2 (± 8.71)
Support Behaviors	40.5 (± 10.47)	39.5 (± 11.24)	40.6 (± 10.05)	40.8 (± 11.82)
Future beliefs	30.4 (± 5.16)	31.5 (± 4.98)	30.3 (± 5.19)	29.9 (± 5.16)

Note: Differences between ethnic groups for these variables were tested using chi-square for categorical variables and one-way analysis of variance for continuous variables.
*$p < .05$
**$p < .001$

and the decision to dichtomize students into "any" substance use in the past versus "no" substance use, logistic regression was chosen as the data analytic tool [17]. Logistic regression, like ordinary least squares regression analysis, is used to examine the relative contributions of a set of independent or predictor variables to variation in a dependent or outcome variable. In the case of logistic regression, that outcome variable is a dichotomy. Logistic regression coefficients provide an estimate of the degree to which an independent variable is associated with a greater or lesser likelihood of being in one or the other category of a dependent variable. Independent variables may be either continuous or categorical. An extremely useful coefficient that can be derived from the logistic regression coefficient is the "risk odds ratio" (also referred to as either the "odds ratio" or the "relative risk"). The risk odds ratio (or ROR) has an expected value of 1.0; that is, if the likelihood of falling into one versus another category is equal at different values of an independent variable, then the ROR = 1.0. If the likelihood of the dependent variable being "present" is increased by increasing values of the independent variable, then the ROR exceeds 1.0. If the likelihood of the dependent variable being "absent" is increased by increasing values of the independent variable, then the ROR is less than 1.0 (with the logical lowest value being 0).

The bivariate associations between the independent variables and substance use are given in Table 2. For the continuous predictor variables, standardized or z-scores are used in this analysis in order to increase the utility of the ROR as an interpretive tool. The RORs can be interpreted as the likelihood that a respondent will (or will not) fall into the substance use category in association with a one standard deviation difference in the independent variable. For example, the

Table 2. Bivariate Risk Odds Ratios between Independent Variables and Substance Use

Independent Variables	Risk Odds Ratio	95% Confidence Intervals	Significance
Ethnic group:			
Hispanics	1.06	0.86, 1.31	n.s.
Anglos	0.93	0.70, 1.24	n.s.
Gender	0.85	0.64, 1.11	n.s.
Socioeconomic status	1.33	1.05, 1.70	.018
Family substance use	2.84	2.30, 3.49	.0001
Friend substance use	4.94	3.79, 644	.0001
Support Orientation	0.49	0.41, 0.66	.0001
Appraisals of Support	0.56	0.48, 0.66	.0001
Support Behaviors	0.85	0.73, 0.97	.022
Future beliefs	0.57	0.48, 0.67	.0001

association of socioeconomic status and substance use is significant, and the ROR indicates that as parental socioeconomic status increases, the likelihood of substance use also increased. Specifically, a one standard deviation difference in socioeconomic status is associated with a 33 percent increase in the likelihood that a student will report having used substances. Also given are the 95 percent confidence intervals for the RORs, indicating the upper and lower limits for the true value of the odds ratios.

Neither ethnic group nor gender is associated with risk of substance use, but all other independent variables are. Substance use by family and friends increases the risk of respondent substance use by factors of nearly three and nearly five, respectively. On the other hand, Support Orientation, Appraisal of Support, and Future Beliefs all reduce the likelihood of respondent substance use by about 50 percent.

Next, a series of multivariate logistic regression models were examined. In these, in addition to the direct effects of the independent variables, interaction effects between each of the social support variables and family and friend substance use, and between future beliefs and family and friend substance use, were included in the analyses. Interaction effects were tested using cross-product terms that were calculated using the standardized scores for the variables. We used a hierarchical modeling strategy suggested by Greenberg and Kleinbaum [18]. When testing a relatively large number of interaction effects, the danger of capitalizing on chance is present. Greenberg and Kleinbaum recommend first testing the contribution of an entire set of interactions to the prediction of category membership; if, as a set, the interactions are significant, there is less danger that any of the individual interaction effects was significant purely by chance. The significant interactions can then more safely be retained in a final model.

Here, separate models were calculated in which the set of interactions between family substance use and the potential moderator variables and friend substance use and the potential moderators were examined separately. The significant individual interaction effects were retained only when the entire set of interaction effects was significant. The final model is shown in Table 3. When the effects are examined in combination, Hispanics are more likely, and females are less likely, to report having used substances, and respondents with higher parental socioeconomic status are more likely to report having used substances. Family and friend substance use are associated with an increased likelihood of use, and Support Orientation and Future Beliefs are associated with a decreased likelihood of use.

The increased substance use associated both with family use and with friend use are significantly modified by Appraisals of Support and Future Beliefs. Respondents with higher scores on the Appraisals of Support scale are more likely to report substance use if they also report use by their families. On the other hand, where respondents have a low score on the Future Beliefs scale, the

Table 3. Multivariate Logistic Regression of Substance Use on
Independent Variables and Interactions

Independent Variables	Logistic Regression Coefficient	Risk Odds Ratio
Hispanic	0.54*	1.71
Anglo	0.57	1.77
Gender	−0.43*	0.65
Socioeconomic status	0.53**	1.69
Family substance use	0.69**	2.01
Friend substance use	1.42**	4.17
Network orientation	−0.38*	0.68
Social support attitudes	0.02	1.02
Future beliefs	−0.46**	0.62
Family substance use × social support attitudes	0.22*	1.25
Friend substance use × future beliefs	−0.74**	0.48

*$p < .05$
**$p < .001$

increase in likelihood of their reporting use if they also report substance use among their friends is greater than for those respondents who have high scores on the Future Beliefs scale. Thus, the influence of friend substance use is greater if one has low future beliefs than if one has high future beliefs. The patterns of these interaction effects are illustrated in Figures 1 and 2.

DISCUSSION

This study examined the degree to which specific dimensions of social support and the variety of other psychosocial factors were related to the substance use of a sample of 779 middle school age adolescents. While approximately half of our sample had used at least one substance, in bivariate analyses we found no statistically significant differences in reported substance use with regard to ethnicity or gender. By far, the most important predictors of whether or not our early adolescent subjects had used alcohol or drugs were the number of their family members or friends who used drugs or alcohol. This finding is consistent with the research literature on teenage substance use.

It is well documented that adolescents are more inclined to use drugs or alcohol if their peers or members of their family also use these substances. Ironically, in the case of adolescents whose families or peers use drugs or alcohol, the same people who provide negative role models also often serve as their major sources

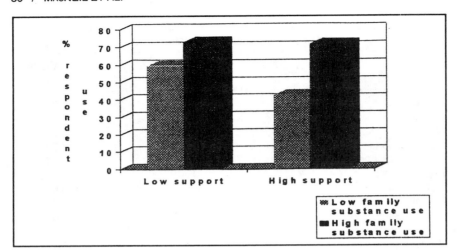

Figure 1. Interaction effects between family substance use and
Appraisals of Support on subject's substance use.

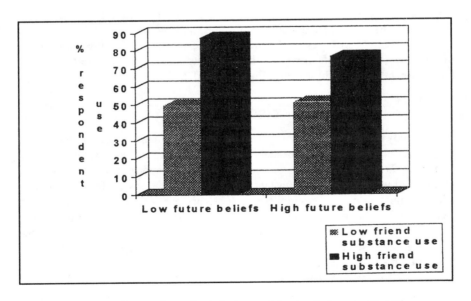

Figure 2. Interaction effects between friend substance use and
Future Beliefs on subject's substance use.

of social support. This paradoxical relationship intrigued us, and suggested that we look at social support in a more explicit manner. We examined the potential influence of three dimensions of social support on the alcohol and drug use behaviors of our subjects. In our multivariate logistic regression analysis we found that the degree to which students actually used parents or friends as sources of advice, guidance, and emotional support (Support Behaviors) had neither a statistically significant main effect or interaction effect on our subjects' substance use.

However, we found that Support Orientation, that is the students' attitudes and willingness to use parents, friends, or teachers as sources of help, had a direct inverse effect on their substance use. This means that the more the adolescents in our sample held positive attitudes toward using significant others in their lives as sources of assistance, the less likely they were to have used drugs or alcohol.

When controlling for other variables, we found no direct relationship between our subjects' substance use and our third social support dimension, Appraisals of Support (AOS), which measured the extent to which the students felt accepted, valued and cared for by parents, school personnel, and friends. However, we did find an interaction effect between AOS and family substance use. Among adolescents whose family members used alcohol or drugs, those who felt more accepted, valued, and cared for by the significant others in their lives, were more likely to use alcohol or drugs than those adolescents who felt less accepted, valued, or cared for. In other words, the influence of family substance use on the substance use of the early adolescents in our sample is exacerbated by higher levels of AOS.

In addition to the social support variables discussed above, we also examined whether the students' beliefs about their future (Future Beliefs) had any relationship with their use of alcohol or drugs. We found that Future Beliefs had a direct effect on the students' substance use and it had a modifying effect upon the substance use of those students whose friends used alcohol and drugs. For those students whose friends used alcohol or drugs, the more optimistic the students were about their future, the less likely they were to use alcohol or drugs themselves.

Because our measures of social support were developed after the data were collected, we were unable to inquire fully about the social support constructs of interest. Therefore, our study can provide only a tentative understanding of the complex relationship between social support and early adolescent substance use. Subsequent research, which uses valid and reliable instruments designed to more fully capture the multidimensional nature of social support, should minimize the limitations we experienced in this area.

Since data for this study were collected in two middle schools in a large city in the southwest, the extent to which our findings are generalizable to adolescents in other locations is limited. Further research on this subject, sampling a broader geographic base, is needed. It will also be important to explore the extent to which findings from samples with SES demographics different from those of our sample are consistent with our findings. Finally, our study is based on data obtained through self-report and is vulnerable to the general limitations of all self-report measurement devices. All of the items in the survey were direct and obvious in their intent so that respondents could easily engage in "impression management" by making themselves appear as problem-free or as problem-laden as they wished. Despite these limitations, we believe that our findings make several important contributions to our knowledge about substance use among early adolescents.

Our findings suggest that complex relationships exist between both adolescents' social support experiences and their beliefs about the future, and their use of alcohol and drugs. A more careful examination of the social network relations of this population is needed, using methods and measures specifically designed for this purpose. For instance, further exploration of the importance of enhancing perceived social support as well as enhancing the actual supportive behaviors from significant others is warranted. If research determines that the manner in which adolescents perceive, experience, and utilize social support has a direct bearing on their use of alcohol and drugs, it can point to new directions for prevention or treatment. Current prevention efforts with this population have primarily used educational and psychological approaches aimed at changing the behaviors of individual adolescents. Our findings suggest that prevention efforts that target the social network relationships of adolescents, focusing specifically on the multidimensional nature of social support, may also be helpful.

"Our findings regarding the influence that adolescents' beliefs about the future may have upon their use of alcohol and drugs also warrant further examination. The popular press has often reported that many of today's youth have extremely pessimistic views about their future and that such views are influencing them to engage in a variety of self-destructive behaviors. Our findings lend support to these disturbing reports and suggest that further knowledge about this complex phenomenon is needed.

REFERENCES

1. J. Dryfoos, *Adolescents at Risk,* Oxford Press, New York, 1990.
2. L. D. Johnston, P. M. O'Malley, and J. G. Bachman, *Drug Use, Drinking, and Smoking: National Survey Results from High School, College, and Young Adult Populations,* U.S. Government Printing Office, Washington, D.C., 1994.
3. J. Falco, *Preventing Abuse of Drugs, Alcohol, and Tobacco by Adolescents,* Carnegie Council on Adolescent Development: Washington, D.C., 1988.
4. J. M. Jensen, Risk and Protective Factors for Alcohol and Other Drug Use in Childhood and Adolescence, in *Risk and Resilience in Childhood: An Ecological Perspective,* M. W. Fraser (ed.), NASW Press, Washington, D.C., pp. 117-139, 1997.
5. R. Loeber, Development and Risk Factors of Juvenile Antisocial Behavior and Delinquency, *Clinical Psychology Review, 10,* pp. 1-41, 1990.

6. R. B. Palmer and H. A. Liddle, Adolescent Drug Abuse: Contemporary Perspectives on Etiology and Treatment, in *Adolescent Dysfunctional Behavior: Causes, Interventions, and Prevention,* G. M. Blau and T. P. Gullotta (eds.), Sage, Thousand Oaks, California, pp. 114-138, 1996.
7. D. Kandel, Parenting Styles, Drug Use, and Children's Adjustment in Families of Young Adults, *Journal of Marriage and the Family, 52,* pp. 183-196, 1990.
8. J. Dacey and M. Kenny, *Adolescent Development,* W. C. B. Brown & Benchmark, Madison, Wisconsin, 1994.
9. J. W. Santrock, *Child Development,* W. C. B. Brown & Benchmark, Madison, Wisconsin, 1994.
10. A. Vaux, *Social Support: Theory, Research, and Intervention,* Praeger, New York, 1998.
11. S. Cohen and T. A. Wills, Stress, Social Support, and the Buffering Hypothesis, *Psychological Bulletin, 98,* pp. 310-357, 1985.
12. M. Barrera, Distinctions between Social Support Concepts, Measures, and Models, *Journal of Community Psychology, 14,* pp. 413-446, 1986.
13. S. Cohen and S. L. Syme (eds.), *Social Support and Health,* Academic Press, New York, 1985.
14. G. Resnick, and M. R. Burt, Youth at Risk: Definitions and Implications for Service Delivery, *American Journal of Orthopsychiatry, 66:*2, pp. 172-188, 1996.
15. A. J. Brooks, J. Stuewig, and C. W. LeCroy, A Family Based Model of Hispanic Adolescent Substance Use, *Journal of Drug Education, 28:*1, pp. 65-86, 1998
16. A. Vaux, *Measures of Three Levels of Social Support: Resources, Behaviors, and Feelings,* Southern Illinois University, Department of Psychology, Carbondale, Illinois, 1982.
17. D. W. Hosmer and S. Lemeshow, *Applied Logistic Regression Analysis,* Wiley, New York, 1989.
18. R. S. Greenberg and D. G. Kleinbaum, Mathematical Modeling Strategies for the Analysis of Epidemiologic Research, *Annual Review of Public Health, 6,* pp. 223-245, 1983.

Direct reprint requests to:

Gordon MacNeil, Ph.D.
The University of Alabama
Box 870314
Tuscaloosa, AL 35487-0314

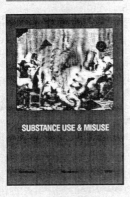

J. DRUG EDUCATION, Vol. 29(1) 41-52, 1999

ATTITUDES OF ISRAELI JEWISH AND ARAB HIGH SCHOOL STUDENTS TOWARD ALCOHOL CONTROL MEASURES

SHOSHANA WEISS, D.SC.

Israel Society for the Prevention of Alcoholism

ABSTRACT

This article describes a study carried out in the winter of 1997 in order to determine the attitudes of 2,186 adolescents of four religions in the north of Israel toward eight alcohol control measures: Taxation on alcohol, age limit for buying alcohol, restrictions on types of outlets which are allowed to sell alcohol to minors, restrictions on opening hours of pubs, restrictions on advertising of alcohol, limit of blood level of alcohol when driving, the authority of policemen concerning the testing of drunk drivers, and restrictions on roadside alcohol outlets. Findings indicate that the majority of the respondents tend to enhance alcohol control measures pertaining to alcohol and driving issues, but only about a third of the participants tend to enhance alcohol control measures in the other domains. In addition, Arabs tend to favor restrictive attitudes toward alcohol control measures in comparison with Jews, and Arab females tend to favor such attitudes more than Arab males. Implications for prevention and effective alcohol policy are discussed.

Most developed countries have policy options for minimizing alcohol-related harm. The European Alcohol Action Plan lays emphasis on the role of legislation as part of a comprehensive policy in addition to national education programs [1-2]. The present study refers to eight legislative measures:

1. Price of alcohol: One of the instruments available to countries to reduce demand for alcohol is to keep the price high by means of taxation. However, in Israel such a policy has not yet been adopted and the real price of

41

alcohol is low. Beer and wine cost about the same as soft drinks, and spirits cost slightly more than fruit juice [3].

2. Age limit for buying alcohol: The age limit in Israel is eighteen years, but it is not at all effectively enforced [4].
3. Types of outlets in which the sale of alcohol to minors is forbidden: In Israel the age limit applies to buying and drinking in pubs, bars, discos, and restaurants, but it is not enforced at all effectively. Adolescents can buy alcohol in supermarkets and grocery stores [4].
4. Hours of sale: In Israel there are no restrictions on hours of sale.
5. Restrictions on advertising: No advertising restrictions are in place in Israel. However, there is one restriction which refers to advertisements aimed at minors or depict minors consuming alcohol, but is not effectively enforced [5].
6. Blood alcohol concentration (BAC): Israel has a permitted BAC of 50 mg/ percent for all drivers, but it is not enforced at all effectively [6].
7. Random breath testing (RBT): Israel does not use RBT at all.
8. Location of outlets: In Israel there are no restrictions on location of alcohol outlets, including roadside outlets.

The aim of the study was to determine the attitudes of Jewish and Arab youth toward the above mentioned eight issues in order to use the results for recommendations for designing effective national alcohol legislative initiatives. This study follows another study, which was conducted in the winter of 1996 among 3,065 adolescents of four religions in the same region, and investigated their opinion toward alcohol beverage warning labels [7]. The present study actually completes the picture concerning attitudes of Israeli teenagers toward legislative measures.

METHOD

Subjects

The subjects were 2,186 adolescents, 1,080 boys and 1,106 girls, age groups sixteen to eighteen. Seventy-one questionnaires were not included due to missing data concerning gender or religion. The sample consisted of 1,387 Jews and 799 Arabs (340 Moslems, 351 Christians, and 108 Druze). Nine hundred forty-five students studied in the tenth grade, 803 studied in the eleventh grade, and 438 in the twelfth grade. The students came from nine locations in the northern region of Israel. Eight hundred seventy-one students were from Haifa (the largest city in the north of the country), 415 came from two developing towns, 436 were from three Arab villages, 137 came from kibbutzim, 175 were from moshavim, and 152 came from a youth village.

No rigorous sampling method was utilized because of difficulties in entering Arab schools, especially Moslem and Druze schools, using an alcohol-related questionnaire. The students came from seventeen schools which had agreed to cooperate. Arabs came from five schools and Jews came from twelve schools, all of which represented a wide range of types of schools: private and public academically-oriented, vocational, comprehensive, agricultural, and specific-education-oriented.

The Questionnaire

Following a pilot-test among forty-eight students, the final anonymous questionnaire included five background variables: gender, grade, religion, name of school and its location, a question which referred to drinking alcohol in the preceding year (not for religious purposes), and the eight above mentioned alcohol control measures with four listed options: enhance, reduce, leave it as it is, do not know.

Procedure

The questionnaire was administered during the winter of 1997. Special attention was paid to measures which increased the validity of the answers. It was anonymously completed, and it was further emphasized to the students that their responses would remain confidential and be used only for research purposes.

RESULTS

A. Drinking Rates

Similar to results of previous studies [8, 9], drinking in the preceding year in the Jewish sector was highest among adolescents from kibbutzim: 71.7 percent among males and 64.4 percent among females. The lowest scores were revealed in developing towns (56.9%, 36.9%, respectively). In the Arab sector the drinking rates were about 10 percent higher among Moslems and Druze than in previous studies [10, 11], because in the present study the subjects were drawn from the large city and three Arab villages well known for their spread of alcoholism, which led to the establishment of alcohol treatment centers there. The rates of drinking in the last year among Christian, Druze, and Moslem males were 67.3 percent, 58.9 percent, 49.9 percent, respectively, and among females 47.9 percent, 23.8 percent, 19.2 percent, respectively.

B. Attitudes of All the Participants toward All Control Measures

Table 1 presents the results concerning the eight alcohol control measures.

As can be seen, about half of the students support reduction in BAC (49.9%), rise in policemen's authority concerning the testing of drunk drivers (56.9%), and

Table 1. Attitudes of the Sample (*N* = 2,186) toward Eight Alcohol
Control Measures, in Numbers

Measure	Enhance	Reduce	Remain	Do Not Know	Missing
Price of alcohol	820	382	528	453	3
Age limit for buying alcohol	693	327	1,078	87	1
Types of outlets forbidden for minors	634	525	803	222	2
Opening hours of pubs	252	639	973	319	3
BAC	212	1,090	661	218	5
Restrictions on advertising	585	448	838	310	5
Policemen's authority	1,243	149	616	175	3
No. of roadside outlets	152	1,249	593	187	5

decrease in roadside alcohol outlets (57.1%). However, only about a third of the subjects support increase in the price of alcohol (37.5%), in the age limit for purchasing alcoholic beverages (31.7%), in the types of outlets in which the sale of alcohol to minors is forbidden (29.0%), or in restrictions on advertising (26.8%), and support reduction in the opening hours of pubs (29.7%).

C. Differences in Attitudes between Jews and Arabs

Table 2 represents differences between Jews and Arabs (Christians, Druze, and Moslems as a group). On the whole, Arabs tend to enhance all alcohol control measures more than Jews.

About two-thirds of Jews (60.1%) do not want to change the age limit for buying alcoholic drinks but more than half of the Arabs (53.3%) support increase in the age limit. About half of the Jewish students (45.0%) do not want to change the possibility to buy alcohol in grocery stores and supermarkets, but more than a third of the Arab students (35.1%) support increase in the types of outlets in which the sale of alcohol to minors is not allowed. More than half of the Jewish subjects (56.4%) do not want to change the opening hours of pubs, in contrast with about half of the Arab students (48.8%) who support reduction in the opening hours. About half of the Jewish participants (46.4%) do not support any changes in restrictions on advertising, but about a third of the Arab participants (31.9%) support more restrictions. About half of the Arab respondents (49.7%) and less than a third of the Jewish respondents (30.5%) support increase in the price of alcoholic beverages. Less than half of the Jews (45.4%) and more than half of the Arabs (57.6%) support reduction in BAC. About half of the Jewish

Table 2. Attitudes of Jews and Arabs toward Eight Alcohol Control Measures, in Numbers

Measure	Jews (N = 1,387)					Arabs (N = 799)					$df = 3$ χ^2
	Enhance	Reduce	Remain	Do Not Know	Missing	Enhance	Reduce	Remain	Do Not Know	Missing	
Price	423	256	387	319	2	397	126	141	134	1	83.42**
Age limit	267	246	834	39	1	426	81	244	48	0	308.12**
Types forbidden	353	293	624	116	1	281	232	179	106	1	112.14**
Opening hours	163	249	782	190	3	89	390	191	129	0	287.35**
BAC	144	630	461	149	3	68	460	200	69	2	39.30**
Restrictions on ads	330	213	643	197	4	255	235	195	113	1	125.04**
Policemen's authority	746	79	456	104	2	497	70	160	71	1	44.24**
No. roadside outlets	94	728	440	122	3	58	521	153	65	2	44.33**

Note: Missing cases are not included in χ^2 calculations.
**$p < 0.01$

subjects (53.8%) and two-thirds of the Arab subjects (62.2%) support strengthening of policemen's authority and reduction in the number of roadside alcohol outlets (52.5%, 65.2%, respectively).

D. Differences in Attitudes between Arab Males and Females

Table 3 shows that Arab females tend to enhance alcohol control measures more than males. For example, 52.2 percent of males support reduction in the number of roadside outlets in comparison with 76 percent of females, 39.5 percent of males do not want any change in the age limit, but 65.7 percent of females support increase in the age limit, 29.8 percent of boys do not support a change in the restrictions on advertising, but 36.1 percent of females support more restrictions.

E. Differences in Attitudes between Jewish Males and Females

Table 4 details the numbers of Jewish boys and girls concerning the attitudes toward the eight control measures. As can be seen, there are differences only concerning half of the control measures. More girls than boys support reduction in roadside alcohol outlets (58.6% vs. 46.8%) and do not want to change the opening hours of pubs (61.6% vs. 51.5%) and the age limit (65.5% vs. 55.1%). More boys than girls support reduction in the price of alcohol drinks (24.2% vs. 12.2%). The findings concerning the opening hours of pubs as well as the age limit are not surprising, because the preferred location of Jewish female drinking is the pub followed by home, whereas males drink at home and in pubs with approximately the same frequency [9, 10].

F. Differences between Christians and the Group of Moslems and Druze

As can be seen in Table 5, differences between Christians and the group of Moslems and Druze exist in half of the control measures. Moslems and Druze, more than Christians, tend to increase the age limit (61.2% vs. 45.6%), and to reduce opening hours of pubs (53.6% vs. 42.7%), BAC (61.4% vs. 52.7%), and the number of roadside outlets (69.4% vs. 59.8%).

G. Differences between Christian Males and Females

In each religion in the Arab sector, girls tend to reveal more strict attitudes than boys. Table 6 presents the findings concerning the Christian group. As can be seen, 57.8 percent of girls support increase in the age limit but 47.1 percent of boys do not support any change, 50 percent of females support reduction in opening hours of pubs but 35.2 percent of males do not want any change. In addition, girls show more strict attitudes concerning alcohol price (49% vs.

Table 3. Attitudes of Arab Males and Arab Females toward Eight Alcohol Control Measures, in Numbers

Measure	Arab Males (N = 362)					Arab Females (N = 437)					$df = 3$ χ^2
	Enhance	Reduce	Remain	Do Not Know	Missing	Enhance	Reduce	Remain	Do Not Know	Missing	
Price	161	88	64	48	1	236	38	77	86	0	39.10**
Age limit	139	60	143	20	0	287	21	101	28	0	72.36**
Types forbidden	109	103	97	53	0	172	129	82	53	1	11.53**
Opening hours	62	139	101	60	0	27	251	90	69	0	40.51**
BAC	35	181	106	39	1	33	279	94	30	1	15.91**
Restrictions on ads	97	89	108	68	0	158	146	87	45	1	28.75**
Policemen's authority	210	46	69	37	0	287	24	91	34	1	15.26**
No. roadside outlets	46	189	91	36	0	12	332	62	29	2	59.24**

Note: Missing cases are not included in χ^2 calculations.
**$p < 0.01$

Table 4. Attitudes of Jewish Boys and Girls toward Eight Alcohol Control Measures, in Numbers

Measure	Jewish Boys (N = 718)					Jewish Girls (N = 669)					$df = 3$ χ^2
	Enhance	Reduce	Remain	Do Not Know	Missing	Enhance	Reduce	Remain	Do Not Know	Missing	
Price	209	174	202	132	1	214	82	185	187	1	41.67**
Age limit	138	169	396	15	0	129	77	438	24	1	37.15**
Types forbidden	184	155	318	61	0	169	138	306	55	1	0.36 n.s.
Opening hours	110	140	370	97	1	53	109	412	93	2	24.36**
BAC	87	309	248	73	1	57	321	213	76	2	7.40 n.s.
Restrictions on ads	177	120	328	92	1	153	93	315	105	3	4.41 n.s.
Policemen's authority	374	52	240	51	1	372	27	216	53	1	7.49 n.s.
No. roadside outlets	75	336	250	56	1	19	392	190	66	2	44.92**

Note: Missing cases are not included in χ^2 calculations.
n.s. = not significant
**$p < 0.01$

Table 5. Attitudes of Christians and the Group of Moslems and Druze toward Eight Alcohol Control Measures, in Numbers

Measure	Christians (N = 351)					Moslems and Druze (N = 448)					χ^2 df = 3
	Enhance	Reduce	Remain	Do Not Know	Missing	Enhance	Reduce	Remain	Do Not Know	Missing	
Price	159	63	71	57	1	238	63	70	77	0	6.78 n.s.
Age limit	160	39	136	16	0	266	42	108	32	0	23.60**
Types forbidden	123	92	88	48	0	158	140	91	58	1	3.79 n.s.
Opening hours	43	150	95	63	0	46	240	96	66	0	9.31*
BAC	34	185	102	28	2	34	275	98	41	0	7.96*
Restrictions on ads	105	107	96	43	0	150	128	99	70	1	4.84 n.s.
Policemen's authority	226	34	59	32	0	271	36	101	39	1	4.36 n.s.
No. roadside outlets	32	210	78	31	0	26	311	75	34	2	9.20*

Note: Missing cases are not included in χ^2 calculations.
n.s. = not significant
*$p < 0.05$
**$p < 0.01$

Table 6. Attitudes of Christian Males and Females toward Eight Alcohol Control Measures, in Numbers

Measure	Christian Males (N = 159)					Christian Females (N = 192)					χ^2 df = 3
	Enhance	Reduce	Remain	Do Not Know	Missing	Enhance	Reduce	Remain	Do Not Know	Missing	
Price	65	46	31	16	1	94	17	40	41	0	27.70**
Age limit	49	28	75	7	0	111	11	61	9	0	30.29**
Types forbidden	45	48	44	22	0	78	44	44	26	0	6.31 n.s.
Opening hours	27	54	56	22	0	16	96	39	41	0	20.42**
BAC	14	73	54	17	1	20	112	48	11	1	7.87*
Restrictions on ads	43	36	56	24	0	62	71	40	19	0	15.17**
Policemen's authority	92	21	27	19	0	134	13	32	13	0	8.21*
No. roadside outlets	25	79	42	13	0	7	131	36	18	0	21.36**

Note: Missing cases are not included in χ^2 calculations.

n.s. = not significant

*$p < 0.05$

**$p < 0.01$

40.9%), BAC (58.3% vs. 45.9%), policemen's authority (69.8% vs. 57.9%), and the number of roadside outlets (68.2% vs. 49.7%). However, as far as restrictions on advertising are concerned, 37 percent of girls support reduction in restrictions and 35.2 percent of boys do not support any change.

DISCUSSION

The involvement of Israeli Jewish and Arab teenagers in drinking alcoholic drinks (not for religious purposes) is relatively high, especially in kibbutzim in the Jewish sector and among males in the Arab sector. In the Islamic faith and in the Druze faith alcohol is presented as a taboo to be avoided and never approached in any way. However, this belief does not result in Israeli Moslem and Druze adolescents refraining from consuming alcohol.

A majority of these teenagers favor restrictive attitudes toward alcohol and driving control measures: reduction in BAC and in the number of roadside alcohol outlets and increase in the policemen's authority in testing drunk drivers. However, only a third of the subjects express strict attitudes toward the other control measures. In addition, Arabs reveal more strict attitudes than Jews.

The study has implications for prevention and for policy makers in the public health domain. The focus should be on three law-proposals for reform in the alcohol and driving domain: the introduction of random breath testing, the introduction of a lower alcohol limit for drivers, perhaps a zero alcohol limit for young drivers and drivers of public service vehicles, and the introduction of restrictions on the sale of alcohol on the roadside.

However, as far as the other measures are concerned, it is necessary first and foremost to emphasize the importance of these less supported measures to public health and safety in the framework of alcohol education programs in schools, workshops for students provided in extracurricular activities in the community and the media, before putting forward law-proposals for reform. This is essential because public health support is crucial for sustained success of alcohol control policies [12].

REFERENCES

1. A. M. Harkin, P. Anderson, and J. Lehto, *Alcohol in Europe—A Health Perspective,* WHO Regional Office for Europe, Copenhagen, 1995.
2. P. Anderson, *Alcohol—Less Is Better,* WHO Regional Publications, European Series, No. 70, 1996.
3. S. Weiss, The Alcohol Scene in Israel, *The Globe, 4,* pp. 14-15, 1996.
4. S. Weiss and P. Eldar, Alcohol Control Policy in Israel 1986-1987: Recognizing the Need for Diverse Primary Prevention Initiatives, *Alcohol and Alcoholism, 23,* pp. 515-520, 1988.

5. S. Weiss and M. Moore, Cultural Differences in the Perception of Magazine Alcohol Advertisements by Israeli Jewish, Moslem, Druze and Christian High School Students, *Drug and Alcohol Dependence, 26,* pp. 209-215, 1990.
6. S. Weiss, What Do Israeli Jewish and Arab Adolescents Know About Drinking and Driving? *Accident Analysis and Prevention, 28,* pp. 765-769, 1996.
7. S. Weiss, Israeli Arab and Jewish Youth Knowledge and Opinion About Alcohol Warning Labels: Pre-Intervention Data, *Alcohol and Alcoholism, 32,* pp. 251-257, 1997.
8. S. Weiss and M. Moore, Nonritual Alcohol Drinking Practices Among High School Students From the Kibbutz Movement in Israel: Implications for Prevention, *Journal of Drug Education, 21,* pp. 247-254, 1991.
9. S. Weiss and M. Moore, Why, Where and With Whom Do Israeli Teenagers Drink? To Whom Do They Turn for Help With Alcohol Problems? *Alcohol and Alcoholism, 29,* pp. 465-471, 1994.
10. S. Weiss and M. Moore, How Do Israeli Adolescents of Four Religions Obtain Alcoholic Beverages and Where? *Journal of Child and Adolescent Substance Abuse, 4,* pp. 79-87, 1995.
11. S. Weiss, Review of Drinking Patterns of Rural Arab and Jewish Youth in the North of Israel, *Substance Use and Misuse,* in press.
12. G. Edwards et al., *Alcohol Policy and the Public Good,* Oxford University Press Inc., New York, WHO Europe, 1994.

Direct reprint requests to:

Dr. Shoshana Weiss
Director of Prevention & Research
The Israel Society for the Prevention of Alcoholism
13 Nordau Street
Ramat Gan, 52464, Israel

J. DRUG EDUCATION, Vol 29(1) 53-62, 1999

FOCUSING ON THE FAMILY IN THE TREATMENT
OF SUBSTANCE ABUSING CRIMINAL OFFENDERS

EVELYN SLAGHT, PH.D.

George Mason University, Fairfax, Virginia

ABSTRACT

Aftercare services are acknowledged in the criminal justice system as critical to enabling drug offenders to avoid relapse and reincarceration, but the content too often is unsupported through research. One program funded under the Department of Justice in Maryland interviewed 150 inmates after three months in the community to determine what environmental influences were having the greatest impact on drug reuse. Findings suggest that more emphasis is needed on family relationships before and after release since satisfaction with family life is strongly correlated with drug abuse.

INTRODUCTION

The objective of most drug treatment programs within the criminal justice system is the reintegration of the offender back into society. The Department of Justice (DOJ) currently pays for intensive programs that provide counseling and support for addicted prisoners to help them return to society as productive citizens. According to Attorney General Janet Reno, "It makes no sense to send somebody to a prison, provide them drug treatment and then dump them back into the world where they got into trouble in the first place without the aftercare and follow up that is so important" [1, p. 8]. Not all programs for criminal offenders have an aftercare component, and those that do offer a range of services not necessarily related to the cause of the individuals' drug involvement.

A number of factors may contribute to the ability of the parolee to remain drug free in the community. Is a suitable job available upon release? Are family members willing to reunite with the offender? Are other resources available at the critical points that they are needed? Persons leaving prison often need health care, educational remediation, job training, social services, and family counseling, as well as services to meet special needs, such as those related to HIV/AIDS or mental health issues.

One DOJ-funded program in Maryland operated out of a prison outside of Baltimore, serving almost exclusively inner city offenders. It consists of a thirty-day cognitive-behavioral inpatient program, similar to that described by Husband and Platt, with an aftercare component that follows the inmates for three to six months after release [2]. In order to examine the experiences of inmates in the community, 150 inmates were interviewed three months after release to determine the factors that effect their success or failure in remaining drug free. A three-month time frame was chosen because most inmates remained accessible at this point. By six months, many were no longer active with the parole service and could not be located. Each inmate was administered a questionnaire which took approximately thirty minutes to complete. The questionnaire focused on the experiences of the inmate in the community that might impact their return to drug use.

The research was not an attempt to evaluate the aftercare program itself. Rather, it was an attempt to weigh the relative impact of different environmental influences. If it could be determined what factors have the greatest influence on drug use, the emphasis placed on different aspects of the program could be modified accordingly. The effort was consistent with the expectation that research should guide practice. For example, if it could be demonstrated that job availability was a major factor in drug reuse, more time could be spent in the inpatient and out-patient programs on vocational preparation and employment counseling. It was also hypothesized that family stability influences drug reuse and abuse. This was consistent with Parole Board expectations that each parolee identify his place of residence upon release. Release was often withheld when the parolee had no where to go. Likewise, parolees were warned to stay away from former friends on the assumption that peers could negatively influence drug use. The influence of family and friends on the parolee was recognized by staff, but it did not effect program content. For example, parole officers rarely met family members, nor were they in any way involved in treatment.

Services rendered by Aftercare workers were determined on an as-needed basis. Support groups were made available, but like other counseling efforts, lacked focus. Participants expressed interest in involving their families in the program, but in lieu of any documented support for a family-focused approach, counselors tended to use more traditional approaches, such as teaching anger management techniques and relapse prevention strategies.

The research was conducted in order to determine how best to direct the aftercare efforts. Family support, avoidance of drug-using friends, employment access and satisfaction, and decreased accessibility to negative neighborhood influences were all expected to impact on avoidance of drug use and correlate with rearrest and reincarceration.

REVIEW OF THE LITERATURE

The literature addressing substance abuse treatment tends to assume that we know what causes relapse or at least have a sense of what constitutes good relapse prevention. A cognitive-behavioral approach to relapse prevention is part of most drug treatment programs today, on the assumption that increased awareness of high risk situations and how to avoid triggers to relapse can prevent a return to drug use. But, according to Wexler, this approach tends to underestimate the harsh realities of the inner-city lives of many ex-convicts.

> It is almost impossible to avoid the easy availability of drugs and drug-using friends when living in the inner city. The relapse-prevention strategy of changing one's lifestyle (e.g., by acquiring new leisure, recreational, social and employment activities that support a drug-free lifestyle) or developing effective coping skills (e.g., exercising instead of going to happy hour, learning to verbally express upsetting feelings instead of using drugs, and the use of cognitive strategies . . . to avoid thoughts of drug craving) often seems unrealistic and out of reach for disenfranchised populations [3, p. 61].

Instead he suggests that more emphasis be placed on basic social and vocational rehabilitation.

The success of cognitively-based interventions has been documented by Husband & Platt [2]. Unfortunately much of the support for these approaches comes from inpatient programs rather than aftercare or outpatient programs. Direct attention to the environmental factors effecting reuse and drug abuse seems more consistent with a community approach. Altering one's life style is seldom accomplished without family support, and whether a job becomes available is an issue for the family since they are rarely in a position to support the parolee indefinitely.

Many factors can interfere with the parolees' success upon release. In many cases, the willingness of the inmate's girl friends or spouse to take them back was the key to their ability to stay drug free.

The role of the family in preventing drug relapse is supported in the literature for juvenile offenders, but there is less documentation of the role of the family in adult relapse and recidivism [4]. In the Maryland aftercare program, inmates who returned to live with parents (often the mother or grandmother who had raised them) usually found themselves facing the same conflicts that contributed to their involvement in crime as juveniles. Using Hirschi's theory, it follows that the inability of parents to apply effective social controls during the teen years does not necessarily change when the teen reaches adulthood; nor is there any evidence to deny the possible continuing effect of the absence of social controls.

In many cases, the ex-convict was not welcomed back to his home, and the *absence* of family support seemingly contributed to relapse. Ragghianti and Glenn, in their pamphlet on *Reducing Recidivism: Treating the Addicted Inmate*, point out that the offender who does not have the advantage of a caring family and support system after treatment returns to society disadvantaged in most respects [5, p. 10]. Gold also emphasizes the importance of being aware of "cues and clues" in the environment that are associated with relapse, especially those triggered by family members and drug-using peers [6].

Much of the research by criminologists relies on Sutherland's long-standing theory of differential association [7]. Negative influences in the immediate environment of the ex-convict would be expected to negatively influence the reuse of drugs and/or return to criminal behavior. Conversely, positive experiences, especially in the form of legitimate opportunities, i.e., education and/or vocational rehabilitation or job availability, would positively impact his resistance to drug use [8]. This approach does not negate the cognitive-behavioral approach, but rather focuses on external influences that bring about behavior change rather than on internal influences. The question is what environmental influences, personal and social, have the greatest impact on an inmates' ability to avoid drug use once back in the community. From a clinical perspective, if family influences can be documented, it suggests a systems approach. Cognitive-behavioral approaches may still be useful, but require more attention to selected environmental influences.

METHODOLOGY

All of the 150 ex-convicts included in the study were males who participated in inpatient drug treatment prior to their release from prison. Aftercare services began with a service-planning module called "Release Preparation," in which aftercare counselors focused on helping inmates anticipate potential problems and service needs as part of planning for their release. Inmates were given career aptitude tests to assist in examining possible job options, and planned living arrangements were discussed. Workers were aware that the "halo" effect often prevailed in these sessions, where inmates tended to fantasize about how great it would be when they got out, rather than discussing realistically what they might encounter. Although similar meetings were available for the inmates after their release, attendance was not mandatory and few responded.

Participants in the program were psychiatrically screened, and any convicts with high scores on the Psychopathology Check List-Revised (PCLR) [9] or with a history of mental illness were not included in the inpatient or Aftercare programs. Very few were rejected for this reason. All were completing relatively short term sentences (3 years, on average), i.e., they were not serious criminal offenders, but found themselves in the criminal justice system as a result of their involvement with drugs. Modifying the program to a more "social" approach seemed justifiable under these conditions.

The 150 inmates involved in the study represented almost 30 percent of the 503 inmates who completed the inpatient program between July 1994 and February

1996. Inmates were contacted by phone three months after release to complete the follow-up interview. Occasionally when inmates could not be reached by phone, they were asked to complete the questionnaire when they attended support group meetings conducted by aftercare staff.

Information was obtained from parole agents as to whether the urinalyses completed weekly for each parolee indicated "never reused," "reused sporadically," or "reused regularly." Urine results were reported for one month, three months, and six months after release. Another indicator of reuse was the self-admission of drug use since release. Reliability of responses to the self-admit item was confirmed by examining the correlation between the self-admit item (DRGUSE) and the urine results (URINE1 after 1 month; URINE2 at the end of three months; URINE3 at the end of six months). There was a positive correlation between all three variables, significant at the $p < .001$ level. A parolee who was clean at one month was highly likely to also be clean at three months. The accuracy of self-admission of drug use may have been related to the parolees awareness that what they said could be substantiated by the urine results.

Urinalysis data was not available for ninety-six of the parolees at the end of six months, requiring the study to focus on reuse at three months. This was preferable to focusing on one month since it allowed more time for the inmate to readjust and provide a better long term predictor of relapse success or failure.

Information was also obtained from parole agents as to whether the ex-convicts had recidivated. Fourteen were rearrested within three months after release; ten were returned to the inpatient program and completed it a second time; four were incarcerated elsewhere. The majority (117 or 89.3%) had no rearrest record, according to the parole agents.

The effects of various forms of treatment were examined by asking the ex-convicts about their personal use of treatments, including AA and NA.

The questionnaire focused on the family and social and environmental conditions they encountered upon release. The independent variables included:

1. Return to the same neighborhood (as an index of the availability of drugs and drug-using friends);
2. Access to educational/vocational training since release;
3. Employment status (whether or not they have been able to secure a job);
4. Living arrangement (same or different from arrangement prior to incarceration);
5. Satisfaction with the living arrangement;
6. Drug/alcohol abuse by others in the household;
7. How well they were getting along with family members (very well, pretty well, not so well, not at all); and
8. How much time they were spending with drug-using friends (a lot, some, none).

These questions were intended to determine whether work, family, friends, or the environment in general were positively or negatively associated with return to drug use. Some other measures of potential influence were also included, such as:

1. Past education achievement (how far they had gone in school);
2. Educational or vocational training since release;
3. Relationship with their parole agent; and
4. Outstanding medical needs.

The scores on the Addiction Severity Index (ASI) were examined as a measure of drug, family, and work history. Inmates with high scores on the drug and alcohol subscales would be expected to be at higher risk for reabuse. (The ASI is routinely administered to inmates coming into any of the treatment programs in this prison.)

RESULTS

All of the respondents were from Baltimore City, and of the 150 inmates in the sample, 130 were African American. Only two respondents were under age twenty-one, and five were forty-one years of age or older; the vast majority were between twenty-one and forty years of age. Age is an important factor since some studies have argued against high investments in treatment based on evidence that many addicts simply "age out" of their substance abuse. As they get older, the hassle of getting drugs and the money for drugs becomes sufficiently burdensome, leading many to stop using. In this study, age is not significantly related to drug reuse. The probability of reuse is not predictable based on knowledge of age of the parolee.

Most of the inmates (110 or 72.8%) return to the same neighborhood in which they lived prior to their arrest, although they do not necessarily return to the same household. Fifteen of those returning to the same neighborhood were not at the same address as prior to arrest. If they could not go back to live with a wife, girlfriend, or mother, they often ended up with other family members living in the same neighborhood. Whether or not they return to the same neighborhood does not correlate significantly with return to drug use, making neighborhood a less useful predictor than anticipated.

It would be expected that a high percentage of drug-using inmates would be HIV+. However, since testing is not currently mandatory for inmates in Maryland, the study relied on self-reported information. Only nine admitted to testing positive; another eight thought it was possible that they had the disease. These seventeen were part of the twenty-nine who indicated they had medical problems. With only twelve having serious medical problems beyond those associated with AIDS, medical reasons do not seem to have much influence on the outcome for this overall sample.

The influence of the availability of technical training and other educational assistance was also less than anticipated. Only thirteen had any educational rehabilitation in the three months after release, and eight reported receiving some kind of technical training, in spite of the fact that many of the men in the sample (60 or 40%) had less than a high school education. Level of education, however, had little direct effect on their ability to stay drug free.

Less than half (62 or 41%) of the respondents were using NA and/or AA, and while most were referred for some kind of community treatment, use of these resources does not significantly relate to reuse of drugs.

Forty-three percent (64) of the respondents were employed at the time of the interview, while 55% (83) were unemployed. Only three were in school full-time or disabled and unable to work.

At the end of the questionnaire, parolees were asked "Are there any problems where you think you could use additional help?" Many indicated that they needed help finding a job.

Most of the variables regarding medical, educational, and vocational accessibility did not relate significantly to the variables measuring drug reuse. Likewise, whether or not respondents were or were not employed did not significantly relate to their reuse of drugs. Their employment status *did* relate significantly to whether or not they are spending time with old friends. Those who were employed spent little or no time with friends, while those who were unemployed or disabled often returned to hanging out with friends on the street.

Current employment is significantly related to whether or not the ex-con is getting along with his family. He is more likely to be getting along with his family if he is employed.

Only *one* independent variable relates significantly to the reuse of drugs at three months, and that is whether or not the ex-convict is getting along at home. If the ex-convict is getting along very well with family members (and this was the case with 84 of the respondents), he is less likely to reuse drugs than if he is only getting along pretty well or not so well (see Table 1).

While getting along with family members is the only direct predictor of drug use, the results suggested that employment status and time spent with friends might indirectly influence drug reuse. Some inmates who get along well with family upon release find that this support disintegrated if they are unable to contribute to the financial survival of the household. As family becomes less supportive, the urge to return to hanging out on the street with drug-using friends may return. In order to test the indirect effects of employment and friends on family relationships (and ultimately on drug reuse), the authors tested several regression equations. None of the results were significant, suggesting that there may be other variables missing from the proposed equations, or the sample may be too small to test these hypotheses adequately.

Table 1. Significant Correlations

	Currently Employed (CUREMP)	Urine Results at 3 Months (URINE3)
Getting along with Family (GTALGFM)	.148 $p = .07^*$	.20 $p = .046^*$
Contact with same Friends (SAMFRDS)	–.226 $p = .017^*$	.07 $p = .60$
Currently Employed (CUREMP)	XXXXX	.12 $p = .25$

*Significant at the $< .05$ level

LIMITATIONS OF THE STUDY

The sample consisted exclusively of short term offenders and cannot be generalized to other offenders. Likewise, results are only useful with offenders who have no major medical or mental health histories. The small sample size is a product of the newness of the program. To delay the study until a larger sample could be secured would risk allowing the program to become entrenched in current methodology. Conducting the study early allows alterations at a point when staff is most flexible.

DISCUSSION

Family influences appear to be a dominant force in whether an ex-convict returns to drug use or not. This may suggest that there is a need for more effort to involve significant family members in the drug treatment, both in the aftercare component as well as in the inpatient activities. Family involvement is more feasible in the aftercare component, directly through such events as "Family Nights," and indirectly by spending more time talking with and about family members and focusing on the role the family plays in the parolees' rehabilitation. Support groups for family members may be as important as these activities are for the parolee. Preparation for release needs to utilize role play and other experiential methods to help the inmate learn how to respond to family conflict. Relapse prevention needs to work not only on identifying family conflicts as frequent "triggers" to reuse, but teach ways of coping with the issues that result in loss of family support.

The relationship between employment and drug-using friends and family relationships needs further exploration, since it is not yet clear what the primary factors are that effect family support. Nor is it clear in what order these events occur. Understanding the dynamics (e.g., employment status) that interfere with successful re-bonding with family members may need to be consistently included in treatment and intervention efforts if relapse is to be avoided.

PROGRAM IMPLICATIONS

The absence of research to guide practice continues to cause problems in the drug treatment field. Program philosophy and content need to consider the environmental factors that play the greatest role in whether a drug addict will reuse upon release. The inmate needs to be encouraged to examine the role that his family plays in his behavior. For inmates without family supports, more emphasis may need to be placed on finding suitable alternatives. Aftercare services are imperative in reconnecting the parolee to his family, and consideration should be given to mandating family-focused services in DOJ Aftercare programs.

Currently, parole officers are assigned to validate the residence that an inmate states will be his residence upon release. While this eliminates bogus addresses, no other responsibility is assumed in spite of the fact that this represents an ideal opportunity to explore family relationships for treatment purposes.

One concern of the aftercare staff was the amount of time parole officers expect releasees to spend in attending treatment programs, especially during the first month. Too little scrutiny of this treatment takes place, and the time spent in these programs detracts from other personal responsibilities the parolee may need to assume. Some of the time spent in treatment might better be utilized by providing concrete job readiness services.

In this age of managed care, services to the substance abuser are diminishing. It is imperative that we have a rationale for the intervention models we are prescribing and be able to document their impact in the context of the environmental factors most heavily influencing recidivism and reuse.

ACKNOWLEDGMENTS

The author gratefully acknowledges the assistance of Faith Storms and Erica Rosen, aftercare workers in the Regimented Offenders Treatment Program at Patuxent Institution in Maryland.

REFERENCES

1. R. H. Feldkamp, DOJ Testing Program to Help Addicts Adjust, *Narcotics Demand Reduction Digest, 6,* 1994.

2. S. D. Husband and J. J. Platt, The Cognitive Skills Component in Substance Abuse Treatment in Correctional Settings: A Brief Review, *Journal of Drug Issues, 23,* pp. 31-42, 1998.
3. H. K. Wexler, The Success of Therapeutic Communities for Substance Abusers in American Prisons, *Journal of Psychoactive Drugs, 27,* pp. 57-61, 1995.
4. T. Hirschi, *Causes of Delinquency,* University of California Press, Berkeley, 1969.
5. M. Ragghianti and T. Glenn, *Reducing Recidivism: Treating the Addicted Inmate,* Hazelden, Center City, Minnesota, 1991.
6. S. Gold, We're All In This Together: Understanding the Interdependence of Prevention and Treatment, *Substance Abuse Policy in a Changing Environment: Summaries of the Proceedings of a Conference for State Policy Makers,* December 5-7, 1991.
7. E. Sutherland, *Principles of Criminology,* Lippincott, Philadelphia, 1939.
8. R. A. Cloward and L. E. Ohlin, *Delinquency and Opportunity,* Free Press, New York, 1960.
9. R. D. Hare and D. Schelling, *Psychopathic Behavior: Approaches to Research,* Wiley, New York, 1978.

Direct reprint requests to:

Evelyn Slaght, Ph.D.
Associate Professor of Social Work
George Mason University
4400 University Drive
Fairfax, VA 22030-4444

J. DRUG EDUCATION, Vol. 29(1) 63-75, 1999

CHILDREN OF ALCOHOLICS:
A SCHOOL-BASED COMPARATIVE STUDY

CONNIE K. MOREY, PH.D.
Seattle University, Washington

ABSTRACT

This study investigates children of alcoholics (COAs) and their cohorts who are not affected by parental alcoholism (non-COAs). Participants include fourth through sixth grade students who are identified as COAs and non-COAs. The study examines differences between COAs and non-COAs on measures of internalized shame, self-esteem, perceived support, and teacher behavior ratings. Results indicate that COAs and non-COAs demonstrate no significant differences on measures of social support and shame. In contrast, self-esteem and teacher ratings for COAs are significantly lower in comparison to ratings for non-COAs. In addition, teacher ratings of male COAs are significantly negatively affected by their COA status, whereas female COA and non-COA teacher ratings do not differ significantly.

INTRODUCTION

According to a National Institute of Alcohol Abuse and Alcoholism report [1], approximately one of every four to five children in a typical elementary school classroom is the son or daughter of an alcoholic. In a classroom of twenty-five students, an average of five students in the class are affected significantly by familial alcoholism. The report estimates that 95 percent of these children are never identified nor do they receive intervention of any kind through the schools. Incidence figures confirm the familial nature of alcoholism. It is estimated that 38 percent of the U.S. adult population has a family history of alcoholism among biological first, second, or third-degree relatives [2]. In summary, although fully a quarter of the children in schools are affected by a parent's alcoholism, the majority of these children are overlooked and under served by the school system.

63

Many negative characteristics have been assigned to children of alcoholics (COAs), based on informal observations of concerned educators and mental health professionals. Robinson lists twenty behavioral and psychological signs for school personnel to notice among children who might be living with alcoholism [3]. These signs, suggested as a result of informal teacher observations, include low self-esteem, anxiety, being easily embarrassed, suppressed anger, a sense that problems are out of control, poor coping skills, depression or frequent sadness, and difficulties adjusting to changes in routine.

Studies of adolescent and college-aged COAs, using self-report measures of depression, self-concept, and behavior problems found that the COAs, compared with non-COAs, reported higher levels of depression, lower self-concept, and more behavior problems, including alcohol-related problems [4, 5]. Johnson, Boney, and Brown compared seventy-two COA and non-COA children, ages eight to fourteen, on self-report measures of depression, anxiety, and a standardized academic test and found that the COAs scored higher on measures of depression and anxiety, and lower on the math portion of the academic test [6]. Stern, Kendall, and Eberhard compared the proportion of COAs in three groups, grades one through five: regular education, emotional disturbance, and learning disabled [7]. In a sample of ninety children these investigators failed to find differences in the proportion of COAs with regard to educational placement. So, even though COAs may be at higher risk for self-esteem and academic problems in later grades, they are not over-represented in special education classes.

Do children of alcoholics in elementary school demonstrate significantly more negative characteristics in comparison with their non-affected cohorts, when they are measured with reliable instruments? This study focuses on providing a preliminary answer to this question. First, this article will provide background in the literature for studying differences between children of alcoholics and their non-affected peers in the areas of shame, self-esteem, social support, and teacher ratings of school behavior. Research questions addressed in this study will then be presented, followed by a description of the method for data collection and results of the study. The article will close with implications of the study results for those who work with children of alcoholics in the schools and in mental health settings.

BACKGROUND

The rationale for examining shame, self-esteem, and social support among children of alcoholics derives primarily from previous research with this population. Cook [8] found an association between alcoholism and internalized shame as measured by the Internalized Shame Scale [9] among adults. Children's shame that may result from living with parental alcoholism has not been studied or measured at this point. The present study used a child's version of the ISS to measure shame among children.

Several studies of children of alcoholics have measured self-esteem with either non standardized or relatively outdated instruments [10]. Both longitudinal [11-13] and cross-sectional studies [14, 15] found that COAs rated their self-esteem as lower than children from families with no reported alcoholism. Harter's Self-Perception Profile For Children [16] was used in this study because it is a current, reliable measure of self-esteem in children.

The area of social support is even less represented in research on children of alcoholics than is shame. Encouragement for seeking social support seems to be a key component that is provided for COAs in school-based groups [10]. Previous research on COAs has not compared perceptions of social support among COAs to those of non-COAs. In the present study, Harter's Social Support Scale For Children [17] was used as a measure of perceived social support.

In the literature evaluating interventions for COAs, teacher ratings are often not utilized [6, 10, 14, 18, 19], and when they are used, they are often informal [15]. The present study used a standardized teacher rating scale of children's behavior [16] that is a part of the Self-Perception Profile For Children. Teacher ratings are used to compare COAs with non-COAs.

The literature on COAs examines only minimally the relationship among self-esteem, perceived support, shame, and school behavior. Results of the Werner longitudinal study suggest that COAs who have high self-esteem as young adults have fewer documented mental health problems as adults than do those with lower self-esteem ratings [12]. The present study investigated the relationship among self-esteem, perceived support, shame, and teacher ratings of behavior for COAs.

The results of two longitudinal studies by Miller and Jang [11] and Werner [12] suggest the following profile for a resilient child: the child is more likely to be a first-born girl who is bright and able to use her intelligence to achieve in both school and extracurricular activities. In addition, the resilient child is likely to demonstrate personality characteristics that draw positive attention, such as a caring for others, good social skills, and the ability to view the family's problems with a certain amount of objectivity [12].

The previous studies certainly point to a pattern of differences between children of alcoholics and their non-affected peers. Generally speaking, these studies suggest that children of alcoholics, when compared with non-COASs, are more prone to have self-esteem problems, lower academic achievement, more behavior problems, and a higher rate of depression. The role of family and personal characteristics in making some COAs more resilient than others is an important mediating factor to consider when looking at research on COAs.

RESEARCH QUESTIONS

Based on previous research findings and what is theorized about children of alcoholics (COAs), it was predicted that COAs in this study would demonstrate lower self-esteem and teacher ratings, higher shame ratings, and lower scores on the social support measure than their non-COA cohorts. Further, it was anticipated that COA males would be more negatively affected by parental alcoholism than their female counterparts. This negative influence would be reflected by lower self-esteem, social support, and teacher ratings, and higher shame scale scores for males in comparison with female participants.

This study focuses on two research questions:

1. Do children of alcoholics differ from children not living with parental alcoholism on measures of shame, self-esteem, perceived social support, and teacher ratings?
2. Among children of alcoholics, what is the effect of the participant's sex, birth order, and number of siblings on measures of shame, self-esteem, feelings of support, and teacher ratings?

METHODS

Participants

The participants for this study ($n = 73$) were drawn from grades four through six and attended one of the eight elementary schools in a suburban public school system in the Midwest. Participants included children of alcoholics ($n = 32$), and a comparison group of children ($n = 43$) who are not children of alcoholics. The actual sample size varied across measurement instruments because some participants did not complete every instrument. Table 1 provides subject characteristics for both COAs and non-COAs.

Children of alcoholics were recruited for the study in two ways, depending on their grade-level. Fourth graders attended a one-hour presentation given by the district's Chemical Health Coordinator in each of eight schools. Shortly after hearing this presentation about how children may be affected by parental alcoholism, all fourth grade children received a letter inviting them to join a support group for children of alcoholics. This letter needed to be signed by one of their parents if the child wanted to participate in a school support group.

Fifth and sixth grade children were recruited for the groups by listening to a ten-minute presentation by the district Chemical Health Coordinator, who came to each classroom separately to discuss the goals of the groups. Letters requesting parent permission for children wishing to participate in the groups were sent home to all children. The COA group for this study consisted of only those children who had both parental permission to be in a COA support group, as well as specific permission to be in this study.

The classification of children as COAs for this study was verified in three ways: by parents, by the children themselves, and by the school psychologists in each building. Parents initially acknowledged the problem of alcoholism in the family by giving their child permission to participate in a group, focusing on

Table 1. Subject Characteristics for COAs and Non-COAs

| | Sample | | | | | |
| | COA | | Non-COA | | Total | |
Characteristic	n	%	n	%	n	%
Age						
9 years	7	21.9	7	17.9	14	19.8
10 years	13	40.6	15	38.5	28	39.4
11 years	10	31.3	13	33.3	23	32.4
12 years	1	3.1	4	10.3	5	7.0
13 years	1	3.1	0	0.0	1	1.4
Sex						
Male	15	46.9	16	41.0	31	43.6
Female	17	53.1	23	59.0	40	56.4
Siblings						
0	0	0.0	3	7.7	3	4.2
1	14	43.8	18	46.2	32	45.1
2	6	18.8	12	30.8	18	25.3
3	3	9.4	6	15.4	9	12.7
4	5	15.6	0	0.0	5	7.1
5 and above	4	12.4	0	0.0	4	5.6
Birth Order[a]						
First	11	34.4	26	66.7	37	52.1
Second	8	25.0	5	12.8	13	18.3
Third	12	27.5	7	17.9	19	26.8
Fourth	0	0.0	1	2.6	1	1.4
Seventh	1	3.1	0	0.0	1	1.4
Child Lives With						
Both Parents	19	59.4	34	87.2	53	74.6
Mother	11	34.4	4	10.3	15	21.2
Father	2	6.3	0	0.0	2	2.8
Someone else	0	0.0	0	0.0	0	0.0
Missing information	0	0.0	1	2.5	1	1.4
Previous Group Involvement						
Yes	10	31.3	1	2.6	11	15.5
No	21	65.5	38	97.4	59	83.1
Missing data	1	3.1	0	0.0	1	1.4
Socioeconomic Status (I = highest, V = lowest)						
I	0	0.0	0	0.0	0	0.0
II	12	37.5	18	46.2	30	42.3
III	18	56.3	18	46.2	36	50.7
IV	2	6.2	3	7.6	5	7.0
V	0	0.0	0	0.0	0	0.0

[a]No subjects had fifth and sixth birth order.

coping with and understanding alcoholism in the family. The parent permission letter clearly stated that the focus of the group was to help children to cope with a parental alcohol problem

Children further substantiated their COA classification by answering three questions about their perceptions and worries regarding parental drinking: 1) Have you ever thought that one of your parents had a drinking problem? 2) Have you ever lost sleep because of a parent's drinking? 3) Have you ever worried about a parent's health because of his or her alcohol use? These questions were taken from the Children of Alcoholics Screening Test, devised by Pilat and Jones [20, p. 28]. The entire thirty-item screening test was not administered because it was not approved by the school board. The three questions selected from this instrument represented a compromise, and were the most direct questions included in this screening device. Eighty percent of the COA participants reported having one or more worries about parental drinking. In contrast with the COAs, 80 percent of the non-COA participants reported no worries about their parent's drinking. Complete results, comparing COA and non-COA participant responses on these three questions, are in the results section.

Final verification of the COA classification was made through the clinical judgment of the eight school psychologists who worked with the COA participants in the treatment portion of this study. Each of these practitioners participated in at least two days of training in identifying COAs, and running groups for them. On the basis of this training, each school psychologist verified that the children in their group were COAs.

Children included in the non-COA sample were chosen by each building school psychologist and matched according to gender and grade with COA children. To assure that there were at least as many non-COAs as COAs, twice as many non-COAs were sent parent permission letters to participate in this study. Forty-three children were classified as non-COAs for this study.

Instruments

The instruments used in this study were as follows: (1) Self-Perception Profile for Children (SPPC) to measure self-esteem; (2) Social Support Scale for Children (SSSC) to measure perceived support; (3) Internalized Shame Scale-Children's (ISS-C) to measure shame; and (4) the Teacher Rating Scale, a classroom behavior rating scale, completed by each student's homeroom teacher to assess in-school behavior. In addition, a fourteen-item questionnaire was used to gather descriptive information about the participants and their families.

Harter's Self-Perception Profile for Children (SPPC)

The purpose of this scale is to measure a child's self-esteem in five domains, as well as in global self-worth [16]. The five domains include Scholastic

Competence, Social Acceptance, Athletic Competence, Physical Appearance, and Behavioral Conduct. The two scores obtained from this scale were the Mean Difference Score and a Global Self-Worth score. The Mean Difference Scores range from +1 to –3, with difference scores closer to zero or above zero reflecting a higher, more positive self-perception. The Global Self-Worth score is the mean rating from the Global Self-Worth sub scale, ranging from 1 to 4, with 1 indicating low self-worth.

Harter's scale was standardized on four samples of third through eighth grade students. Students (a total of 1,543) were drawn from lower-middle to upper-middle class neighborhoods in Colorado. Harter reports internal consistency reliabilities for each subscale [16]. Alpha coefficients ranged from .71 for the Behavioral Conduct subscale to .86 for the Athletic Competence subscale. Content validity for each subtest was determined by factor analysis. This analysis revealed that factor loadings for each subtest domain are substantial, suggesting that the five subscales do in fact define distinctly separate domains.

Harter's Social Support Scale For Children (SSSC)

The SSSC was developed to measure the perceived support and regard that significant others demonstrate toward the child [17]. Harter's SSSC consists of four subscales which emphasize the degree to which others treat individuals like a person, like them as they are, care about their feelings, listen to them, and understand them as unique individuals. Perceived support is assessed on this scale from four groups of significant others in the child's life: parents, teachers, classmates, and friends. The answers on this scale are rated from 1 to 4, with 4 representing the highest level of perceived support.

This scale was standardized on 2,338 students, grades three through eight, drawn from lower-middle to upper-middle class neighborhoods in Colorado. Alpha coefficients ranged from .88 and .86 for the middle school sample for the Parent subscale to .72 and .74 for the Friend subscale at the elementary school level. The validity of content in these scales was supported by a factor analytic study done by Harter [17]. This analysis revealed that there are four separate sources of support for middle school samples and three separate sources of support at the elementary level: peer (classmate and friend at the middle school level), teacher, and parents.

Internalized Shame Scale-Children's Version (ISS-C)

Cook's Internalized Shame Scale was adapted for use with children in this study [9]. Wording was changed on the ISS-C so that it would be at the fourth grade reading level. The ISS-C measures shame, i.e., the sense of self as worthless and deficient at the core [21]. An adapted version of the ISS-C, consisting of twenty-five of the original thirty items, was used in this study. Five items related to self-worth were not used in the final data analysis because self-worth was measured, using the Harter scale (SPPC). The possible range of mean item scores is 0 to 4, with 0 representing the least amount of shame.

Cook reported an alpha coefficient of .94 for the twenty-four-item shame scale administered to a non-clinical college student sample of 472 students who were given the adult version of the ISS [9]. A test-retest reliability coefficient over a period of nine weeks using graduate students ($n = 44$) was .84. The ISS scores (adult version) correlated .77 and .79 with the Janis-Field Feelings of Inadequacy Scale and the Ineffectiveness scale from the Eating Disorder Inventory [21-23].

Teacher Rating Scale of Child's Actual Behavior

This scale was developed as a part of the Self-Perception Profile for Children to obtain teachers' ratings of children in five areas: scholastic competence, social acceptance, athletic competence, physical appearance, and behavioral conduct [16]. These same five areas are rated by the children taking the self-report portion of this rating scale. A score of 4 indicates that the child rates favorably in the area, from the teacher's point of view, and a score of 1 indicates an unfavorable teacher rating. Internal consistency for this scale, using the alpha coefficient, was .92, as reported in Table 2.

Data Collection

Administration of the student-completed instruments took place outside of the classroom in February 1990. All items were read orally to the children to assure that participants understood questions. COA students were tested together with non-COAs in rooms/offices within each of the eight schools participating in the study. Data was collected for this study by the author. The COA or non-COA status of students was not known by this author. Teacher Rating Scales were placed in teacher mailboxes with instructions, and returned to building school psychologists when completed.

Table 2. Alpha Coefficients for Study Instruments

Measures	Alpha Coefficients
Internalized Shame Scale-Children's Version	.94
Self-Perception Profile for Children	
Difference Score	.93
Global Score	.63
Social Support Scale for Children	.91
Teacher Rating Scale	.92

RESULTS

Responses of COAs and Non-COAs to Questions About Parental Drinking

Within the COA sample, 80 percent ($n = 24$) of the participants reported having one or more worries about parental drinking. One-third ($n = 10$) of the COA sample reported having three worries, 26.7 percent ($n = 8$) reported having two worries, and the remaining 20 percent ($n = 6$) reported one worry about parental drinking. In contrast with the COA participants, 80% ($n = 32$) of the non-COA sample reported no worries about their parent's drinking. Within this sample only 12.5 percent ($n = 5$) and 7.5 percent ($n = 3$) of the children reported one or two worries, respectively, about parental alcohol use. None of the children in the non-COA sample reported three concerns about their parent's use of alcohol.

Reliability Data from Present Sample

Table 2 provides internal consistency coefficients for all measures used in this study. Estimates of internal consistency for all instruments used in this study ranged from .63 to .94 (alpha coefficients). The reliability of the SPPC Global was lower than the other measures because it consists of only six items within the SPPC. Other measures have relatively more items, ranging from fifteen items on the Teacher Rating Scale to thirty-six items on the Social Support Scale for Children.

Effects of Gender, Birth Order, and Number of Siblings

An analysis of variance revealed no significant main effects for gender, birth order, or number of siblings on measures of self-esteem (SPPC), social support (SSSC), or shame (ISS-C). There was, however, a significant main effect for gender on ratings from the teachers (Teacher Rating Scale), $F(1,29) = 10.19$, $p < .004$. Males received lower behavior ratings ($x = 2.64$) than females ($x = 3.34$) by their teachers. For subsequent analyses with the Teacher Rating Scale, gender effects are examined.

COA versus Non-COA Group Differences

COAs and non-COAs were compared on the ISS-C, SPPC Difference, SPPC Global, and SSSC using an independent t-test. Significant group differences were found only on the SPPC. The COA sample earned significantly lower mean difference scores (–0.68) on the SPPC than did the non-COA sample (–0.41), $t(67) = -1.88$, $p < .05$.

A 2 (Group) by 2 (Gender) ANOVA was used to examine for differences between COAs and non-COAs on the Teacher Rating Scale by gender. This analysis revealed main effects for both group ($p < .001$) and gender ($p < .005$). There was also a significant Group $\times$ Gender interaction, $F(1,71) = 10.03$ ($p < .002$). The mean ratings for COAs versus non-COAs by sex revealed that male COAs received lower behavior ratings from teachers compared to female COAs and non-COAs. In terms of teacher ratings, COA status seemed to affect males more negatively than females.

DISCUSSION

This study examined differences between COAs and non-COAs on measures of shame, self-esteem, perceived support, and teacher behavior ratings. No differences were found between COA and non-COA participants in their perceived social support or self-reported shame. Self-esteem was significantly lower for COAs in comparison to non-COAs. Teacher ratings on the Teacher Rating Scale were lower for male COAs in comparison to male non-COAs. Female COA teacher ratings were not significantly different in comparison to female non-COA teacher ratings.

Lower scores among COAs on self-esteem are consistent with research [3, 5, 11, 12] which indicates that COAs have generally lower self-esteem than their non-COA counterparts. COA boys in this study fared more poorly than girls in teacher ratings, suggesting a perceived vulnerability of boys who are in alcoholic families in comparison to girls. This is consistent with findings in Werner's [12] longitudinal study which also found that male COAs were more likely than female COAs to demonstrate negative behavior. However, it should be noted that results from this teacher rating are tentative, at best, because the teacher rating, although demonstrating acceptable internal consistency alpha coefficients in this study, has not been validated in a larger study.

There are several plausible explanations for the findings that COAs did not differ from non-COAs in their feelings of shame or perceived support from others. First, it may reflect a lack of awareness and sensitivity to feelings of shame or perceived support on the part of the COAs. Since it is hypothesized that COAs may block feelings and thoughts that reflect negatively on them and/or their family, it is possible that this defense has rendered the COA sample less able to express their true needs for support from significant others. Second, with its strongly-worded negative language, the shame scale may have triggered COAs' defenses, and thus not accessed their underlying feelings of shame. In contrast, the self-esteem scale may have been less likely to trigger a defensive reaction since it is written in more positive or neutral language. Finally, it is possible that the COA participants in this study did not experience higher levels of shame, or nor more of a need for support from others than their non-COA cohorts.

SUMMARY AND CONCLUSIONS

This study was done on a relatively small sample of children from one school district in the midwest. For these reasons, implications of these findings need to be seen as preliminary, and interpreted cautiously. However, this author would like to make some modest suggestions, based on the current findings and with the hope that future research will examine these issues in more depth, and add suggestions to the ones offered here. It would be especially helpful if a future researcher did a large study establishing the reliability and validity of Harter's teacher rating scale [16].

Results of this preliminary study revealed that COAs and non-COAs differed significantly in their self-esteem ratings and in their teachers' ratings of their behavior in school. As suggested in the literature comparing COAs with the non-COAs, it was found that having a parent with alcoholism did affect children's self-esteem in a negative manner. The relationship between COA status and teacher rating of school behavior appeared somewhat more complex. The study results indicated that teacher ratings for male COAs were significantly lower than ratings for female COAs or non-COAs. This may indicate that male COAs who have exhibited socially unacceptable behavior in school would benefit from more specific intervention efforts which increased their socially acceptable school behavior.

Since this study suggested that children of alcoholics were negatively affected in the area of self-esteem, schools and agencies that provide services for school-aged COAs would be well-advised to provide support for this high-risk group of youngsters. Support could focus on bolstering the skills that enhance self-esteem in the areas investigated in this study: scholastic and athletic competence, social skills that lead to social acceptance, and positive behavior. Peer coaching and tutoring are examples of practical, relatively inexpensive methods for providing large numbers of children with positive, pro-social models in the school setting. Since the self-esteem rating used in this study is skill-based, improving the skills of COA children would be likely to increase their self-esteem.

Since teachers viewed male COA behavior more negatively than female COA behavior in this study, schools might provide indirect support for COAs by providing teachers with information regarding alcoholism, and the potential positive affects of skill-based programs for these high-risk children. Teachers and school personnel need to know that this group of children could benefit from extra teacher help and attention in both scholastic and athletic areas. Nastasi and DeZolt report extensively on substance abuse preventive programs, and point out that problem-solving and drug abuse resistance skills, paired with personal-social competence, seem to be most effective in preventing alcohol problems with high-risk populations [24].

On a broader scope, McNamara, suggests that preventive measures in schools need to include clear school policies that provide consequences for drug use and educate students about risks of use; they need to provide education regarding effective coping skills for resisting drug use; and finally, schools need to foster and support protective factors that have been found to strengthen a student's ability to resist drug abuse [25]. Some factors that McNamara cites as fostering student ability to resist drugs include positive peer affiliations, bonding/ involvement in school activities, relationships with caring adults, opportunities for school success and responsible behavior, and availability of drug-free activities.

The present study, although preliminary in its results, clearly points to the need for preventive programs for COAs in the schools. Recommendations such as peer coaching and support for student drug resistance and social competence skills, as suggested by McNamara [25] and Nastasi and DeZolt [24], need to be studied to determine their effectiveness in providing support for vulnerable youngsters, such as the children of alcoholics in this study.

REFERENCES

1. National Institute on Alcohol Abuse and Alcoholism, Alcoholism and Co-Occurring Disorders, *Alcohol Alert,* pp. 1-4, October 1991.
2. T. Harford, Family History of Alcoholism in the United States: Prevalence and Demographic Characteristics, *Health Education Quarterly, 87,* pp. 931-935, 1992.
3. B. E. Robinson, *Working with Children of Alcoholics: The Practitioner's Handbook,* Lexington Books, Lexington, Massachusetts, 1989.
4. J. Gross and M. McCaul, A Comparison of Drug Use and Adjustment in Urban Adolescent Children of Substance Abusers, *International Journal of the Addictions, 25:*4A, pp. 495-511, 1990-91.
5. A. Jarmas and A. Kazak, Young Adult Children of Alcoholic Fathers: Depressive Experiences, Coping Styles, and Family Systems, *Journal of Consulting and Clinical Psychology, 60:*2, pp. 244-251, 1992.
6. J. Johnson, T. Boney, and B. Brown, Evidence of Depressive Symptoms in Children of Substance Abusers, *International Journal of the Addictions, 25:*4A, pp. 465-479, 1990-91.
7. R. Stern Kendall and P. Eberhard, Children of Alcoholics in the School: Where Are They? Their Representations in Special Education, *Psychology in the Schools, 28,* pp. 116-123, 1991.
8. B. E. Cook, Measuring Shame: The Internalized Shame Scale, *Alcoholism Treatment Quarterly, 4,* pp. 197-215, 1987.
9. D. R. Cook, *Internalized Shame Scale (ISS),* General Information for Directions and Use, unpublished manuscript, 1989.
10. J. Riddle, J. Bergin, and C. Douzenis, Effects of Group Counseling on the Self-Concept of Children of Alcoholics, *Elementary School Guidance & Counseling, 31,* pp. 192-203, 1997.
11. D. Miller and M. Jang, Children of Alcoholics: A 20-Year Longitudinal Study, *Social Work Research and Abstracts, 13,* pp. 23-29, 1977.
12. E. E. Werner, Resilient Offspring of Alcoholics: A Longitudinal Study from Birth to Age 18, *Journal of Studies on Alcohol, 47:*1, pp. 34-40, 1986.

13. S. A. Weintraub, Children and Adolescents at Risk for Substance Abuse and Psycho-pathology, *International Journal of the Addictions, 25*:4A, pp. 481-494, 1990-91.
14. L. A. Bennett, S. J. Wolin, and D. R. Reiss, Cognitive, Behavioral, and Emotional Problems among School-Age Children of Alcoholic Parents, *American Journal of Psychiatry, 145,* pp. 185-190, 1988.
15. A. L. Kearney and M. H. Hines, Evaluation of the Effectiveness of a Drug Education Program, *Journal of Drug Education, 10*:2, pp. 127-134, 1980.
16. S. Harter, *Manual for the Self-Perception Profile for Children,* University of Denver, Denver, 1985.
17. S. Harter, *Manual for the Social Support Scale for Children,* University of Denver, Denver, 1985.
18. S. Kim, J. McLoed, and Palmgren, The Impact of the "I'm Special" Program on Students Substance Abuse and Other Related Student Problem Behavior, *Journal of Drug Education, 19,* pp. 83-85, 1989.
19. A. A. Riddell, "I Never Knew There Were So Many of Us." A Model Early Inter-vention Alcohol Program, *Alcohol Health and Research World, 12*:2, pp. 110-124, 1987-88.
20. J. M. Pilat and J. W. Jones, Identification of Children of Alcoholics: Two Empirical Studies, *Alcohol Health and Research World, 36,* pp. 27-33, 1984-85.
21. D. R. Cook, *The Measurement of Shame: The Internalized Shame Scale,* unpublished manuscript, 1989.
22. D. M. Garner and M. P. Olmsted, *Eating Disorder Inventory Manual,* Psychological Assessment Resources, Odessa, Florida, 1984.
23. R. Crandall, The Measurement of Self-Esteem and Related Constructs, in *Measures of Social Psychological Attitudes,* J. P. Robinson and P. R. Shaver (eds.) Institute for Social Research, University of Michigan, Ann Arbor, Michigan, 1973.
24. B. K. Nastasi and D. M. DeZolt, *School Interventions for Children of Alcoholics,* The Guilford Press, New York, 1994.
25. K. M. McNamara, Best Practices in Substance Abuse Prevention Programs, in *Best Practices in School Psychology–III,* A. Thomas and J. Grimes (eds.), National Asso-ciation of School Psychologists, Washington D.C., pp. 369-382, 1995.

Direct reprint requests to:

Connie K. Morey, Ph.D.
180 E. Cty. Rd. B2
Apt. 24
Little Canada, MN 55117

J. DRUG EDUCATION, Vol. 29(1) 77-94, 1999

TRENDS FROM 1987 TO 1991 IN ALCOHOL, TOBACCO, AND OTHER DRUG (ATOD) USE AMONG ADOLESCENTS EXPOSED TO A SCHOOL DISTRICT-WIDE PREVENTION INTERVENTION

TINA M. YOUNOSZAI
University of Maryland, College Park

DAVID K. LOHRMANN
Academy for Educational Development, Washington, D.C.

CAROL A. SEEFELDT
University of Maryland, College Park

ROBERT GREENE
Troy School District, Michigan

ABSTRACT

This study involved a school-based prevention program initiated to reduce alcohol, tobacco, and other drug (ATOD) use among adolescents in the Troy School District in the Detroit area. One purpose was to describe the current ATOD situation by investigating changes in reported ATOD use from 1987 to 1991. Another purpose was to explore and identify the most salient risk and protective factors present. In 1987, 1,490 students (comprising grades 8 and 11) and in 1991, 3,171 students (comprising grades 8 to 12) completed questionnaires. Significant decreases were found for use of most drugs with the exception of alcohol. Involvement in problem behaviors was identified as the most salient risk factor, while having a member of a non-using peer group was the most salient protective factor. Implications for the design of subsequent intervention programs are discussed.

Adolescence is a period of experimentation, exploration, and curiosity. Nationally, 70 percent of eighth graders reported having tried alcohol, 25 percent have used it

77

during the preceding thirty days, and 13 percent consumed five or more drinks on a single occasion during the previous two weeks [1]. In addition, 57 percent of high school seniors have tried an illicit drug, and more than a third have tried an illicit drug other than marijuana [1]. These statistics suggest that alcohol, tobacco, and other drug (ATOD) use is a part of many adolescents' need for exploration and experimentation. It may even be seen by adolescents as a normal part of the transitional process from adolescence to adulthood [2].

Adolescents are at particular risk due to the increased opportunities to use ATOD [1, 3]. During this period, they must sort out the many messages received about ATOD and make decisions regarding their own use [3, 4]. In forming attitudes and beliefs, and in defining appropriate behavior, adolescents draw from the past actions, attitudes, and norms of significant others (e.g., parents, other family members, sports heroes, or other adult role models), as well as from characters depicted in the media [5].

In an effort to prevent ATOD use among adolescents, ATOD prevention intervention programs have been initiated in schools. To understand ATOD use, and to more effectively develop and initiate interventions, school districts need to consider ATOD prevalence for particular drugs over time and factors which may be related to ATOD use.

Changes in adolescent ATOD use have been monitored at the national level annually since 1975 through studies funded by the National Institute on Drug Abuse [1]. Reports summarize prevalence of ATOD use, trends in ATOD use, and other related factors, such as grade level when ATOD were first used, intensity of ATOD use, attitudes and beliefs about ATOD use, and the social milieu of ATOD use. Distinctions are made among important demographic subgroups (e.g., gender, race, socioeconomic status, college plans, region, and population density) in these populations. Findings serve to guide policy making in resource allocation and early detection and localization of emerging ATOD problems [1]. Yearly reports have shown that changes in ATOD use occur as particular drugs rise or fall in popularity (e.g., since the 1980s, there have been steady declines in the proportion of high school students who report actively using any illicit drug; alcohol use has remained widespread, and past month cigarette use has remained around 30% [1].

While national data are useful for providing an overall picture of drug use and changes from year to year across the United States, they do not necessarily accurately depict trends in a particular state or school district within a state. To better target prevention efforts toward a specific population, ATOD prevalence within a particular school district should also be monitored.

Additionally, school districts need to be aware of risk and protective factors that exist in their student population so that the effectiveness of intervention programs is maximized [4, 6]. In a comprehensive review, Hawkins, Catalano, and Miller identified risk factors found in previous studies to be associated with ATOD use [7]. Factors comprised those existing within the broad society and culture (e.g., laws and norms favorable to use, high availability, extreme economic deprivation, and neighborhood disorganization) and those that lie within individuals (e.g., problem behavior, rebelliousness, and attitudes favorable toward use) and their interpersonal environment of family (e.g., high parental use and attitudes favorable toward use, negative family management practices, and low family bonding), school (e.g., academic failure and low commitment to school), and peer group (e.g., association with drug-using peers).

Since many risk factors may be resistant or impossible to change, ATOD interventions should also address protective factors that mediate risk for ATOD use and abuse [7, 8]. Protective factors that have been found to be related to non-ATOD use include prosocial values, high commitment to school, family cohesion, clear parental expectations, and perceived parental punishment for ATOD use [8-10].

School districts need to address risk and protective factors in their student population and surrounding community and develop intervention programs which target those that are most salient [7]. Strategies that target multiple factors, in an effort to reduce factors placing an individual at risk while enhancing those that serve as protective, will be more effective in prevention efforts [7].

The current study described the initiation of an ATOD prevention intervention program that was based on a needs assessment of students enrolled in an upper-Midwest, suburban school district in the United States. The needs assessment included a community ATOD prevalence survey and the school district's assessment of risk and protective factors present in this population of students. Findings revealed that adolescents in this school district are involved in ATOD use and suggested that they may differ in their involvement from other communities [11].

Adolescents from suburban communities may be at greater risk than other communities due to the hidden nature of ATOD use; ATOD use in suburban communities is less likely to occur in plain view and contribute to neighborhood blight, and families with money and power may harbor secrets about drug abuse that contribute to shame and guilt [12]. Adolescents from these types of families may resist intervention, and without continual monitoring and community-wide prevention efforts, the ATOD problem is likely to go unnoticed [12].

One purpose of this study was to describe the current ATOD situation in the school district by investigating eighth and eleventh grade students' reported ATOD prevalence and changes in ATOD use from 1987 (the start of the intervention) to 1991. Another purpose was to explore and identify the most salient risk and protective factors for students in grades eight through twelve. Three research questions were addressed: 1) Did adolescents' self-reported use of ATOD change between 1987 and 1991? 2) What risk factors seem to be related to higher reported ATOD use in adolescents? 3) What protective factors appear to serve as buffers for reported ATOD use in adolescents? Results from these analyses were used to monitor the current ATOD situation and initiate subsequent intervention efforts in the school district.

METHOD

Participants

All schools in the Troy School District in the Detroit area received the ATOD prevention intervention. The population in the school district was 72,884 persons [13]. The median income of the 19,591 families in the district was $63,187 [13]. Fifty-two percent of families had related children (47% dual-parent families and 5% single-parent families) [13].

The school district involved 11,287 students in two high schools (serving 3,297 students), four middle schools (serving 2,540 students), and twelve elementary schools (serving 5,450 students). Student distribution by racial-ethnic group was: 90.0 percent White, 7.6 percent Asian American, 1.6 percent Black, 0.6 percent Hispanic, and 0.3 percent were classified as Other. Graduation rate was 96.0 percent, dropout rate was 1.0 percent, and 1.9 percent of the school district's students were on free or reduced lunch.

Students from the surveyed grades (i.e., 8 to 12) completed questionnaires in 1987 and in 1991. 1987 data were collected from 1,490 students (51% male and 49% female) in grades eight (50%) and eleven (50%). 1991 data were collected from 3,171 (47% male and 53% female) in grades eight (24%), nine (21%), ten (20%), eleven (19%), and twelve (16%). Of students surveyed in 1991, 57 percent indicated that they had attended school in the district throughout their schooling. Only 8 percent indicated that they had attended school in the district for one year or less. Eighty-five percent of the 1991 participants indicated that they had taken a middle or high school health education course in the school district.

ATOD Prevention Efforts in School District

ATOD use prevalence data were used to demonstrate the need for a prevention program in the school district. The program was initiated in 1988 through the use of a health education planning model that accounted for multiple predisposing, enabling, and reinforcing factors [14]. As suggested by Hawkins et al., an attempt was made to reduce or buffer the effects of risk factors while enhancing protective factors in a variety of social domains (e.g., school, family, peer, etc.) [7]. Specific factors related to the causes of ATOD use among adolescents in the school district were identified and targeted in the intervention.

To increase effectiveness of the intervention in reducing reported ATOD use, prevention education was provided via several approaches (e.g., direct instruction through a comprehensive school health education program, student assistance programs, alternative programs, and school policy) cited in the literature [4, 15, 16]. The Kindergarten through grade twelve curriculum was revised to include *Growing Healthy* at the elementary level and *Teenage Health Teaching Models* at the secondary level, two curricula shown to be effective for ATOD prevention [17, 18]. Student assistance programs were offered to middle and high school students who were identified "at risk" for academic and personal difficulties due to major life changes (e.g., groups in each school building met about chemical dependence, bereavement, divorce, stress, and adjustment to new school). Parent and community components, as suggested in the literature, were included to further support prevention efforts by sending a unified message that ATOD use among adolescents is unacceptable [4, 7, 19].

Components focused on the ATOD, the environment relative to ATOD use, and the user. Goals of the intervention were to: 1) increase knowledge about ATOD use and its effect; 2) improve decision-making and peer refusal skills in regard to ATOD use; 3) improve family bonding and communication; 4) improve school values, commitment to school, and academic success; 5) improve neighborhood cohesion and organization; 6) limit ATOD consumption through legal restrictions and lower availability; and 7) prevent and/or decrease ATOD use among all students, including those individuals identified as "at risk" for ATOD use and other problem behaviors.

Measures

Measures included student self-report questionnaires. Items on all questionnaires were selected from a variety of previously used standardized instruments that deal with ATOD usage, as well as social conditions and attitudes which are perceived to be related to such ATOD behaviors.

At Year 1, a questionnaire used by Fors and Rojek was administered to participants [20]. The 122-item questionnaire included a standard set of background items relating to the respondent's demographic and socioeconomic status (parents' occupation, marital status, education, living arrangement, religious involvement, academic achievement, and employment or allowance status) and sixteen ATOD prevalence questions soliciting respondent's past year involvement (e.g., how often ATOD used) in a wide array of drugs ranging from cigarette and alcohol usage to cocaine, psychedelics, and narcotics. Intensity of alcohol use was captured in one prevalence item which asked participants to report how often they had "gotten really drunk." Response options for the ATOD prevalence questions included a 5-point Likert-type scale ranging from 1 (*never*) to 5 (*nearly every day*). Other items included on the questionnaire, but not used for this study, measured respondents' attitudes toward school, parents, and the law; respondents' perceptions of the seriousness of using each of the drugs in the prevalence questions, availability of drugs, why people their age use drugs, and where drugs are used; and respondent's perception of their parents' and friends' involvement in several drugs.

At Year 4, questionnaires included sixteen drug prevalence items from the Monitoring the Future Survey, developed and administered yearly by the University of Michigan's Institute for Social Research, and some of the demographic questions used at Year 1 [21]. Additional items, developed by Wayne State

University's Center for Urban Studies, were added to the Year 2 questionnaire in order to gather data about ATOD risk and protective factors [22].

For each of the ATOD prevalence questions, respondents were asked about ATOD use in their lifetime, during the last year, and during the last month. Response options included a 7-point Likert-type scale ranging from 1 (*0 occasions*) to 7 (*40 occasions*). For drugs that may have been unfamiliar to the respondents, brief excerpts preceded each question describing the drug's main use and legal ways of obtaining the drug (e.g., doctors prescribe). Daily cigarette use was measured with an item asking respondents to report the amount of cigarettes smoked in the past month. Response options ranged from 1 (*not at all*) to 7 (*2 packs or more per day*). To capture intensity of alcohol use, prevalence items asked students about the number of times they consumed enough alcohol to feel "pretty high" and the number of times during the last two weeks where five or more drinks in a row were consumed.

The survey was divided into A and B forms to reduce survey length. Both forms contained 120 items and included the standard set of background and drug use prevalence items used on the Year 1 questionnaire; Form A contained items related to rebellion, problem behaviors, prosocial values, school values, family involvement, family cohesion, parental expectations, and parental punishment. Form B contained items about perceived risk, parental use, availability, legal consequences, and peer group. Internal consistency of risk and protective scales (Cronbach's alpha) averaged .70, and most had a Lilliefors K-S value under .10, indicating less deviation from normality. Approximately half of the respondents completed Form A (N = 1,598) and half (N = 1,572) completed Form B.

Comparable items from Year 1 and Year 2 surveys, involving eight drugs, were used in the analysis. Prevalence rates were derived from rescaling items to dichotomous categories (0 = no use, 1 = any use past year/past month/daily). Analyses included reported past year use of alcohol, inhalants, marijuana, cocaine, stimulants, depressants, and narcotics; past month use of alcohol, cigarettes, inhalants, and marijuana; daily use of cigarettes; and intensity of alcohol use. Past year use data captured regular users as well as experimentation with particular substances, while past month and daily use data tended to reflect more frequent or regular use of a substance. Intensity of alcohol use served as an indicator of those who may be more likely to abuse ATOD.

Procedure

The prevention intervention was initiated during the 1987-1988 school year. Questionnaires were administered to eighth and eleventh grade students in November 1987 by school personnel as a baseline measure. In November 1991, school personnel administered questionnaires to students in grades eight and eleven, and additionally to students in grades nine, ten, and twelve. Letters informing parents about the study and requesting parental permission through passive consent were sent home prior to administering surveys. All students in attendance during the day of questionnaire administration were asked to participate. Upon receiving the surveys, students were told that their participation was voluntary and anonymous. To encourage accurate reporting, great care was taken to protect student confidentiality. Students were asked not to write their names anywhere on the survey, and no identifiers were used to try to match surveys.

Data Analysis

For purposes of this study, pre-existing data were obtained from the school district. To investigate changes in self-reported ATOD use from 1987 to 1991, proportions of adolescents' reported ATOD use (e.g., past year, past month, daily, and intensity of alcohol use) for survey years were compared using chi-square analyses. Differences between years were computed overall for all adolescents (both eighth and eleventh grade students), and separately for each grade and for gender within grade.

To investigate risk and protective factors for self-reported drug use, correlations and logistic regression analyses were conducted using 1991 data. Adolescents were placed into "risk" categories based on their reported alcohol and marijuana use. Categories included abstainers, low risk users, moderate risk users, and high risk users. Scaled risk and protective factors were entered as predictors for membership in risk category. Two basic analysis models were used in investigating Research Questions 2 and 3. One model used risk factors as predictors for membership or nonmembership in the high risk user group. A second model used protective factors as predictors for membership or nonmembership in the abstainer/low risk group. Separate analyses were conducted for Form A and Form B risk and protective factors.

Of the 1991 students surveyed, 32 percent (n = 944) were classified as abstainers, 34 percent (n = 1,015) as low risk, 19 percent (n = 574) as moderate risk, and 15 percent (n = 461) as high risk. Six percent (n = 177) did not provide enough information to be classified and were omitted.

Prior to addressing Research Questions 2 and 3, analyses were computed to determine whether students who completed Form A differed significantly from those who completed Form B on demographic variables. Significant differences were found among grade and risk category. Students completing Form B tended to be enrolled in higher grades (Form A, M = 9.76, SD = 1.14 and Form B, M = 9.88, SD = 1.37), $F(1,3069)$ = 5.70, p < .05) and had more students falling in a higher risk category (Form A, M = 1.13, SD = 1.04 and Form B, M = 1.24, SD = 1.05), $F(1,2993)$ = 7.95, p < .01.

RESULTS

Trends from 1987 to 1991 in ATOD Use

Trends in reported ATOD use from 1987 to 1991 are reported below for each drug studied. They include comparisons for adolescents overall (both eighth and eleventh grade students), by grade, and gender within grade that are statistically significant (see Tables 1 and 2).

Alcohol Use

Reported past year alcohol use increased overall from 1987 to 1991. These increases were found among both eighth and eleventh grade adolescents and for eighth grade males, eighth grade females, and eleventh grade females. Increases were also found for reported past month use for both grades and for both males and females within each grade. Adolescents reporting "getting really drunk/high" showed slight decreases; however, these were not significant.

Cigarette Use

Decreases from 1987 to 1991 were found for reported past month and daily cigarette use. Decreases in past month use occurred for both eighth and eleventh grade adolescents and for both males and females within those grades, and decreases in daily use occurred for each grade; however, decreases by gender only occurred for eleventh grade males.

Inhalant Use

Reported past year inhalant use decreased overall from 1987 to 1991. Decreases were found for eighth and eleventh grade adolescents and for both males and females. No differences were found for reported past month use.

Marijuana Use

Reported past year marijuana use decreased overall from 1987 to 1991. Decreases were found for eighth and eleventh grade adolescents and for eighth grade females, eleventh grade males, and eleventh grade females. No differences were found in eighth grade males. Decreases for reported past month marijuana use were only found among eleventh grade adolescents; these differences were found for both males and females.

Cocaine, Stimulants, Depressants, and Narcotics Use

Overall decreases from 1987 to 1991 in reported past year use of cocaine, stimulants, depressants, and narcotics were found among adolescents for past year use. Decreases only occurred among eleventh grade students and, with the exception of narcotics, were found for both males and females.

Table 1. Trends in ATOD Use from 1987 to 1991 in Eighth- and Eleventh-Grade Adolescents (Percentages)

	Total			8th-Grade			11th-Grade		
	Nov 1987	Nov 1991	χ^2	Nov 1987	Nov 1991	χ^2	Nov 1987	Nov 1991	χ^2
Alcohol									
Past Year	64.9	73.9	21.60***	49.7	64.4	24.60***	80.2	83.2	1.71
Past Month	23.6	41.7	88.88***	7.6	26.3	78.64***	39.6	56.8	34.21***
"Really Drunk"	40.0	37.9	0.78	18.4	15.7	1.43	61.5	60.0	0.26
5+ Drinks	—	19.5		—	8.2		—	30.8	
Cigarettes									
Past Month	29.2	15.7	70.83***	18.5	7.8	35.51***	39.6	25.2	30.83***
Daily	13.9	9.7	14.84***	6.1	3.6	4.74*	21.4	15.8	6.83***
Inhalants									
Past Year	19.4	8.9	60.80***	20.5	9.1	36.59***	18.2	8.6	25.07***
Past Month	3.5	4.7	2.49	3.9	4.9	0.77	3.1	4.5	1.77
Marijuana									
Past Year	22.0	7.7	108.12***	6.1	2.4	12.11***	37.8	14.1	91.81***
Past Month	10.7	4.3	39.76***	2.4	1.3	2.71	18.9	7.9	32.49***
Cocaine									
Past Year	4.6	2.0	13.39***	1.6	1.7	0.01	7.5	2.4	16.55***
Stimulants									
Past Year	14.1	5.5	55.67***	4.5	4.6	0.01	23.6	6.6	69.49***
Depressants									
Past Year	6.4	3.3	13.87***	3.4	2.6	0.83	9.4	4.2	13.29***
Narcotics									
Past Year	2.8	1.6	3.99*	1.8	1.4	0.25	3.8	1.9	4.03*

*$p < .05$ **$p < .01$ ***$p < .001$

Table 2. Trends in ATOD Use from 1987 to 1991 by Gender Within Grade (Percentages)

	8th-Grade Males			8th-Grade Females			11th-Grade Males			11th-Grade Females		
	Nov 1987	Nov 1991	χ^2	Nov 1987	Nov 1991	χ^2	Nov 1987	Nov 1991	χ^2	Nov 1987	Nov 1991	χ^2
Alcohol												
Past Year	51.6	65.0	9.90**	47.8	62.4	11.09***	81.1	80.2	0.07	79.1	86.1	4.60*
Past Month	6.4	25.9	44.83***	8.6	25.2	29.02***	42.0	58.0	14.13***	37.2	55.3	18.84***
"Really Drunk"	18.5	16.3	0.67	18.2	14.3	1.45	61.5	60.6	0.04	61.6	58.4	0.62
5+ Drinks	—	8.3		—	7.9		—	36.2		—	24.4	
Cigarettes												
Past Month	15.8	8.0	10.02**	21.0	7.2	26.64***	38.6	22.6	18.84***	40.8	27.0	13.55***
Daily	6.6	4.3	0.59	5.4	2.7	1.41	21.7	12.8	14.97***	21.2	18.8	0.80
Inhalants												
Past Year	15.4	9.2	6.10*	25.5	8.1	36.19***	18.9	9.2	11.47***	17.6	7.7	13.48***
Past Month	4.3	6.0	0.97	3.3	3.4	0.01	4.5	5.0	0.10	1.7	3.8	2.79
Marijuana												
Past Year	6.2	4.0	1.68	5.8	0.9	12.24***	42.0	13.9	58.58***	33.2	13.8	32.54***
Past Month	3.0	2.2	0.44	1.7	0.3	3.14	24.0	6.8	33.20***	13.4	8.3	4.17*
Cocaine												
Past Year	2.2	2.8	0.29	0.8	0.9	0.01	9.9	2.7	12.60***	4.8	1.7	4.61*
Stimulants												
Past Year	4.8	5.3	0.07	3.9	4.0	0.01	25.5	4.6	48.07***	21.8	8.3	21.73***
Depressants												
Past Year	3.8	3.8	0.00	2.8	1.5	1.22	10.3	4.6	6.90**	8.5	3.8	5.65*
Narcotics												
Past Year	2.2	2.5	0.10	1.1	0.3	1.50	5.2	2.7	2.58	2.3	0.7	2.54

*$p < .05$ **$p < .01$ ***$p < .001$

Risk and Protective Factors

The strongest relationship was found between the risk factor problem behaviors (r = .692, p .0005) and the protective factor peer group (r = .576, p .0005). In this school district, adolescents who took part in moderate to high ATOD use were more likely to report a higher level of problem behaviors, and adolescents who abstained from or had a low use of ATOD were more likely to report that their peer group was in support of no or low use. Other factors were significant; however, their magnitude was not as strong (absolute r values ranged from .199 to .369).

Five risk factors were entered as predictors for membership in the high risk user group versus the non-high risk user group: Rebellion and problem behaviors (Form A Analysis), and perceived risk, parental use, availability, and legal consequences (Form B Analysis). From Form A, problem behaviors (Odds Ratio = 9332.25) was the only variable that was found to differentiate between the two groups (see Table 3). The high risk group consisted of members who had more problem behaviors. This model was able to correctly classify 89 percent of the cases.

All of the Form B risk factors were found to differentiate between the two groups. Parental use (Odds Ratio = 6.33) appeared to be the most salient. The high risk group consisted of members who had a lower perception of risk associated with drug use, perceived availability to be high, reported higher parental use of drugs, and perceived legal consequences in using drugs to be low. This model was able to correctly classify 85 percent of the cases.

Six protective factors were entered as predictors for membership in the abstainer/low risk user group versus the non-abstainer/low risk user group: Prosocial values, school values, family involvement, family cohesion, parental expectations, and parental punishment (Form A Analysis), and peer group (Form B Analysis). Protective factors from Form A that were found to differentiate between the two groups included prosocial values, school values, family involvement, family cohesion, and parental punishment (Odds Ratio's ranged from .40 to 1.88). The abstainers/low risk groups consisted of members who had higher prosocial values, higher school values, higher family involvement and cohesion, and lower levels of parental punishment. The model was able to correctly classify 72 percent of the cases.

The protective factor on Form B, peer group (Odds Ratio = 6.24), also was found to differentiate between the two groups. The abstainer/low risk groups consisted of those who were more likely to have a peer social circle with social norms against drug use. This model was able to correctly classify 75 percent of the cases.

Table 3. Risk and Protective Factors Found to Differentiate between
Risk Categories on the Basis of Logistic Regression Analyses

	B	Odds Ratio	Overall % Correct
Risk Factor			
Form A			
Problem Behaviors	6.8376	932.2539	
			88.79
Form B			
Perceived Risk	–0.0395	0.9612	
Availability	0.0347	1.0354	
Parental Use	1.8454	6.3304	
Legal Consequences	–0.0434	0.9575	
			84.59
Protective Factor			
Form A			
Prosocial Values	0.2012	1.2229	
School Values	0.6320	1.8813	
Family Involvement	0.0198	1.0200	
Family Cohesion	0.2168	1.2421	
Parental Punishment	–0.9042	0.4049	
			72.05
Form B			
Peer Group	1.8314	6.2424	
			74.66

DISCUSSION

ATOD prevalence rates and changes in ATOD use from 1987 to 1991 provide the school district valuable data about the ATOD situation in their student population. For all adolescents, significant decreases during this time period were found in all drugs studied except alcohol; however, these decreases may not have occurred for both grades or for both male and females within a grade. Patterns found were consistent with findings reported nationally which show that certain drugs are more prevalent among certain grades and/or a particular gender [1]. It should be noted that ATOD use data from this study, with the exception of alcohol, compare favorable with national data (see Table 4).

When examining differences by grade in reported ATOD use, it is important to consider the progression of initiation. Use of legal drugs, such as cigarettes and

Table 4. Comparisons of 1991 ATOD Use in this Sample (Grades 8 and 11) with National Data (Grades 8, 10, and 12) (Percentages)

	Sample	National	Sample	National	
	8	8	11	10	12
Alcohol					
Past Year	64.4	54.0	83.2	72.3	77.7
Past Month	26.3	25.1	56.8	42.8	54.0
"Really Drunk"	15.7	*	60.0	*	*
5+ Drinks	8.2	12.9	30.8	22.9	29.8
Cigarettes					
Past Month	7.8	14.3	25.2	20.8	28.3
Daily	3.6	7.2	15.8	12.6	18.5
Inhalants					
Past Year	9.1	9.0	8.6	7.1	6.6
Past Month	4.9	4.4	4.5	2.7	2.4
Marijuana					
Past Year	2.4	6.2	14.1	16.5	23.9
Past Month	1.3	3.2	7.9	8.7	13.8
Cocaine					
Past Year	1.7	2.8	2.4	5.2	8.2
Stimulants					
Past Year	4.6	6.2	6.6	8.2	8.2
Depressants					
Past Year	2.6	NA	4.2	NA	3.4
Narcotics					
Past Year	1.4	*	1.9	*	*

*Data not comparable
NA = Data not measured

alcohol, is most likely initiated at an early age, with inhalants and marijuana likely to come next, followed by other illicit drugs [23]. Decreases were found in reported use among eighth and eleventh grade adolescents for the drugs typically initiated early in the drug progression sequence (e.g., cigarettes, inhalants, and marijuana) with the exception of alcohol. The most dramatic differences were seen in reported past month and daily use of cigarettes and past year inhalant and marijuana use, which had significant differences among both grades. Decreases in cigarette use in eighth grade could have been the result of exposure to the health education curriculum previously shown to be effective in reducing initiation of tobacco use [17].

Similarly, decreases were found in reported use among eleventh grade adolescents for the drugs typically initiated in later grades (e.g., cocaine, stimulants, depressants, and narcotics). The lack of decrease among eighth grade adolescents, in part due to low prevalence, suggested that there was a small percentage of adolescents who initiated those drugs earlier than others, and that small percent did not change from 1987 to 1991. In the literature, this small percent has been classified as adolescents "at risk" for ATOD abuse and other problem behaviors [24]. These "at risk" adolescents start using drugs early, continue to do so at a higher level, and take part in multiple drug use [24].

Findings from the eleventh grade analyses suggest that some of these "at risk" adolescents may reduce their drug use by eleventh grade while others may not. Perhaps, the intervention was effective in helping those adolescents in the school district who were identified as being "at risk"; in particular, those adolescents who had been caught using ATOD and required to attend the school's student assistance program. The remaining percent of those "at risk" adolescents may not have been identified and, subsequently, were not reached through the intervention.

Trends also suggested that benefits from the intervention existed for both genders. The most dramatic difference was seen in use of cigarettes. Males and females within both grades reported reduced past month use by between 8 to 16 percent, and daily use was reduced by 9 percent for eleventh grade males. These findings suggest that eleventh grade females, who use cigarettes daily, were not as easily influenced by the intervention. These findings are not consistent with national data which showed declines for twelfth grade females and increases for twelfth grade males [1].

With regard to reported inhalant use, decreases from 1987 to 1991 were found for eighth and eleventh grade males and females. These results suggest that all groups got the message regarding the dangers of inhalant use. For reported marijuana use, the only group not showing a decrease was eighth grade males. Perhaps, these eighth grade males were those who are "at risk" for subsequent drug use and who had not been reached by the intervention. For other illicit drug use (only year differences found among eleventh grade adolescents), both eleventh grade males and females reported lower use of stimulants, depressants, and cocaine from 1987 to 1991; however, no decreases were found by gender in reported use of narcotics, perhaps due to the low prevalence in the school district.

Of great concern were the findings about alcohol use. Results, showing increases in reported use, suggested that alcohol use is widespread among adolescents in the school district (especially among females) and that initiation of alcohol use occurred earlier in 1991 than in 1987. Results, although not statistically significant, showing slight reductions in intensity of alcohol use (i.e., Gotten "Really Drunk"/"High") add promise, but are still higher than desirable. These findings differ from national trends among twelfth grade adolescents which showed steady decreases in past year alcohol use from 1987-1991 [1].

In this study, both grades accounted for this increase, and this difference was seen for eighth grade males, eighth grade females, and eleventh grade females. The lack of a significant decrease in eleventh grade males suggests that alcohol use in that group was already at its peak in 1987. It would appear that adolescents were shifting from other "more serious" drugs to alcohol, which may not be viewed as serious since it is often used by adults. This "displacement effect" was not seen in the national data with twelfth grade adolescents [1].

It is noteworthy to point out that eleventh grade females exceeded eleventh grade males in their alcohol use by 6 percent. This is consistent with national data which have shown the gap among males and females with regard to alcohol use narrowing since 1987. However, national findings still suggest that males exceed females in their alcohol use [1].

In an attempt to explore risk and protective factors, eighth through twelfth grade students were classified into ATOD use categories. Consistent with the literature reviewed by Hawkins et al., all protective and risk factors measured in this study were found to be significantly related in the expected direction with ATOD use [7].

Unlike most studies reported in the literature, this study additionally looked at multiple risk and protective factors in an effort to identify the most salient factors to target in subsequent interventions. Findings suggest that problem behaviors and parental use were the most salient risk factors, and that peers was the most salient protective factor. Other risk and protective factors (perceived risk, availability, legal consequences, prosocial values, school values, family involvement, family cohesion, and parental punishment) entered the models, but were not as salient.

Considering the school district population and surrounding community, results were not surprising. Students who were classified in higher risk categories tended to have a high level of problem behaviors and were more likely to have parents who also took part in ATOD use. Individuals who abstained or rarely used ATOD were more likely to have peers who did the same and who were supportive of nonuse. Findings suggested that ATOD use in this community is determined, in part, by the perceived availability of ATOD and legal consequences resulting from use, with alcohol and, perhaps, inhalants being more available and having fewer legal consequences, and by an individual's perceived risk in using a particular drug, with cigarettes, marijuana, and other illicit drugs perceived as more risky to some.

The models with protective factors were not as successful as the risk factor models in classifying cases correctly. Protective factors in this school district exist to some extent, and may even contribute to lower levels of reported ATOD use; however, some adolescents who have protective factors may still take part in moderate to high levels of ATOD use. It is likely that those individuals have protective factors within the community (e.g., norms against ATOD use), but not within their families or peer group (e.g., high parental use of ATOD and peer support of ATOD use). It is also likely that these individuals are the same small percent who are involved in multiple ATOD use.

By monitoring ATOD prevalence and trends in ATOD use over time, a school district can more accurately assess the ATOD situation and develop intervention programs which directly target specific problem areas. Findings like these highlight patterns of ATOD use among adolescents, with particular emphasis on trends by grade and gender, and pinpoint drugs which are "popular" among the student population.

In this study, a broad range of risk factors was identified, and a few were identified as being more salient than others. For now, program planners know which risk factors should be targeted for the most promising results; however, research is still needed to explore which are causal and which are spurious in the etiology of drug abuse.

In designing prevention interventions, there is an assumption that all adolescents are "at risk" for drug use and that a small percent of them are "at risk" for drug abuse. In this study, protective factors for all adolescents were explored. Future research should explore protective factors in only those individuals who are "at risk" and who did not take part in higher levels of ATOD use. Future intervention programs in this school district need to continue to address risk factors for marijuana, inhalant, and cigarette use, with greater emphasis on reducing alcohol use, and additional efforts need to be made to reach those "at risk" adolescents who may take part in more serious drug use. Further research is needed to explore "at risk" adolescents in this school district.

Findings provide a school district with an indication of how well prevention efforts are doing. Although cause and effect conclusions cannot be drawn regarding the intervention's effectiveness in producing the desired changes from 1987 to 1991, it is likely that the intervention made some contribution. Additionally, it is impossible to determine what the ATOD situation would have been without the intervention. It is quite probable that national trends in ATOD use contributed both positively and negatively. Comparisons with national data allow this to be put in perspective. To look at the intervention's effectiveness, more research is needed comparing these data with school districts comprising similar populations without such an intervention.

Even when considered in light of these inherent weaknesses in determining the intervention's effectiveness, findings strengthen the concept of using a multi-component approach to ATOD prevention interventions and add support to the benefit of targeting specific risk and protective factors. An intervention such as this should start early in a child's life and be part of a larger school and community health program. Efforts must be made to involve parents and the community in all aspects of health promotion, especially for ATOD prevention. Finally, a mechanism should also be put in place for early identification and referral for intervention services of children and adolescents who are susceptible to problem behaviors and ATOD abuse.

The approaches taken in developing this intervention and the components initiated may be beneficial to other school districts. In designing the ATOD prevention intervention, efforts were made to address the unique needs of children and families in the school district. By regularly monitoring ATOD prevalence rates and changes in ATOD use over time, school district prevention specialists will be attuned to the current ATOD situation and better prepared to respond to potential problematic trends.

ACKNOWLEDGMENTS

The authors gratefully acknowledge the contributions made by Drs. Charles Flatter and Robert Marcus.

REFERENCES

1. L. D. Johnston, P. M. O'Malley, and J. G. Bachman, *Smoking, Drinking, and Illicit Drug Use Among American Secondary School Students, College Students, and Young Adults, 1975-1991: Volume 1. Secondary School Students*, U.S. Government Printing Office, Washington, D.C., NIH Publication No. 93-348, 1992.
2. R. Jessor, Problem Behavior Developmental Transition in Adolescence, *Journal of School Health, 52:*5, pp. 295-300, 1982.
3. S. P. Schinke and L. D. Gilchrist, Preventing Substance Abuse With Children and Adolescents, *Journal for Consulting and Clinical Psychology, 55*, pp. 596-602, 1985.
4. Office for Substance Abuse Prevention, *Prevention Plus II*, U.S. Government Printing Office, Washington, D.C., DHHS Publication No. ADM 89-1649, 1990.
5. A. Bandura, *Social Learning Theory*, Prentice-Hall, Englewood Cliffs, New Jersey, 1977.
6. U.S. Congress, Office of Technology Assessment, *Adolescent Health Volume II: Background and the Effectiveness of Selected Prevention and Treatment Services*, U.S. Government Printing Office, Washington, D.C., OTA Publication No. OTA-H-466, 1991.
7. J. D. Hawkins, R. F. Catalano, and J. Y. Miller, Risk and Protective Factors for Alcohol and Other Drug Problems in Adolescence and Early Adulthood: Implications for Substance Abuse Prevention, *Psychological Bulletin, 112:*1, pp. 64-105, 1992.
8. B. Bernard, *Fostering Resiliency in Kids: Protective Factors in the Family, School and Community*, Northwest Regional Educational Laboratory, Portland, Oregon, 1991.
9. P. Nelson, Involving Families in Substance Abuse Prevention, *Family Relations, 38*, pp. 306-310, 1989.
10. J. D. Hawkins, D. M. Lishner, and R. F. Catalano, Childhood Predictors and the Prevention of Adolescent Substance Abuse, in *Etiology of Drug Abuse: Implications*

for Prevention, C. L. Jones and R. Battjes (eds.), U.S. Government Printing Office, Washington, D.C., DHHS Publication No. ADM 85-1385, 1985.

11. Troy Community Coalition, *A Report on the Results of the Comprehensive Assessment of the Behaviors and the Attitudes of Troy Residents Concerning the Use and Abuse of Drugs and Alcohol*, Troy, Michigan, 1992.

12. Think Tank for Action on Substance Abuse Prevention in Southeastern Michigan, *Action Strategies for Preventing Substance Abuse: A Resource Manual for Southeastern Michigan*, Community Foundation for Southeastern Michigan, Detroit, Michigan, 1990.

13. U.S. Bureau of the Census, State Profile, Statistical Abstracts for the U.S., 1990.

14. L. W. Green, M. W. Kreuter, S. G. Deeds, and K. B. Partridge, *Health Education Planning a Diagnostic Approach*, Mayfield Publishing Co., Palo Alto, California, 1980.

15. M. D. Newcomb and P. M. Bentler, Substance Use and Abuse Among Children and Teenagers, *American Psychologist, 44:2*, pp. 242-248, 1989.

16. N. S. Tobler, Meta-Analysis of 143 Adolescent Drug Prevention Programs: Quantitative Outcome Results of Program Participants Compared to a Control or Comparison Group, *The Journal of Drug Issues, 16:4*, pp. 537-567, 1986.

17. R. L. Andrews, *Summary Analyses Growing Healthy: A Longitudinal Study Kindergarten-Grade 9*, American Lung Association, New York, 1987.

18. M. T. Errecart, H. J. Walberg, J. G. Ross, R. S. Gold, J. L. Fiedler, and L. J. Kolbe, Effectiveness of Teenage Health Teaching Modules (THTM), *Journal of School Health, 61:1*, pp. 26-30, 1991.

19. Lindblad, A Review of the Concerned Parent Movement in the United States of America, *Bulletin on Narcotics, 35:3*, pp. 41-49, 1983.

20. S. W. Fors and S. D. Rojek, The Social and Demographic Correlates of Adolescent Drug Use Patterns, *Journal of Drug Education, 13:3*, pp. 205-222, 1983.

21. Institute for Social Research, *National Senior High School Survey*, University of Michigan, Ann Arbor, Michigan, 1991.

22. Northwest Regional Educational Laboratory, items used on 1991 surveys, Center for Urban Studies, Wayne State University, 1991.

23. D. Kandel and J. Logan, Patterns of Drug Use From Adolescents to Young Adulthood: I. Periods of Risk for Initiation, Continued Use, and Discontinuation, *American Journal of Public Health, 74*, pp. 668-672, 1984.

24. J. G. Dryfoos, *Adolescents at Risk*, Oxford University Press, Inc., New York, 1990.

Direct reprint requests to:

Tina M. Younoszai
Institute for Child Study
University of Maryland
3304 Benjamin Building
College Park, MD 20742-1131
e-mail: tinay@wam.umd.edu

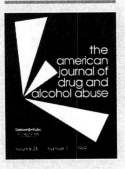

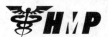

Journal of DRUG EDUCATION

INSTRUCTIONS TO AUTHORS

Submit manuscript to: Dr. Seymour Eiseman, Editor
Department of Health Science
California State University, Northridge
Northridge, CA 91330

Manuscripts are to be submitted in triplicate. Retain one copy, as manuscript will not be returned. Manuscript must be typewritten on 8-1/2" × 11" white paper, one side only, double-spaced, with wide margins. Paginate consecutively starting with the title page. The organization of the paper should be indicated by appropriate headings and subheadings.

Originality   Authors should note that only original articles are accepted for publication. Submission of a manuscript represents certification on the part of the author(s) that neither the article submitted, nor a version of it has been published, or is being considered for publication elsewhere.

Abstracts of 100 to 150 words are required to introduce each article.

References should relate only to material cited within text and be listed in numerical order according to their appearance within text. State author's name, title of referenced work, editor's name, title of book or periodical, volume, issue, pages cited, and year of publication. Do not abbreviate titles. Please do not use ibid., op. cit., loc. cit., etc. In case of multiple citations, simply repeat the original numeral. Detailed specifications available from the editor upon request.

Footnotes are placed at the bottom of page where referenced. They should be numbered with superior arabic numbers without parentheses or brackets. Footnotes should be brief with an average length of three lines.

Figures should be referenced in text and appear in numerical sequence starting with Figure 1. Line art must be original drawings in black ink proportionate to our page size, and suitable for photographing. Indicate top and bottom of figure where confusion may exist. Labeling should be 8 point type. Clearly identify all figures. Figures should be drawn on separate pages and their placement within the text indicated by inserting: —Insert Figure 1 here—.

Tables must be cited in text in numerical sequence starting with Table 1. Each table must have a descriptive title. Any footnotes to tables are indicated by superior lower case letters. Tables should be typed on separate pages and their approximate placement indicated within text by inserting: —Insert Table 1 here—.

Authors will receive twenty complimentary reprints of their published article.
Additional reprints may be ordered.

SUBSTANCE ABUSE PREVENTION:
A Multicultural Perspective
Edited by Snehendu B. Kar

Alcohol, tobacco, and other drugs (ATOD) abuse is a major threat to our health and quality of life. In this volume, nationally recognized substance abuse specialists, public health researchers, and community-based practitioners undertake an in-depth state-of-the-art review of substance abuse prevention intervention from a multicultural perspective.

Special emphasis is on the application of the lessons learned from fields of substance abuse and the new public health paradigm as a modus operandi for ATOD prevention in multicultural communities. The book further makes specific recommendations for prevention policy, research, professional preparation, and effective intervention strategies.

In thirteen chapters, twenty-four authors share their analyses, concerns, and conclusions in several domains including the: meaning and dynamics of multiculturalism affecting prevention intervention, relative risks and knowledge gaps across ethnic groups, social trends affecting health risks and substance abuse, lessons learned from substance abuse research and prevention, role of the media, promises and limits of the new public health paradigm for assessment, policy development, assurance of preventive services, and social action and empowerment for prevention in partnership with the public.

This pioneering volume will serve as a valuable resource to researchers, policy makers, educators, professionals and organizations interested in the health and quality of life of our communities as we approach the 21st century.

Format Information: 6" x 9", 336 pages, ISBN: 0-89503-194-9, $42.00 plus $4.00 postage and handling

Baywood Publishing Company, Inc. 26 Austin Avenue, Amityville, NY 11701
Call (516) 691-1270 Fax (516) 691-1770 **Orderline** (800) 638-7819
e-mail: baywood@baywood.com● **web site:** http://baywood.com

Volume 29, Number 2 — 1999

JOURNAL OF

DRUG EDUCATION

CONTENTS

Executive Editor:

SEYMOUR EISEMAN, DR.P.H.

Baywood Publishing Company, Inc.

ISSN 0047-2379

Journal of DRUG EDUCATION

EXECUTIVE EDITOR
SEYMOUR EISEMAN, DR. P.H.
Department of Health Sciences
California State University, Northridge

The *Journal of Drug Education* is a peer-refereed journal.

Journal of Drug Education is noted in: *Abstracts on Criminology and Penology; Academic Abstracts; Adolescent Mental Health Abstracts AGRICOLA; ALCONARC: ASSIA: All-Russian Institute of Scientific and Technical Information; Applied Social Sciences Index & Abstracts; Cambridge Scientific Abstracts; Cancer Prevention and Control Database; Counseling and Personnel Services Information Center; Criminal Justice Abstracts; Criminology, Penology and Police Service Abstracts; Cumulative Index to Nursing & Allied Health Literature (CINAHL);Current Contents; Current Index to Journals in Education; Dokumentation Gefahrdung durch Alkohol, Rauchen, Drogen, Arzneimittel; Drug Abuse and Alcoholism Review; EMBASE/Excerpta Medica; Health Promotion and Education Database; International Bibliography of Periodical Literature; International Bibliography of Book Reviews; International Pharmaceutical Abstracts; Kindex Medicus; MEDLINE; NCJRS Catalog; National Institute on Alcohol Abuse and Alcoholism's Alcohol and Alcohol Problems Science Database, ETOH; Psychological Abstracts; Smoking and Health Database; Safety and Health at Work ILO-CIS Bulletin;* and *Sociological Abstracts, Inc.*

The *Journal of Drug Education* is published by the Baywood Publishing Company, Inc., 26 Austin Ave., P.O. Box 337, Amityville, NY 11701. Subscription rate per Volume (four issues): Institutional—$160.00 Individual—$45.00 (prepaid by personal check or credit card). Add $6.50 per volume for postage inside the U.S. and Canada and $11.75 elsewhere. Back list volumes are available at $149.60. Subscription is on a volume basis only and must be prepaid. Copies of single issues are not available. No part of this journal may be reproduced in any form without written permission from the publisher.

J. DRUG EDUCATION, Vol. 29(2) 95-96, 1999

EDITORIAL: CONSENSUS STATEMENT, 14TH JULY 1997 OF THE FARMINGTON CONFERENCES

The purpose of *this statement* is to define the basis for shared identity, commitment and purpose, among journals publishing in the field of psychoactive substance use and associated problems. Our aim has enhanced the quality of our endeavors in this multi-disciplinary field. We share common concerns and believe that we do well to join together in their solution. To that end we accede to this document as a statement of our consensus and as basis for future collaboration.

1. *Commitment to the peer review process*
   1.1 We are committed to peer review and would expect research reports and scientific reviews to go through this process. As regards the extent to which other material well be so reviewed, we see that as a matter for editorial discretion, but policies should be declared.
   1.2 Referees *should be told* that their access to the article on which they have been requested to comment is in strict confidence. Confidentiality should not be broken by pre-publication statements on the content of the submission. Manuscripts sent to reviewers should be returned to the editor or destroyed.
   1.3 Referees *should be asked* to declare to the editor if they have a conflict of interest in relation to the material which they are invited to review, and if in doubt they should consult the editor. We define "conflict of interest" as a situation in which professional, personal, or financial considerations, could be seen by a fair-minded person as potentially in conflict with independence of judgment. Conflict of interest is not in itself wrong-doing.

2. *Expectations of authors*
   2.1 **Authorship:** All listed authors on an article should have been personally and substantially involved in the work leading to the article.
   2.2 **Accordance of double publication:** Authors are *expected to ensure* that no significant part of the submitted material has been published previously

95

and that it is not concurrently being considered by another journal. An exception to this general position may be made when previous publication has been limited to another language, to local publication in report, or publication of a conference abstract. All such instances, we would expect authors should consult the editor. Editors are encouraged to develop policies concerning electronic publication. Authors are asked to provide the editor at the time of submission with copies of published or submitted reports that *are related to that submission.*

2.3 **Sources of funding for the submitted paper must be declared** *and will be published.*

2.4 **Conflicts of interest experienced by authors:** *Authors should* declare to the editor if their relationship with any type of funding source might fairly be construed as exposing them to potential conflict of interest.

2.5 **Protection of human and animal rights:** *Where applicable* authors *should* give an assurance that ethical safeguards have been met.

2.6 **Technical preparation of articles:** We will publish guidance for authors on the technical preparation of articles with the form of instruction at the discretion of individual journals.

3. *Formal response to breach of expectations be an author*

3.1 Working in collaboration with our authors, we have a responsibility to support the expectations of good scientific publishing practice. To that end each journal will have defined policies for response to attempted or actual instances of *duplicate* publicatplagiarismarism, or scientific fraud.

4. *Maintaining editorial independence*

4.1 *We are committedmited to independence in the editorial process. To the extent the owner or another body may influence the editorial process, this should b.? declared, and in that case any sources of support from the alcohol, tobacco, pharmaceutical, or other relevant interests should be published in the journal.*

4.2 *We will publish declarations on any sources of support received by a journal, and will maintain openness in regard to connections which a journal or its editorial staff may have established which could reasonably be construed as conflict of interest.*

4.3 **Funding for journal supplements:** When we publish journal supplements, an indication will be given of any sources of support for their production.

4.4 **Refereeing journal supplements:** An editorial note will be published to indicate whether it has or has been peer reviewed.

4.5 **Advertising:** Acceptance of advertising will be determined by, or in consultation with, the editor of each journal.

Seymour Eiseman

J. DRUG EDUCATION, Vol. 29(2) 97-114, 1999

ILLEGAL DRUG ABUSE AND THE COMMUNITY CAMP STRATEGY IN CHINA

WEN WANG PH.D.
California State University, Northridge

ABSTRACT

Since the 1980s, China has experienced major changes in its traditional drug use patterns which included mostly tobacco and alcohol use. The introduction of opium, marijuana, heroin, and cocaine is the most noticeable change. In 1995, there were about 520,000 reported drug users in China and the rate of increase was about 200 percent. During the 1990 Strictly Against Illegal Drug Campaign (Yan Da), the Chinese government implemented a compulsory detoxification plan and a Community Drug Rehabilitation Camp strategy to deal with the diverse aspects of the illegal drug control. This article provides an initial evaluation of the community camp approach to drug detoxification and rehabilitation. Open-ended interviewing schedules were given to two samples from two government sponsored rehabilitation community camps in 1994. These interviews reveal that: 1) the social and cultural reorientation of drug addicts is facilitated by an intensive mass media propaganda; 2) there is a mobilization of the health care and social security systems to provide detoxification, rehabilitation, and employment to drug addicts in a relatively short period of time; 3) "recidivist" addicts and drug traffickers are condemned to a long-term incarceration in work camps; and 4) the camp strategy experiences some problems. Results show that in the two community camps, an average of twelve month's training yielded a rehabilitation rate of 80 percent.

INTRODUCTION

Different from almost every single country in the world, People's Republic of China had experienced a thirty-year period (1949 to 1979) of no illegal drug using and dealing, thanks to its effective and strict governmental control program under the socialist regime [1]. Since the 1978 Economic Reform, China has

97

re-opened its door to the outside world and the country's economy has been affected not only by foreign technology, but also by the international illegal drug market [1]. Consequently, China has experienced major changes in its traditional drug use patterns which so far included mostly tobacco and alcohol abuse. The introduction of opium, marijuana, heroin, and cocaine is one of noticeable change. According to the Chinese Security Bureau, in 1990, there were about 70,000 reported drug users in the countryside and in cities. This number doubled in 1991, tripled in 1992, and reached 520,000 in 1995. The rate of increase was about 200 percent [2].

Drug using and dealing heavily disturbed the Chinese people's lives. For examples, in Shengzhen City, Mr. Zhang and his younger brother spent 1,400,000 RMB to purchase drugs, which led the family to the brink of poverty and pushed the mother to commit suicide. Mr. Hong had been married for three years and had to sons. He spent all the family savings, and his wife left him with their two sons. In Shanwei City, a young couple with two children worked very hard during the Economic Reform. They saved money, bought two grocery stores and one fish farm on the seaside. Once they started using drugs, they had to sell their properties one by one in order to pay for the drugs. Finally they went bankrupt. Loosing patience with her son who was a drug user, another women tried to get help from her relatives, then killed her son out of despair. She reported herself to the police and said that she would rather see her son dead than using drugs [2].

Drug use is often related to crime. Many teenagers, who start using drugs when they are twelve or thirteen, end up in gangs. Some drug users are arrested more than twenty times by the local police officers and some stay in prison for more than ten years. Male drug users are sometimes found guilty of robbing banks, burning public properties, and murdering merchants. A majority of female drug users turn to prostitution to support their habit [2].

As the number of illegal behaviors related to drugs continued to increase, the unity and solidarity of the Chinese were severely hurt [2]. Since the 1990 Strictly Against Illegal Drug Campaign (Yan Da), the Chinese government implemented a compulsory detoxification plan and a Community Drug rehabilitation Camp strategy to deal with the diverse aspects of the illegal drug control.

This study provides descriptive data gathered in 1994 in two government sponsored rehabilitation camps—one in the suburbs of Xian city and one in Shenzhen city—to gain insight into the effects of the ideological, psychological, and educational control of the camp strategy designed to curb illegal drug use in China.

TREATMENT MODALITIES

During the past twenty years, drug research and drug literature have expanded almost exponentially. The bulk of this research focuses on two primary aspects of drug use. First, the examinations of the prevalence, frequency of drug use, and description of the progression of use [3-8]. Second, following more than a decade of the "war on drugs," attention appears to be shifting toward issues surrounding prevention, termination, and treatment of drug use [9-14].

In the United States, treatment modalities are approached according to one of three viewpoints. The medical model views addiction as a disease, for which the patient receives an out-patient or open-ward hospital medical treatment, such as chemical blockade, including methadone maintenance. According to the psychological model, the client goes under psychotherapy (individual, family, and group therapy), in an attempt to uncover the reasons why he or she became chemically dependent, so that his or her behaviors could be corrected. The social model treats the client within a social group such as a community camp or a boot camp. The chemical dependency is assumed to be a primary condition which can be overcome by a combination of insight and behavior modification. Many other types of counseling services are available to drug addicts such as crisis counseling on the street and in day clinics. Over the years, the boundaries among the three models have become fluid and most treatment approaches present a combination of at least two models.

Drug problems can be treated by prevention, treatment, and legal sanction. This article focuses on the community treatment model since it is the tool that generates all three revenues and displays a variety in its forms. In the United States, Synanon was one of the earliest residential treatment communities. Its therapy has provided the inspiration for many rehabilitation programs throughout the country, including Daytop Village (New York), Phoenix House (Arizona), Delancey Street (California), Tuum Est (California), and Cedu (California) [15]. However, the earlier evaluations of these therapeutic communities deemed them as ineffectual, based on the logic that aggregate outcomes should be more encouraging if these programs were worthwhile [16].

In comparison, the Chinese community detoxification and rehabilitation camps combined the medical model, the psychological model, and the social model into one—Jie Du Swo. This three-in-one approach reshaped and rehabilitated millions of drug users' body, mind, and behavior [1]. The Chinese community rehabilitation camps are not limited to certain counties and cities; they are all over the country especially where illegal drug use is prevalent. In the two camps under study, drug users undergo an average of twelve months of intense education on the damaging nature of illegal drugs, dispensed by political leaders and police officer trained in detoxification. Studies show that the camp strategy in China obtains a higher rehabilitation rate and costs less, when we compare it to the results obtained by therapeutic communities in the West [17].

THE RATIONALE

The rationale for the community camp approach of detoxification is not based on the typical method of isolating the drug users from the community in which they live for long periods of rehabilitation, but without connecting them with their local community to increase social interaction on a daily basis. The mechanism of the camp approach is to reinforce existing positive social bonds in the community to facilitate the process of rehabilitation. As this process develops, the chance for medical detoxification emerges. Thus, the drug user is not suddenly detoxified before rehabilitation, but rather, detoxified after the dual process of community empowerment and rehabilitation.

In reviewing the historical background and the approaches to treatment and rehabilitation in the region, Spencer and Navaratnam concluded that multiple needs exists:

> the need for developing a more extensive provision of treatment, the need for adequate after-care and out-reach, the need for the proper evaluation of those programs which have been undertaken. A further need to achieve an overall policy on the mixture of traditional and modern practices . . . the dependent individual needs considerable more than just medical treatment [18].

Spencer and Navaratnam, by analyzing the camp approach in Singapore, suggested multiple treatment and rehabilitation approaches in response to the diverse needs of drug users in the community. In 1979, there were six such rehabilitation centers in Singapore, where 3,698 males and 143 females were treated mostly for heroin addiction [19]. Drug users were detoxified without medication and then subjected to an intensive campaign on "the evils" of drugs. After the nine weeks induction, a military style training was provided in order to instill discipline and restore physical fitness. The final three months were devoted to industrial training, such as working in factories. After the drug users were released from the centers, a compulsory after-care supervision of two years was required [17].

Although a systematic evaluation of the Singapore programs was never performed, the rehabilitation rate at 44 percent was interpreted as a promising outcome [20]. The Singapore approach became widely discussed in the drug literature as a feasible new modality. Often, law enforcement alone is unable to achieve a dramatic reduction in the supply of drugs, once a drug distribution network has been established. Also, the typical medical treatment facility is depressing in its atmosphere and can be very expensive. On the other hand, the community camp approach allows the drug dependent person to live in a family/community atmosphere and to continue to work or to go to school. It also provides social support, thanks to optimistic staff members and to participation in an ex-user activist group. Thus, the outcome of such strategy is substantially improved [21].

In assessing the applicability of the camp approach across a range of cultures and settings, its Asian origins were recognized. China, as it is well known, had the largest prevalence of opiate addiction in the nineteenth century. However, the Qing dynasty was able to control this problem in a few years [1]. The famous burning of the nation's entire stock of opium in Hu Men, China, was organized by General Zexu Lin [1]. Again, during the establishment of New China, in the early 1950s, the socialist government effectively controlled the nation's illegal drug problem in just a couple of years [22]. As previously noted, since the Economic Reform, China imported not only foreign technology, but also unhealthy habits, such as drug use, which increased dramatically, especially among people along the southern and northern borders of China [2]. By using the community rehabilitation camp strategy in the 1990s, the Chinese embarked on a second wave of massive campaigning against illegal drug use.

DATA

The Chinese government has not revealed any information to the outside world regarding its camp approach treatment until very recently. It is very difficult even for Chinese citizens to collect data from these rehabilitation camps, due to the security measures imposed by the Chinese Security Bureau.

I will provide an analysis of open-ended questionnaire interviews showing the attitudes of drug users and user-dealers (users who had minor drug dealing histories) toward the rehabilitation camp approach. The study population is defined as those drug abusers in China who have been treated at least once in the rehabilitation and detoxification camps. Two samples totaling 243 individuals (N1 = 135, N2 = 108) were selected from two rehabilitation camps in Xian and Shenzhen in 1994, by Professor Shao Qin and others of Beijing University. The purpose of open-ended interviewing is to gain insight from the drug users into the effects of the community camp strategy designed to provide drug rehabilitation and detoxification.

The open-ended interviews reveal the following: 1) social and cultural reorientation of drug addicts make use of intensive mass media propaganda; 2) there is a mobilization of the health care and social security systems to provide detoxification, rehabilitation, and employment in a relatively short period of time to drug addicts; 3) "recidivist" addicts and drug traffickers are condemned to a long-term incarceration in work camps; and 4) the Camp strategy experiences some problems.

THE CAUSES OF THE SPREADING DRUG USAGE

The rapid spreading drug usage in China can be traced to socioeconomic factors, both domestically and internationally. First, after China opened its door to the outside world in 1979, foreign drug dealers not only managed to smuggle drugs into China, but also to use China border-territories as a transit area to sell drugs to other parts of the world. Second, northwestern and southwestern China had a long history of drug use before 1949, and the new conditions rekindled the traditional drug habits. Third, the high profitability of drug dealing easily convinced some greedy Chinese to take the risk of breaking the law. The gangsters who are involved in this illegal activity try to seduce and even threaten those young men who are the most vulnerable to the temptation of illegal drugs. Fourth, foreigners who are drug users and reside in China have an influence on Chinese social life. Fifth, the economically new upstarts in China take drugs as a luxurious and "fashionable" entertainment. There is a saying among the new upstarts: "If you want to be in Paradise, use drugs to lead you there." Gambling, prostitution, and drugs function as indicators of one's wealth. Sixth, these decadent and corrupted attitudes poison young people's souls. Many of them lack a moral sense and use drugs out of curiosity. Others use drugs as a palliative to depression. On the onset of drug use, many young people are convinced that they will do drug only once—"give it a try and give me a high," but many of them end up becoming drug addicts [23].

The spreading drug usage is a severe threat to China's social stability and security. Drug dealing and using are linked with crimes such as gambling, prostitution, pilfering, ammunition smuggling, gold and cultural relics smuggling, and other illegal activities [23]. Supported by intensive campaigning against drug use in the early 1990s (Yan Da), lawmakers strengthened their positions to reduce drug supply in the country. Severe penalties, including lifetime in prison and death sentencing, are now imposed on most of the drug traffickers who are arrested. This helps reducing the in-flow and sale of drugs on the market. Drug demand reduction is carried out through drug preventive education, the arrest and detention of drug abusers for treatment and rehabilitation, and after-care services.

DEMOGRAPHIC CHARACTERISTICS OF THE DRUG USERS AND USER-DEALERS

Gender: among the 243 drug users, 87 percent are male, and 13 percent are female. This is similar to the statistics provided by a northern China police bureau in 1991. Among the 1,881 arrested drug users in northern China, there were 289 females (15%) and 1,592 males (85%).

Age: drug users are young and middle aged people. About 1.3 percent of them are under age twenty; 63.6 percent of them are between the ages of twenty and thirty; 34.3 percent of them are between the ages of thirty-one and forty; and only .85 percent are over forty. The youngest drug user is only fifteen years old, and the oldest drug users is forty-two. These figures are similar to the Xian City Police Department's 1991 data which reported that in north-western China, about

85 percent drug users were under age forty. However, the mean age of the drug user-dealers is higher than the mean age of drug users. The reason might be that to engage in drug selling and smuggling, one must benefit from a certain social and criminal experience. Most of the drug user-dealers had a criminal history, before they got involved in drug selling and smuggling. For drug users, such experience is not necessary.

Table 1 shows that 31.6 percent drug user-dealers are under the age of twenty-five, and that 51.9 percent of them are between the ages of twenty-six and thirty-five. Those below seventeen and above sixty-one years old are only 3 percent.

Education: most drug users from big cities have a junior high school education, and those from small to medium size cities normally have below junior high school education. Drug user-dealers are more likely to have a high school education, no matter where they came from.

The information in Table 2 is similar to a 1992 statistic which revealed that most of the drug users have a junior high or a high school education. In large cities such as Lanzhou and Xianyang, the percentages of drug users who have high school degrees are 84.1 percent and 70 percent respectively. Twenty-five percent of them have elementary school education, and only about 5 percent of them have a university or college degree.

Table 1. Age

Below 17	3	1.1%
18-25	74	30.5%
26-35	126	51.7%
36-60	35	14.5%
61 above	5	2.2%
Total	243	100%

Table 2. Education

Illiteracy	13	5.3%
Elementary school	31	13.0%
Junior high school	153	62.9%
High school	44	18.3%
College and above	2	0.1%
Total	243	100%

Table 3. Occupation

Technician	12	4.9%
Office clerk	7	2.9%
Sales/serviceman	26	10.7%
Farmer	1	0.4%
Local cadre/leader	1	0.4%
Factory worker	125	51.4%
Self-employed	42	17.3%
Craftsman	3	1.2%
Manual labor	2	0.8%
Unemployed	24	9.9%
Total	243	100%

Occupation: The drug users are mostly young and have a low level of education, so they can easily be seduced by the drug traffickers. In the two camps, about 64 percent of the drug users are factory workers and self-employed salesman and servicemen. Others are unemployed and belong to the category "wait-for-job" (Dai Ye Qing Nian). The illegal drug network in these cities attracts unemployed young people.

Table 3 provides similar results to the 1992 Lanzhou University survey, showing that among 335 drug users, 51.3 percent were blue-collar workers, 17 percent were self-employed, 10.7 percent were store salesmen, clerks, and servicemen, and 5.1 percent were specialized technicians. This indicates that intellectuals as well as skilled workers indulge in drug use.

THE CAMP STRATEGY TO DRUG REHABILITATION AND DETOXIFICATION

The rehabilitation rate in the camps indicates the number of rehabilitated individuals per hundred drug users being treated. When a drug abuser is rehabilitated, the individual not only recognizes his/her addictive behavior, but also decides not to use these drugs again. He/she will be graduated from the camp and will be monitored by his/her family members or the work units' leaders, to prevent him or her to use drugs or to get involved into deviant actions.

The rehabilitation camp basically offers ways to achieve deterrence, supervision, and structural care. It is the tough-love system needed to incorporate delinquents back into the society, while providing them with a new life chance through healthy daily practices.

1) Social and Cultural Reorientation Using Intensive Mass Media Propaganda

During the period of intense campaigning against drugs in the early 1990s, the Chinese government exercised a central controlled political ideology which emphasized that correct thoughts led to correct human behaviors. This ideology has a wide range of applications: it represents a new culture, a new way of life, through purposeful, collective means [24]. Deviant individuals are being taught that they lost their positive energy and that they destroyed the balance necessary to both the individual and society. The drug education in the two camps underlines the key-issue that in order to be maintained, China's social order needs morality, cooperation, obedience, as well as the rejection of violence and sinful behaviors among individuals [25]. Social conflicts of all kinds with individuals and groups can be powerfully affected by this general worldview: it is important to merge conflicting and deviant elements into a unified harmony [26]. Under these guidelines, delinquent individuals are considered as being able to change, once they recognize their deviant behaviors, through ideological education, psychological/medical treatments, military training, and social production.

Just as Western psychologists and sociologists believe that the mind determines people's behavior and expands the individual's psychic consciousness, Chinese believe that ideology holds the same functions. "Correct thought is the key to correct action." This famous saying of Mao is as old as Confucianism [24]. Drug users and minor drug dealers are treated as people who lost the correct thought—Zheng Que Si Xang, subsequently engaging in incorrect social behaviors—Cuo Wu Xing Dong. Therefore, they are prime candidates to receive a Correct Thought Education—Si Xiang Jiau Yu. In 1993, the Correct Thought Education was applied to drug detoxification and rehabilitation in the two community camps.

Through the open-ended interviews, the respondents disclosed some of the teaching that they received. According to Chinese Correct Thought, there are three basic kinds of human actions: first, we do something that can benefit both ourselves and others—this is the most desired; second, we do something that can benefit ourselves but damage others—this is selfish and undesired; and third, we do something that can damage both ourselves and others—this is the least desired. The drug addicts claimed having realized that drug dealing and using belonged to the third category, carrying the most damaging effect.

About 56 percent of the drug users answered positively when asked if the camp-education was helpful and necessary. One male user said:

> The community camp provides me with education, work, army training, and
> health examination and treatment. Without the camp, many of us would have

no place to go. We would simply drift on the streets and cause problems. No work place or school accept us, even our families reject us. When I came here, I found out that against all my fears, the camp was not comparable to a jail. Indeed, I had many kinds of contacts with the local folks. I learned the government's documents, read newspapers, and listened to radio broadcasts . . . People like me have to write 'Thought-Change Report' every week. We gradually learned to quit using and selling drugs. In the beginning, these tasks and requirements were very difficult to me, and I wanted to run away. However, several months later, things started to change, . . . I mean, my mind started to change. I realized that I made a mistake and that I almost destroyed my life. I began to appreciate what they (camp leaders and workers) are doing for us.

Another male drug user/dealer said:

Here I communicate with individuals similar to myself. I observe people like myself, and I see changes in people when they go through the training here. I didn't understand much about the bad influences of the drugs before I came in. I learned it both from the organizers' lectures and the ex-users' talks, from watching relevant documentary movies, from listening to the radio broadcasts, and from hard work training.

A female drug user said:

The political leaders, teachers, medical workers, and army officers here are warm-hearted people who sympathize with us and are willing to help us. I thought that they were going to punish us and to treat us badly like in a prison, but I was wrong. They repeatedly emphasized the dangerous and the damaging nature of illegal drugs, and let us perceive our problems. I learned that I lost the 'yin' and 'yang' (positive and negative) balance in my mind and body. I lost the spirit of life. I didn't know the meaning of 'the spiritual achievement' which is promoted by our government and I had sunk into my own 'good world' when I was using drugs. The doctor examined me and gave me a medical treatment. The political worker talked to me over and over. He also let me talk to some other users and ex-users, and finally I realized my problems. This rehabilitation camp really helped people like me who had a drug problem.

Of the 243 people interviewed, 62 percent responded positively to the question asking them if the camps provided both mental and physical help. They were taught to think positively and to try to re-shape their lives. Regarding the question whether the government detoxification campaign was necessary, 43 percent of the respondents responded again positively.

2) Mobilization of the Health Care and Social Security Systems to Provide Detoxification, Rehabilitation, and Employment to Drug Addicts, in a Relatively Short Period of Time

Similar to other types of government controlled programs, community rehabilitation camps in China are set up by the government welfare program and are organized by the political leaders and the police officers of local counties. In the two camps, the political leaders and police officers attend drug detoxification and rehabilitation education seminars before they start working in the camps. They are aware of the sources and the types of illegal drugs; the variety of their damaging effects on individuals; the socioeconomic and demographic background of the drug abusers; the possible behavioral and personality changes of the drug users and dealers; the existing drug network in China, and its connection with the international drug market.

Medical workers, such as doctors and nurses from the local hospitals, come to the camps on different schedules and provide the drug abusers with all necessary medicine such as imported methadone and domestic made herb medicine. The "patients" of these two camps are examined to detect physical illnesses such as stomach problems, liver disease, high blood pressure, heart problems, and tuberculosis, all associated with drug abuse.

The normal length of stay in the camp is about six to twelve months, depending on the individuals' progress. Originally, drug users are either arrested by policemen or reported to the camp by their family members and/or local community leaders. They may enter the camp by their own will or be forced to leave their homes, streets, or gang to enter the rehabilitation program. While in the camp, they follow the daily scheduled activities, such as continuing their education, learning about the damaging nature of illegal drugs, taking medical examinations and treatments, working in the local factories, and receiving training to increase self-control, discipline, and physical fitness.

One drug user in Weinan city, Shanxi province said:

> A black snake sneaked into my stomach, it sucked all my energy away and burned off all of my organs. My body turned thin, my face turned yellow, and finally the ghost sent me to the hell. . . . After 3 months' studying and working here, I want to quit using drugs, and they (leaders) will arrange for me to get a job in a lumber factory as soon as I receive my camp-graduation certificate.

Sixty-one percent of the respondents claimed having lost a job or a spouse or both as a consequence of drug use. Deprived of economic support from a job or their family, many turned to street crime to satisfy their habit. During the detoxification and rehabilitation program, they realized their mistakes.

A former factory worker in Lanzhou explained:

> I started to use drugs three years ago. In the beginning, I was curious about the effect of marijuana and heroin. I just tried several times with a fellow worker and I felt good after I used them. Later, I found out that by selling them, I would not have to work so hard in my factory everyday and that I could make much more money, compared to my salary. Two years ago, I contacted a gang, and we smuggled illegal drugs from the Xinjiang border to the northern cities of China. Although I got some "easy" money from selling drugs, I was almost killed by a gang member who was fighting with me about my profit, and my wife divorced me after she found out what I was doing. Now, after two months here, I realize the "evil" nature of drugs and I will 'wash my hands' and quit it.

According to the camp organizers, this worker had made rapid progress and will be able to work in a factory soon. Twenty-two percent of the drug dealers left their farms and villages, hoping to become rich through selling drugs.

A farmer said:

> I wanted to have a better life, I mean, a better material life. I left my poor village, traveled several provinces, and finally I found a guy who told me I could help him sell drugs and he would pay me lots of money for helping him. He gave me a 'magic' smoke and asked me if I liked it. It was very different from smoking cigarettes and I felt like in heaven. I said I would like to smoke more. He said that I could get more if I helped him. We got some drugs from the Kasakthan border and transferred them secretly into Xian. When we were selling these drugs, I was able to smoke for free, but he always told me that I would get the money later. One day he disappeared and I was arrested by a policeman while I was smoking inside my motel room. . . . My dream of getting rich is gone and I have been cheated by this guy. After I was arrested and sent here, I went through a study program and learned that we were the people who messed our country. I regret, I shouldn't have thought of getting money this way. I hope to return to my village and start to work at home again.

About 32 percent of the drug users in both camps made rapid progress and the leaders promised to help them return to their original school/work places, or to get new jobs once they "graduated" from the camps.

3) Long-Term Incarceration in Work Camps for "Recidivist" Addicts and Drug Traffickers

The head drug dealers in China are often sentenced to the death penalty. This is a convenient way for the Chinese government to get rid of its social "evils." However, if one is not the head dealer, and yet is classified into the "recidivist addict" or the "drug trafficker" category, then he/she will be condemned to a long-term incarceration in the work camps. Typical of these categories are people who spent a tremendous amount of money on buying drugs, went bankrupt, and yet could not quit using drugs. They substituted one drug for another, or got involved in criminal activities such as stealing, burglary, child/spouse abuse, or street violence.

In the two camps, there are about 9 percent of "recidivist drug addicts" or drug traffickers. They were arrested by police officers and will be incarcerated for almost three years in the camps. These people have no regrets as far as their actions were concerned and they manifest very negative attitudes toward the camps. A women who was a cocaine addict said that the rehabilitation training was very painful for her, and that the camp felt like a jail.

The camp organizers admit that about two-thirds of the "recidivists" are uncooperative: they either refuse to talk to the doctors and educators, or stay in bed all day, complaining of being sick. Some individuals even attempt suicide. The "recidivist" and the most problematic individuals are under special supervision, away from the rest of the camp population. In addition, they are not allowed to contact their family nor their local community members. This group of people is alienated from society. Usually, after graduation, it is still difficult for them to obtain jobs, and they are stigmatized as bad social elements.

4) The Existing Problems of the Camp Strategy

Although the Camp strategy shows some positive results in the battle against illegal drugs in China, it is not completely successful. The various faults of this approach are also reflected in the interviews. About 17 percent of the respondents made negative comments (27% are neutral or have no answer) when asked if the camp-education was helpful and necessary to control drug addiction. A woman said:

> The economic condition of this camp is terrible. The facility is almost like a jail. Besides the beds and tables in the room, we have absolutely nothing (see attached photo). There are no TV set, no newspapers, and no magazines in our rooms, We are allowed to have only a few pieces of our personal clothes. When I was sick, I was sent to a far-away hospital which was about 45 Kilometers from here, and the rough drive made me even sicker. The education that we receive here is only at the junior high school level and many of us were high school students. I can't contact my family members and I can't go home when I want to. There's absolutely no freedom here.

A man said:

> I and many others like me are forced to admit our mistakes. We have to pretend that we will quit using drugs, but I doubt that it will be the case once we get out. The political studies and training here are forced upon us and I don't think that many of us will change as a result. Smoking Opium is not

harmful, just like smoking cigarettes . . . and I don't understand why I can't use drugs if I work normally and don't commit crimes.

Of the 243 people interviewed, 19 percent responded negatively when asked if the camps helped them both physically and mentally. They said that the political leaders, as well as the therapeutic workers, were prejudiced and discriminatory toward them. In turn, this often made them feel depressed and even caused them to have hostile feelings toward the political leaders and the therapy workers.

One female recidivist said that she was frustrated with the camp system because the only thing she heard was the camp leader's yelling voice. She said that there was no advocacy program in the camp to deal with her case. She unsuccessfully attempted suicide by hanging herself with shoe laces.

About 15 percent of the respondents told the interviewer that the spiritual/ mental rehabilitation was conducted in such a simplistic manner, that it could not fit individual needs.

A male user said:

I and seventeen other people were sitting in one rehabilitation session the other day. The social worker asked us to tell each other how we began to use drugs. One woman had a terrible relationship with her family. Her father wanted her to become a prostitute in order to earn some extra income for the family. She refused and was kicked out of her home. She started to use drugs to release her anger and sadness. In another case, a man began to sell drugs after he hit a pedestrian with his truck, and was not able to pay for the medical fees. I myself was a factory worker, and I just felt curious about drugs so I started to use them two years ago . . . You see, we are all different. But the social worker told us that we all lost the balance of positive and negative thoughts, that we were blind, that we took a wrong road and that this road would lead us to commit national crimes, which was not true. We have to agree with him, otherwise we will be punished and forced to stay here longer.

When asked if the government detoxification campaign was necessary, 13 percent of the respondents expressed negative feelings. Eighteen percent of the drug users voiced doubt that it would change their behavior.

A man who had to follow military discipline training at the time of the interview said:

The training and education are useless for many people. They participate in these programs but when they are among themselves they claim that as soon as they will be out, they will use drug again. Personally, I don't believe in the government propaganda. The propaganda is just a way to control individual freedom. I don't mean that using drug is a good thing. But if we are told to quit drugs, then the local county leaders should quit using drugs too. Many high-rank officials' sons and daughters and some high-rank officials themselves use drugs and no one dares to touch them. Discipline and rules only apply to folks like us.

This person claimed that several people went back to drugs as soon as they graduated from the camp.

About 9 percent of the individuals interviewed explained that the camp rehabilitation education was superficial. A drug user does not change behavior because of the full spiritual realization of his or her mistakes, but because political leaders exert a firm ideological control. Also, because of the increasing number of offenders compared to the limited space and resources of the camps, it happens that leaders and organizers "graduate" those individuals who stayed there for some time, even though they did not change their attitudes and behaviors completely.

RECOMMENDATIONS

Through the analysis of these interviews, several recommendations emerge regarding the camp strategy. First, at the macro level, a policy approach of a much wider scope is needed. The policy agenda envisioned here suggests a perspective in which structural issues are key components in the development of the camp strategy. The structural issues include poverty, educational access, and job opportunity in the nation. To reduce the demand for drugs, the government needs to improve individual opportunities.

Second, at the individual level, treatment and prevention must be approached in a broader sense than with the constrained "Correct Thought Education" model. Most drug abusers are currently offered a narrow range of options. All of them often the same treatment, regardless of their individual needs. Similarly, after-care is prescribed by the camp leaders with the same level of intensity for all, again regardless of the individuals' situations.

Third, an optimistic and non discriminatory work ethic should be encouraged among the political leaders and the social workers in both the camps and the local communities, to increase the effectiveness of the treatment.

Fourth, the facilities need some improvement, in order to make living arrangements more agreeable. People would certainly be less inclined to run away if their conditions were more pleasant.

DISCUSSION

Thus far, none of the community rehabilitation programs in China have been completely successful. In both camps under study, an average twelve-month training results in a rehabilitation rate of about 80 percent.

In the work camps, drug users are first forced to learn about their behaviors, then to participate in the rehabilitation program, and eventually are led to change their deviant behaviors. In their eyes, other deviants are mirrors of themselves. Their behaviors are re-shaped under the political persuasion first, and under the establishment of self-esteem and positive attitudes toward life later. They experience rejection from the society first, then regain acceptance once they have completed the rehabilitation programs. Their lot is substantially improved as they live with individuals who are similar to themselves, as they continue their education and participation in the work force, and as they receive social support both from the staff members and from their involvement with an ex-user activist group.

China, as it is well known in the world, had the largest prevalence of opiate addiction in the past. It was remarkable that, in the 1860s and in the 1950s, Chinese governments were able to eliminate opiate addiction and to solve this massive problem in just a couple of years. Such a success was a great motivation for the future governmental control of illegal drugs.

The camp approach is comprehensive in its scope. It integrates treatment, rehabilitation, and primary prevention, all as a part of the community effort, with voluntary medical and social assistance. On the other hand, it clearly represents the compulsory and legal pressure characteristics found in boot camps within other Asian regions.

REFERENCES

1. X. Guo, Drug Related Crimes in China, in *From Hu Men Burning Opium to Drug Detoxification in Contemporary China*, Q. Ling and Q. Shao (eds.), Sichan People's Publisher, pp. 112-119, 1977.
2. H. C. Zeng, The Detoxification Thought of Lin Zexu and Its Influence to Against Illegal Drug Use Movement, in *From Hu Men Burning Opium to Drug Detoxification in Contemporary China*, Q. Ling and Q. Shao (eds.), Sichan People's Publisher, pp. 5-59, 1977.
3. J. S. Brook, M. Whiteman, and A. Scovell Gordon, Stages of Drug Use in Adolescence: Personality, Peer, and Family Correlates, *Developmental Psychology, 19*, pp 269-277, 1983.
4. D. B. Kandel and J. A. Logan, Patterns of Drug Use From Adolescence to Young Adulthood: Periods of Risk Initiation, Continued Use, and Discontinuation, *American Journal of Public Health, 74*, pp. 660-666, 1984.
5. K. Yamaguchi and D. B. Kandel, Patterns of Drug Use From Adolescence to Young Adulthood: Sequences of Progression, *American Journal of Public Health, 74*, pp. 668-672, 1984.
6. L. Lanza-Kaduce, R. L. Akers, M. D. Krohn, and M. Radosevich, Cessation of Alcohol and Drug Use Among Adolescents: A Social Learning Model, *Deviant Behavior, 5*, pp. 79-96, 1984.

7. B. H. Raveis and D. B. Kandel, Changes in Drug Behavior From the Middle to the Late Twenties: Initiation, Persistence, and Cessation of Use, *American Journal of Public Health, 77,* pp. 607-611, 1987.
8. O. Ray and C. Ksir, *Drugs, Society, and Human Behavior,* Mosby, St. Louis, 1990.
9. R. T. Jones, D. W. McDonald, M. F. Fiore, T. Arrington, and J. Randall, A Primary Prevention Approach to Children's Drug Refusal Behavior: The Impact of Rehearsal-Plus, *Journal of Pediatric Psychology, 15*:2, pp. 211-223, 1990.
10. G. Botvin, E. Baker, A. Filazzola, and E. Botvin, A Cognitive-Behavioral Approach to Substance Abuse Prevention: One-Year Follow-Up, *Addictive Behaviors, 15,* pp. 47-63, 1990.
11. R. Kadden and I. Mauriello, Enhancing Participation in Substance Abuse Treatment Using an Incentive System, *Journal of Substance Abuse Treatment, 8*:3, pp. 113-124, 1991.
12. M. W. Fourcier, Substance Abuse, Crime and Prison-Based Treatment: Problems and Prospects, *Sociological Practice Review, 2*:2, pp. 123-131, 1991.
13. J. A. Morris, Jr., Alcohol and Other Drug Dependency Treatment: A Proposal for Integration with Primary Care, *Alcoholism Treatment Quarterly, 13,* pp. 345-355, 1995.
14. M. Sealock, D. C. Gottfredson, and C. A. Gallagher, Drug Treatment for Juvenile Offenders: Some Good and Bad News, *Journal of Research in Crime and Delinquency, 34*:2, pp. 210-236, 1997.
15. R. D. Mann and J. Wingard, A Cross-Cultural Field Study of Drug Rehabilitation Methodologies in Sweden and the U.S., *Journal of Drug Education, 11*:3, pp. 245-260, 1981.
16. D. Frans, Social Work, Social Science, and the Disease Concept: New Directions for Addiction Treatment, *Journal of Sociology and Social Welfare, 21*:2, pp. 71-87, June 1994.
17. C. D. Kaplan, R. Shiota, J. Sell, and B. Bieleman, *The "Camp" Approach to Drug Detoxification: The Community Strategy to Drug Abuse Control,* paper prepared for Director, Program on Substance Abuse, WHO, Geneva, 1993.
18. C. P. Spencer and B. Navaratnam, *Drug Abuse in East Asia,* Oxford University Press, Oxford, pp. 161-162, 1981.
19. *Commonwealth Regional Working Group on Illicit Drugs,* Singapore Country Report, Kuala Lumpur, 1979.
20. B. C. Ng., *Review of Treatment and Rehabilitation Measures for Drug Users in Singapore,* in Proceedings, Colombo Plan Workshop, Penang, 1978.
21. W. H. McGlothin, The Singapore Heroin Control Program, *Bulletin of Narcotics, 32*:1, pp. 1-14, 1980.
22. P. Lowinger, The Solution to the Narcotic Addiction in the People's Republic of China, *American Journal of Drug and Alcohol Abuse, 4*:2, pp. 165-178, 1977.
23. Q. Shao, *An Initial Research Report on Drug Use and HIV Infection in P.R. China,* Beijing University Bulletin, March 1994.
24. J. C. Hsiung, *Ideology and Practice, the Evolution of Chinese Communism,* Praeger Publishers, New York, Washington, London, 1970.
25. C. R. Hallpike, *The Principles of Social Evolution,* Clarendon Press, Oxford, 1988.

26. D. Bodde, Harmony and Conflict in Chinese Philosophy, *Essays on Chinese Civilization*, C. LeBlanc and D. Borei (eds.), Princeton University Press, pp. 237-298, 1981.

Direct reprint requests to:

Wen Wang, Ph.D.
Department of Sociology
California State University, Northridge
18111 Nordhoff St.
Northridge, CA 91330

J. DRUG EDUCATION, Vol. 29(2) 115-138, 1999

CORRECTION OF NORMATIVE MISPERCEPTIONS: AN ALCOHOL ABUSE PREVENTION PROGRAM*

GEORGE STEFFIAN, PH.D.
University of Wyoming

ABSTRACT

Normative misperception refers to the tendency of college students to misperceive campus drinking norms to be more liberal than they actually are. Initial investigations have demonstrated the effectiveness of normative education on reduction of alcohol use in primary and secondary education settings. This study examined the utility of a group program designed to challenge seventy-one male college students' misperceptions of college drinking norms. Participants were enrolled into either a normative education group or a control group representing traditional alcohol education efforts. Participants in the normative education groups demonstrated more accurate perceptions of campus drinking norms and a significant reduction in consequences of alcohol use while those in the control group did not. Changes in normative perceptions were among the strongest contributors to a function discriminating between those who decreased their drinking and those who did not. Results suggest that normative education may be an effective approach to modifying drinking behaviors.

For several decades, alcohol use by college students has been a serious concern of university administrators and public health officials. A number of studies [1-4] have documented the attempts of college drug educators to influence the attitudes and behaviors of college students regarding alcohol. Traditional prevention programming has employed a number of strategies ranging from increasing

---

*This research is based on the author's dissertation completed in partial requirement for his Ph.D. in Clinical Psychology at the University of Wyoming.

knowledge about the effects of alcohol and raising awareness of the possible consequences of drinking, to training resistance against peer pressure to drink.

Despite the determined efforts of drug and alcohol educators, it has become increasingly apparent that such traditional models of prevention have relatively little effect on student's attitudes and behaviors related to alcohol [5-9]. As such, researchers are continually searching for new, more effective techniques for encouraging more conservative use of alcohol on college campuses. An area of the literature which seems to hold potential for alcohol abuse prevention focuses on student's misperceptions of drinking norms. Several studies have documented that students often over-estimate both the quantity and frequency of their friends' drinking compared to their own consumption [10, 11]. Perkins and Berkowitz administered a drinking attitudes survey which measured both the students' personal attitudes toward their drinking as well s their perception of the average student's attitudes toward drinking [8]. The results demonstrated a significant misperception of the campus' normative attitude toward drinking by the students. While most students endorsed a moderate personal attitude toward drinking, they misperceived the campus norm as being more liberal. In a follow-up survey, Perkins and Berkowitz found that students perceived close friends, housing peers, and the general student population as being more liberal in their attitudes toward alcohol use than themselves [12]. These results also held for ratings of actual number of drinks per party, providing a behavioral correlate for the attitudinal findings.

CONSEQUENCES OF NORMATIVE MISPERCEPTIONS

Findings from recent studies suggest that the consequences of such widespread misperceptions may be substantial. Marks, Graham, and Hansen found that misperceptions of alcohol use prevalence influenced alcohol use in seventh- and eighth-grade adolescents [13]. Controlling for levels of use at baseline, participants' estimates of prevalence of alcohol use predicted level of own use one year later. Similar results were found when predicting onset of use. These findings coincide with the general association between level of friends' alcohol use and one's own use [14, 15].

As normative misperceptions may influence level of alcohol use, it is critical to examine their impact on negative consequences for the user. Inaccurate perceptions of attitudinal and behavioral norms may serve to excuse risky behaviors and increase resistance to prevention programming. Students are likely to ignore warning signs of their behavior if they believe others behave more liberally and suffer more serious consequences than themselves. Baer and Carney found that students tend to rate the average member of their residence and the average student as encountering significantly more negative consequences due to alcohol use than themselves [16].

APPLICATION

The literature cited above suggests that normative misperception is a powerful phenomenon which may not only affect students' attitudes, but also their behaviors concerning alcohol use and negative consequences related to level of use. Therefore, it behooves drug and alcohol educators to incorporate this knowledge into a coherent prevention strategy which helps to correct these erroneous assumptions. If normative misperception can enable dangerous use of alcohol to be justified and to continue unquestioned, then accurate perception of campus drinking norms can have the reverse effect. If a student recognizes that his attitudes are more conservative than those of his peers and then becomes more liberal, then recognition that his attitudes are more liberal than the norm may have the reverse effect.

The approach of correcting students' perceptions of campus drinking norms has recently been implemented by Perkins and Berkowitz [12]. Their program consisted of collecting descriptive and perceived data from campus-wide surveys and organizing these data into presentations to specific student groups. If as it seems, students' attitudes toward drinking are already more conservative than thought, then it may be that these attitudes lose their significance in the face of misperceived normative environments. Although the authors' summary of these efforts is enthusiastic, no specific research has been conducted to document the efficacy of their programming.

Hansen and Graham compared the effectiveness of normative education and peer pressure resistance training in preventing the onset of alcohol abuse, cigarette use, and marijuana use among junior high school students [17]. They found that correcting students normative misperceptions resulted in significant reductions in onset for all three variables while resistance training had no significant effects on these variables.

More recently, Agostinelli, Brown, and Miller recruited twenty-six heavy drinkers, and provided a subset of them with normative feedback through the mail [18]. The feedback consisted of providing participants with a comparison of their level of alcohol use to population norms. The researchers noted that those who received the feedback reported greater reduction in weekly consumption and estimated level of intoxication per week than those who did not.

ATTITUDES TOWARD DRINKING

Social psychologists have demonstrated that attitudes play a significant role in determining behavior [19]. In particular, attitudes have been shown to predict drinking behavior [20-22]. Given the importance of attitudes in determining alcohol consumption, a question regarding the correction of normative perceptions is raised. What variables are responsible for changes in drinking behaviors seen as a result of programs directed at normative misperceptions? Do more accurate perceptions of campus drinking norms affect drinking behavior directly, or is a subsequent attitudinal change or combination of the two responsible for changes in drinking behavior? If abstainers are seen as more normative and heavy drinkers as more deviant, perhaps a change in attitudes toward these categories would be an important factor in a subject's resulting change in drinking patterns.

Based on the previous research, the present study sought to investigate the effectiveness of an education group aimed at correcting normative misperceptions of first-year college students. To determine the extent and relevance of changes in attitudinal variables, subjects' attitudes toward drinking and different categories of drinkers were also assessed. It was hypothesized that at one-week and one-month follow-up intervals, students in the normative education groups would exhibit decreased estimates of weekly and heavy alcohol consumption by the average student relative to baseline estimates. Subjects in the experimental condition were also expected to demonstrate decreased weekly and heavy consumption of alcohol at one-week and one-month follow-up periods. It was further hypothesized that relative to baseline levels, subjects in the experimental condition would report a decrease in negative consequences due to drinking at the one-month follow-up periods. Subjects in the control condition were not expected to exhibit significant changes on any of these variables.

DISCRIMINATING VARIABLES

It was expected that students' perceptions of campus drinking norms would discriminate between the prevention and control group subjects. Subjects' attitudes toward abstainers and heavy drinkers were also expected to discriminate between the two groups. In addition, all three of these variables were expected to discriminate between those subjects who reduced their drinking and those who did not.

METHOD

Participants

Due to the gender differences in drinking patterns and experienced consequences [23-25] only males were included in the sample. Subjects were seventy-one male undergraduate volunteers enrolled in introductory level psychology courses at the University of Wyoming.

Procedures

Each subject was required to sign up for three sessions, the second at a one-week interval, and the third at a one-month interval. Because of the extensive time commitment required, participants were allowed to sign up for the series of sessions which best accommodated their schedules. Sessions were then assigned to either the experimental or control condition based on which sessions fit with the schedules of the group facilitators. Before beginning, subjects provided informed consent to participate in the study.

Participants assigned to the prevention group were first required to fill out three questionnaires. Students were asked to give the name and phone number of someone who could be contacted to verify their reported drinking behavior; these individuals were never actually contacted. This procedure, the "bogus pipeline" [26], has been used to increase the accuracy of self-report data. This technique entails asking participants to report their behavior under conditions where they are led to believe that their responses will be subject to "objective" external validation. Students then completed the Core Alcohol and Drug Survey (Core) [27], a supplemental questionnaire with items mirroring those on the Core and a questionnaire assessing attitudes toward alcohol use and toward different categories of drinkers. Participants were then engaged in a group task to establish consensus regarding an estimate of the average student's weekly consumption, frequency of binge drinking, and frequency of consequences due to alcohol use. Upon reaching consensus, participants were presented with the actual self-report data of University of Wyoming students. Data from previous collections of the Core (1989 through 1995) were used to reference actual campus-wide reports of alcohol use. Students were then involved in a discussion concerning possible explanations for and consequences of their misperceptions. Group facilitators covered the general theoretical assumptions with reference to the reasons given by students to support their opinions in the consensus exercise. During this discussion, the results of the Core (completed by participants) were tabulated, creating means for the group's weekly alcohol consumption as well as frequency of consequences of alcohol use. In addition, the group's estimates of weekly consumptions and frequency of consequences for the "average student" were also tabulated. After the group discussion regarding campus-wide norms was completed, subjects were then presented with the results of their responses on the Core survey. The aim of this presentation was to demonstrate that among the group, there was a self-reported mean for weekly alcohol consumption and frequency of consequences which was much lower than the mean of their individual and consensus estimates of these variables for the "average student." This finding was then shown to be representative of the campus-wide pattern of overestimation of drinking norms. Thus, the students were presented with not only statistics indicating a pattern of misperception at their university but were confronted with their own misperceptions. Students were then led in a discussion concerning the impact of normative education on their self-perception, attitudes toward alcohol use, and future decision making regarding alcohol use. Finally, students were provided with pamphlets containing the conservative, campus-wide statistics discussed in the presentation. At a second session, one week later and a third session, one month later, subjects were required to complete the Core, supplemental questions and attitude questionnaire.

Subjects assigned to the control group were first required to fill out the Core, supplemental questions, and attitude questionnaire. They then viewed a thirty-minute educational film documenting the physiological effects of alcohol. After watching the film, subjects were dismissed. One week and one month later, subjects were again required to complete the same measures to assess for any short term changes in normative perceptions, attitudes, and drinking behavior as a result of viewing the film or merely being involved in the study.

Materials

The Core Alcohol and Drug Survey is a twenty-three-question self-report measure developed by a committee of grantees of the U.S. Department of Education's Fund for the Improvement of Post-Secondary Education (FIPSE). Its primary purpose has been to aid universities in assessing the effectiveness of substance abuse prevention efforts. The Core was designed to assess a number of content areas including: perception of campus substance abuse policies and their enforcement, frequency of binge drinking episodes number of drinks per week, and perceptions of others' use of alcohol [27].

The supplemental questions for the Core survey consisted of the following: Four existing questions regarding estimates of personal weekly usage and frequency of consequences were converted to have subjects also estimate these variables for the "average student." One question from a later version of the Core was also included requesting students to give an over-all rating of change in their alcohol use at each follow-up period.

The supplemental questionnaire compiled by the investigator includes two sections: "attitudes toward alcohol use," and "attitudes toward others." The "attitude toward alcohol use" section contains seven items requiring subjects to rate their attitudes toward drinking on 5-point Likert scales. This section yields a composite score ranging from 7 (most liberal) to 35 (most conservative). The "attitudes toward others" section requires subjects to rate their attitudes toward four different categories of drinkers: "non-drinker, "light drinker," "moderate drinker," and "heavy drinker." This section uses on fourteen adjective pairs with a 7-point Likert scale for each adjective pair. Responses range from −3 (least approval) to +3 (most approval) creating a continuous scale between each adjective pair. These scales represent a version of the Semantic Differential Scale [28].

The pamphlet given to the subjects in the experimental condition contains statistics regarding the conservative use of alcohol and other drugs as reported by University of Wyoming students. The pamphlet was created by the University of Wyoming Drug Education Resource Center using data collected from campus-wide administrations of the Core Alcohol and Drug Survey between 1989 and 1993. The educational film viewed by the subjects in the control condition was titled: Understanding Alcohol Use and Abuse (Disney Productions, 1979). This film documents the physiological and psychological effects of alcohol, specifically the subjective states accompanying different blood-alcohol content levels.

Statistics

Six one-way Analyses of Variance (ANOVAs) were conducted to test the following hypotheses. In all six cases, the independent variable was group (experimental or control) and the repeated measure was set at three intervals (baseline, 1-week follow-up, and 1-month follow-up).

The first ANOVA tested the hypothesis that students in the experimental condition would exhibit decreased estimates of weekly consumption by the average student at both follow-up periods. The dependent variable was estimated number of drinks per week for the average University of Wyoming student (measured by students' response to question #1 on the Core supplement).

The second ANOVA was used to examine the effect of the intervention on students' perception of the average student's heavy consumption of alcohol. The dependent variable was students' estimate of the frequency of binge drinking for the average U. W. student (measured by the students' response to question #2 on the Core supplement).

In order to test the hypothesis that students in the experimental group would demonstrate decreased weekly consumption of alcohol at one-week and two-month follow-up periods, a third one-way ANOVA with a repeated measure was performed. The dependent variable was students' reported average number of drinks per week (measured by students' response to question #15 on the Core).

The fourth one-way ANOVA was used to examine the effect of the prevention program on heavy consumption of alcohol. The dependent variable was students' reported frequency of binge drinking (measured by the students' response to question #14 on the Core).

The fifth one-way ANOVA was employed to test the hypothesis that subjects in the experimental condition would report a decrease in negative consequences due to alcohol at the two-month follow-up period. The dependent variable was subjects' scores on question #21 on the Core.

To examine the effect of the presentation on students' attitudes toward drinking at both follow-up periods, a final one-way ANOVA was performed. The dependent variable was subjects' composite scores from the "attitude toward alcohol use" section of the supplemental questionnaire.

A one-way ANOVA with two repeated measures was conducted to determine the effect of the presentation on subjects' attitudes toward the four different categories of drinkers. The independent variable was group (experimental or control) the within subject variables were category rated (non- light-, moderate-, and heavy-drinker) and collection time (baseline, 1-week follow-up and 1-month follow-up) and the dependent variable was degree of approval (measured by subjects' responses on the Attitudes Toward Others Questionnaire).

In order to determine which variables best discriminate between the experimental and control groups, a discriminant analysis was conducted using the following variables: perception of average student's # of drinks per week, perception of average student's # of binges per two weeks, perception of average student's frequency of alcohol use, attitudes toward alcohol use, approval of abstainers, approval of light drinkers, approval of moderate drinkers, and approval of heavy drinkers (change scores for these variables were used). A discriminant analysis was also performed to establish which variables best discriminate between those subjects who reduced their alcohol use at one month follow-up and those who did not.

RESULTS

Repeated Measures ANOVAs

The first hypothesis addressed the effect of the intervention on participants' estimates of the average student's weekly consumption of alcohol and average student's frequency of binge drinking. Group means can be found in Table 1. With regard to perception of drinks per week, a main effect was observed for collection time, $F(2,68) = 7.64$, $p < .001$, suggesting an overall decrease in participants' perceptions of the number of drinks per week consumed by the average University of Wyoming student. Closer examination of the data indicates that this effect was far more pronounced for subjects in the experimental condition, as shown by the significant interaction of group and collection time, $F(2,68) = 11.05$, $p < .0001$. Subjects' perceptions of the average student's number of binges per week also decreased across collection periods, $F(2,68) = 8.47$, $p < .001$. An interaction between group and collection time reveals that this effect was more robust for subjects in the experimental group, $F(2,68) = 8.47$, $p < .001$. See Table 1 for group means and Figures 1 and 2 for graphical representation of these results.

The second hypothesis addressed the impact of the intervention on participants' reported drinking behavior. An overall trend for collection time was noted, with subjects tending to report a decrease in number of drinks per week across collection times, $F(2,68) = 2.95$, $p = .059$. Membership in the experimental condition had no differential effect on this trend, $F(2,68) = 2.01$, $p > .05$. As for frequency of binge drinking, a main effect was found for collection time, with subjects reporting a decrease in frequency of binge drinking across collection periods, $F(2,68) = 3.93$, $p < .05$. A trend was observed for the interaction between group and collection time, $F(2,68) = 2.95$, $p = .059$. As can be seen in Table 1, participants who received the intervention tended to report a greater decrease in binge episodes than those who did not. Data for both these hypotheses are displayed graphically in Figures 3 and 4.

Table 1. Group Means for Repeated Measures ANOVAs

Variable	Time	Group Experimental	Control
P.D.W.[a]	1	10.69	9.20
	2	6.11	9.26
	3	5.94	9.74
P.BIN.[b]	1	3.24	2.17
	2	1.62	2.11
	3	1.47	1.82
DRINK.W[c]	1	11.67	8.71
	2	9.06	8.43
	3	8.36	8.69
BINGE[d]	1	2.65	1.73
	2	1.75	1.66
	3	2.31	1.69
CONSQ.[e]	1	13.66	12.09
	2	11.64	11.71
	3	11.28	11.94
A.ALC[f]	1	21.56	22.09
	2	21.50	21.89
	3	21.58	21.00
A.NON[g]	1	48.36	47.94
	2	49.33	48.09
	3	49.22	48.37
A.LIGHT[g]	1	46.58	48.26
	2	47.69	48.94
	3	49.11	50.03
A.MOD[g]	1	41.28	42.20
	2	40.75	42.83
	3	43.44	42.83
A HEAV[g]	1	31.72	33.06
	2	33.08	33.94
	3	34.31	35.20

[a]Perception of average student's # drinks/week
[b]Perception of average student's # binges/week
[c]# drinks/week
[d]# binges/week
[e]# and weight of consequences in last month
[f]Attitude toward alcohol (higher scores denote healthier attitudes)
[g]Approval of each category of drinker (higher scores denote greater approval).

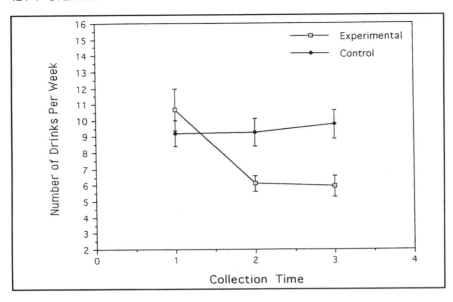

Figure 1. Perception of the number of drinks consumed per
week by the average student.

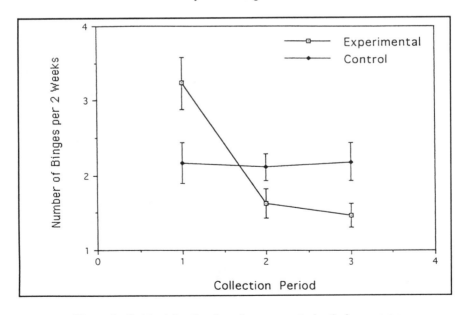

Figure 2. Subjects' estimates of average student's frequency
of binge drinking episodes.

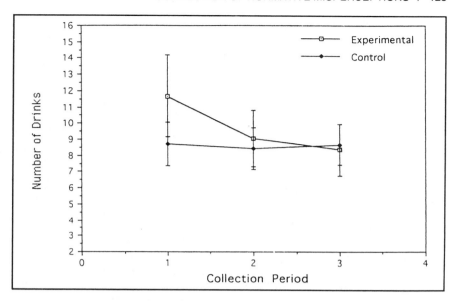

Figure 3. Subjects reported number of drinks consumed per week.

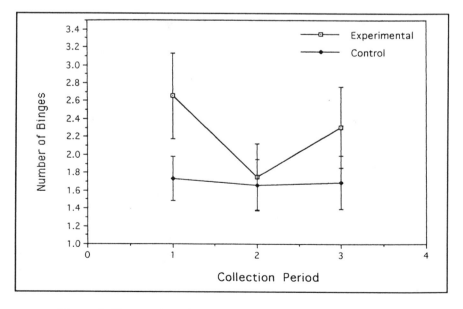

Figure 4. Reported number of binge episodes in past two weeks.

Hypothesis three examined the influence of the intervention on subjects' report of the number of consequences experienced as a result of alcohol use. As can be seen in Figure 5, a main effect was found for the repeated measure, indicating that regardless of group, subjects reported a decrease in the number of experienced consequences across collection times, $F(2,68) = 3.47$, $p < .05$. No interaction was found between group and collection period, $F(2,68) = 2.17$, $p > .05$. Means can be found in Table 1.

Hypothesis four addressed the effect of the intervention on subjects' attitudes toward alcohol use. As can be seen in Table 1, participants attitudes toward alcohol use remained fairly stable across time. As such, no main effect was found for the repeated measure, $F(2,68) = .506$, $p > .05$, and no interaction was observed between group and collection time, $F(2,68) = .419$, $p > .05$.

The fifth hypothesis examined the impact of the intervention on subjects approval of four categories of drinkers (non, light, moderate, and heavy). For this hypothesis, a one-way ANOVA with two repeated measures was performed. The independent variable was group, the within subject variables were category rated and collection time, and the dependent variable was degree of approval. One significant finding yielded by this analysis was a main effect for category, $F(3,67) = 41.99$, $p < .0001$, suggesting that across groups and collection times, the mean ratings for all three drinking categories were not equal. The second finding was a main effect for collection time, $F(2,68) = 5.98$, $p < .004$. As can be

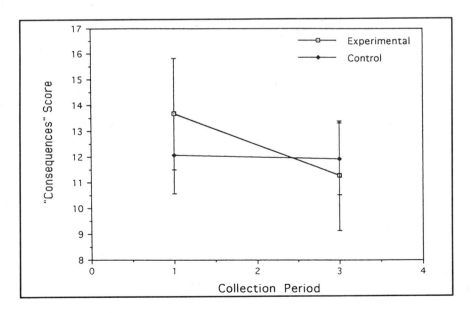

Figure 5. Subjects' score on CORE #21; consequences due to alcohol use.

seen in Table 1, mean approval ratings for the four drinking categories seemed to increase over time. Treating each category as a separate analysis yielded three main effects for time for the categories of light, moderate, and heavy. In other words, there was a significant increase in approval ratings over time for the categories: light, moderate, and heavy. Group membership did not influence this pattern.

Although there was no direct hypothesis regarding participants' perceptions of the average student's frequency of alcohol use, this variable was measured and analyzed post hoc, using a one-way ANOVA with a repeated measure. Results of this analysis yielded a significant effect for collection time, $F(2,68) = 10.07$, $p < .001$. This effect was more pronounced for the experimental group as indicated by a significant interaction between group and collection time, $F(2,68) = 5.84$, $p < .005$. Means can be found in Table 2 and are displayed graphically in Figure 6.

A similar post hoc analysis was conducted on subjects' self-reports of their own frequency of alcohol use. While there was no main effect for collection time, $F(2,68) = 1.16$, $p = .32$, the interaction between collection time and group was significant, $F(2,68) = 3.48$, $p < .05$. Closer inspection of the simple effects for each group did not yield significant effects for collection time, control: $F(2,33) = 2.01$, $p = .14$; experimental: $F(2,33) = 1.75$, $p = .19$. Thus, while the difference in trends between experimental and control groups was significant as a whole, there was no significant change across collection time for either group when each was examined separately. Means can be found in Table 2 and are displayed graphically in Figure 7.

Discriminant Analyses

To determine which variables would best discriminate between control and experimental groups, a discriminant analysis was performed. The grouping

Table 2. Group Means for Post Hoc Repeated Measures ANOVAs

Variable	Time	Group	
		Experimental	Control
P.F.USE.[a]	1	10.03	8.01
	2	4.90	7.36
	3	5.49	7.73
F.USE[b]	1	7.19	6.31
	2	6.58	5.76
	3	5.65	6.77

[a]Perception of the average student's frequency of alcohol use in past thirty days.
[b]Subjects' reported frequency of alcohol use in past thirty days.

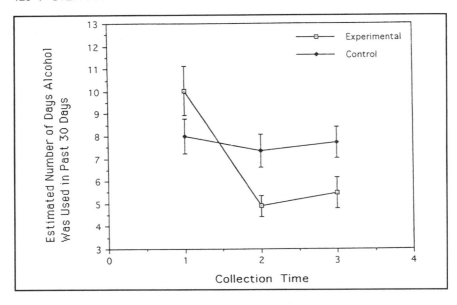

Figure 6. Perception of frequency of alcohol use by the average student.

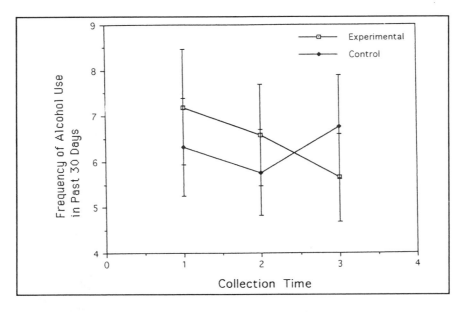

Figure 7. Subjects' reported frequency of alcohol use.

variable was group (experimental or control) and the discriminating variables used were change scores from baseline to one-month follow-up for the following variables: perception of the average student's number of drinks per week; perception of the average student's number of binges per two weeks; perception of the average student's frequency of alcohol use; attitudes toward alcohol use; approval of non drinkers; approval of light drinkers; approval of moderate drinkers; approval of heavy drinkers.

On the basis of four discriminating variables, the discriminant function generated was found to be significant, $\chi^2(4) = 26.62$, $p < .0001$. Structure coefficients, function statistics, and group centroids can be found in Table 3. Examination of the structure coefficients, revealed three variables with positive correlations to the discriminant function. As hypothesized, change in perception of the average student's number of drinks per week ($r = .83$), change in perception of the average student's number of binges every two weeks ($r = .71$) and, change in perception of the average student's frequency of alcohol use ($r = .43$) all had positive loadings in the function. Lower values for these variables correlated with lower function scores and thus greater likelihood of classification in the

Table 3. Discriminant Analysis Results for Experimental and Control Groups

Variable	Function 1 Structure Coefficients
Perception of average student's # drinks/week	.83
Perception of average student's # binges/week	.71
Perception of average student's frequency of alcohol use	.44
Attitudes toward alcohol use	−.33

Function Statistics		Centroids	
Chi Square:	26.62	Experimental:	−.68
df:	4		
Probability:	<.0001	Control:	.70
Canonical Corr:	.57		
Variance accounted for between groups:	.32		

Note: Change scores for all variables were used for discriminant analysis.

experimental group. One variable, change in attitudes toward alcohol use, correlated negatively with the discriminant function. Higher values for this variable (shift toward healthier attitudes) correlated with lower function values, and thus greater likelihood of classification in the experimental group. The hypothesis that change in approval of abstainers would load on the discriminant function was not supported. This variable did not contribute to the discrimination between experimental and control subjects.

The above function was the result of the combination of variables which yielded the greatest discrimination power without high correlations between the discriminating variables. Variables with high correlations to other variables in the function were run separately to avoid problems associated with multicolinearity.

To determine which variables would best discriminate between those subjects who reported a decrease in weekly alcohol consumption and those who did not, a second discriminant analysis was conducted. The grouping variable was decrease or same/increase in drinking from baseline to one-month follow-up. The discriminating variables entered were group (experimental or control) and change scores from baseline to one-month follow-up for the following variables: perception of the average student's number of drinks per week; perception of the average student's number of binges per two weeks; perception of the average student's frequency of alcohol use; attitudes toward alcohol use; approval of non drinkers; approval of light drinkers; approval of moderate drinkers; and approval of heavy drinkers.

On the basis of four discriminating variables, a discriminant function was generated and found to be significant, $\chi^2(4) = 17.51$, $p < .001$. Structure coefficients, function statistics and group centroids can be found in Table 4. Examination of the structure coefficients reveals that scores for all four contributing variables correlated positively with discriminant function scores. The loading of perception of average student's drinks per week gave some support to the hypothesis that changes in perceptions of campus drinking norms would help discriminate between subjects who decreased their drinking and subjects who did not. The hypothesis that change in approval of abstainers would help discriminate between those who decreased their drinking and those who did not, was not supported. This variable did not contribute the discriminant function for these two groups.

Due to moderate correlations between some discriminating variables, variables with higher correlations were entered in separate functions. Results, however, did not yield functions which were able to discriminate between groups significantly. Thus, the first discriminant function was retained as the most useful in describing the data.

DISCUSSION

This study investigated a number of questions addressing the utility of a small group intervention designed to challenge college students' normative

Table 4. Discriminant Analysis Results for Groups Defined
by Reduction Drinking

Variable	Function 1	
		Structure Coefficients
Perception of average student's # drinks/week		.92
Approval of moderate drinkers		.88
Approval of heavy drinkers		.21
Attitudes toward alcohol use		.21

Function Statistics		Centroids
Chi Square:	17.51	Decreased: −.92
df:	4	
Probability:	.001	Equal or
		Increased: .31
Canonical Corr:	.48	
Shared Variance:	.23	

Note: Change scores for all variables were used for discriminant analysis.

misperceptions regarding alcohol use. Generalization of these findings should be cautious as subjects were males sampled from undergraduate psychology courses and may not be representative of the general population of college students.

Perception of Campus Drinking Norms

For the most part, the normative education was associated with hypothesized perceptual changes. Compared to traditional alcohol education efforts this program was associated with a significantly greater decrease in participants' estimates of the average student's quantity of alcohol consumed per week and frequency of binge drinking episodes. In this respect, the group appeared to accomplish its objective of helping students incorporate more accurate information regarding campus drinking norms and retain this information over a month's time.

Drinking Behavior

The impact of the intervention on participants' behavior was less clear. While a trend was noted for reduction of quantity of alcohol consumed for both groups, there was no evidence to suggest that correction of normative misperceptions performed any better than traditional educational efforts in reducing students' weekly use of alcohol. With regard to curtailing misuse of alcohol, both approaches were effective. The experimental intervention, however, resulted in marginal gains over the control condition. Both programs resulted in a reduction in the number of negative consequences reported by the subjects as a result of alcohol use. Correction of normative misperceptions, however, did not surpass the traditional educational approach in its reduction of these consequences.

It is possible that these results accurately represent the relative efficacy of both approaches in reducing alcohol use and misuse. A thoughtful interpretation however, needs to take into account several contextual and methodological issues. First, the problems encountered with subject assignment may have resulted in unequal group characteristics. Due to the length of the time commitment required by the study, subjects were allowed to sign up for the sessions which best fit their schedules. Random assignment of sessions to either condition was also difficult due to the limited availability of group rooms and rigidity of group leaders' schedules. As seen in Figures 3 and 7, initial differences in drinking behavior between the two groups may have obscured the significance of outcome trends.

The directive nature of the experimental group could have mediated its effectiveness. Berkowitz and Perkins noted that some subjects in their study reported that completing the Core was a valuable experience in itself because it made them think about their own drinking patterns and extent of consequences resulting from alcohol use [12]. If the Core promotes this kind of introspection and self-evaluation, then the less threatening control group environment may have been better at priming subjects for these benefits. The control groups certainly produced less arousal and potentially less resistance than the experimental groups. It is unlikely, however, that the subtle benefits from completing the Core substantially affected the results. Inspection of means in Table 1 reveals little if any benefit resulting from the control intervention.

Attitudinal Measures

Participants' attitudes toward alcohol use were not influenced much by the interventions and remained fairly stable across collection periods. Attitudes toward certain categories of drinkers did shift across time. Approval of light, moderate, and heavy drinkers increased throughout the course of the study. For those subjects in the experimental condition, the increase in approval of light drinkers was expected. In other words, if subjects see that light drinkers are more representative of the norm than are moderate and heavy drinkers, it would follow that the stigma associated with being "deviant" would lessen, and approval ratings would increase. The increase in approval ratings for moderate and heavy drinkers was unexpected as these categories were intended to be seen as more deviant as a result of the intervention. Interestingly, the increase in approval for all three categories was present across both groups indicating that the perceptual shift was not necessary for this phenomenon to occur. An alternative explanation would be that as participants became more familiar with the experimenter and came closer to receiving credit for the study, their general attitude toward the study became more positive, and had a similar effect on approval ratings.

The proximity of the first two collection periods (1 week) may have affected the apparent stability of attitudes toward alcohol use. The questions used for this index were of a 5-point Likert scale format and this may have facilitated subjects' memory of responses given at baseline. Although the composite score for this index seems to have room for variation, the increments between scores on the 5-point scales within the index may have been too large and thus less sensitive to more subtle attitudinal shifts that may have occurred. Using seven 7-point (or greater) Likert scales might increase the overall sensitivity of the index.

One potential confound affecting approval ratings of the different drinking categories may have been subject fatigue. These indices were located at the end of subjects' questionnaire packets and answers given by subjects, particularly in evening groups may have suffered from this phenomenon. Ratings for moderate and heavy drinkers may have been impacted most by subject fatigue as these categories were rated last. In scoring these indices, the investigator noted that a few subjects became more indifferent in their approval ratings (endorsing scores indicating no preference for either adjective on the Semantic Differential Scale) as they neared the end of their questionnaires. Whether this trend reflected their true attitudes or weariness is debatable. A simple solution to this problem would be to choose a scale with no center score so that subjects would be required to endorse one adjective to some extent. Varying the order of questions could result in more confusion among subjects, but may have some utility in reducing the impact of fatigue on certain questions. Ideally, participants would have less paperwork to complete but this is probably unrealistic considering the amount of information required to make meaningful statements about one's hypotheses.

Discriminant Analyses

As was expected, the variables representing changes in perception of campus norms had the highest loadings on the discriminant function for group (experimental or control). The contribution of the variable "attitudes toward alcohol use" to this function was slight but in the opposite direction. That is, a shift toward healthier attitudes about alcohol could add slightly to the probability of a subject's classification in the experimental group. As a whole, however, the function most accurately represented a conservative shift in perceptions of campus drinking norms.

The second discriminant function was computed to determine which variables best discriminate between subjects who decreased their drinking over the course of the study and those who did not. While "group" was hypothesized to be one of these discriminating variables, it correlated highly with "change in perception of drinks per week" and when run separately, did not combine with other variables to generate a significant discriminant function. The fact that the first loading on the function was "change in perception of drinks per week" seems to indicate that the shift toward more conservative perceptions of campus drinking norms may have played a part in the reduction of drinking for those subjects who did demonstrate this reduction.

The loadings of "change in approval of moderate drinkers" and "change in approval of heavy drinkers" may represent the decrease in approval of these categories associated with a reduction in drinking behavior. It is possible that the difference in magnitudes of the variables' loadings was due to the fact that approval ratings for heavy drinkers were already lower than those for other drinkers and thus less likely to decrease even further. Another possible explanation for the higher loading of "change in approval of moderate drinkers" is that subjects are more likely to identify with this category. If subjects identify more strongly with this category, then a reduction in approval of moderate drinkers would dictate a reduction in drinking in order to move toward a more acceptable category.

The positive correlation between "change in attitudes toward alcohol use" and the discriminant function is counterintuitive to what would be expected for this variable. A shift in the direction of having less healthy attitudes toward alcohol use increased probability of membership in the group of subjects who decreased their drinking. This finding, in conjunction with the relative stability of this variable across collection periods, might suggest that attitudes toward alcohol have little to do with actual drinking behavior.

This second discriminant analysis demonstrated that the targeted changes in perceptions as well as accompanying decreases in approval of more liberal drinkers were important factors in decreasing alcohol use. Unfortunately, only a subset of the sample decreased their drinking. Taken together with the marked decrease in perceptions of drinking norms among experimental subjects, and no significant difference in approval ratings between experimental and control groups, this analysis may contribute to the interpretation of the behavior results.

Inspection of the group means in Table 1 reveals that for the most part, approval ratings for moderate and heavy drinkers remained the same or increased slightly for both groups across collection times. Thus, while only a small proportion of subjects demonstrated decreases in approval of these categories this pattern seemed to be associated with a greater likelihood of a decrease in their alcohol consumption. Based on anecdotal observations from the treatment and follow-up sessions, the increase in approval ratings may have reflected a reactive defensiveness to the information presented in the intervention. If this is at all true, it may be that while most subjects reacted to the intervention defensively, those who did not were more likely to question their drinking and make a behavioral change.

This explanation would point to the motivational importance of normative misperceptions. Since subjects who did not reduce their drinking were able to maintain some combination of increased normative estimates and approval of heavier drinkers, it would seem that these cognitions would have some functional value in protecting the perceived validity of their behaviors.

Implications for Future Research

The results of this study raise questions about the efficacy of challenging the normative misperceptions of male college students. The observation that those who reduced their drinking were likely to report decreased estimates of campus drinking norms and decreased approval of moderate and heavy drinkers seems to suggest that the intervention was beneficial to a subset of the sample. An important question to address would then be: What types of students are more likely to benefit from this type of intervention? A study employing extensive baseline measures of subject characteristics including personality traits could use these as discriminating variables to assess which interact most effectively with the intervention to reduce alcohol use and misuse. The results of this type of study could help drug and alcohol educators chose the approach most effective for their target population.

Future studies in this area would also benefit from having subjects rate the believability of the information presented to them. It would seem that credibility of normative data is an important mediator of the impact of this type of intervention and should be assessed. Using trained peer leaders for the groups in this study may have also increased the credibility of the information presented. Regardless of the age and status of the group leaders, more extensive training and practical experience in running alcohol education groups would increase their confidence which might add to the perceived legitimacy of the intervention.

It is the investigator's opinion that the addition of a discussion covering the reasons some students might have for not drinking would help legitimize the conservative data presented. Coed groups might also increase the credibility of this information. As females have demonstrated lower quantity and frequency of alcohol use [25] and fewer consequences due to alcohol use [23], their presence may give a greater voice to the segment of the campus population with healthier approaches to alcohol use. Haines (personal communication) noted that students at Northern Illinois University rated media sources such as the campus newspaper and campus radio station to be the most believable sources of information regarding campus health and substance use statistics. Future studies might also benefit from using these in conjunction with the primary intervention.

If the tenuousness of behavioral change was in fact due to the intervention's activation of subjects' defenses, a more subtle approach may be indicated. Embedding this intervention into a larger program with a health-oriented focus, might help to disguise it somewhat or at least reduce its abrasiveness. This may in turn induce less arousal of subjects' defenses.

Finally, the intervention may simply not have been powerful enough to promote significantly greater behavior change than a traditional educational approach. Recommendations for increasing its impact are: extending the intervention to include discussions at each follow up period, giving homework assignments requiring participants to interview a light or non-drinker, and using normative education as a component in a broader, more comprehensive intervention.

In conclusion, the results of this study suggest that normative education has the potential for influencing drinking behavior. Changes in perceptions of campus drinking norms can play a role in reducing the drinking behavior in certain students. The role of future research should be to identify the characteristics which predispose those students to benefiting from normative education and address methods for making normative information a more credible and powerful component to alcohol education programming.

REFERENCES

1. W. H. Bruvold and T. G. Rundall, A Meta-Analysis and Theoretical Review of School Based Tobacco and Alcohol Intervention Programs, *Psychology and Health, 2,* pp. 53-78, 1988.
2. C. A. Flynn and W. E. Brown, The Effects of a Mandatory Alcohol Education on College Student Problem Drinkers, *Journal of Alcohol and Drug Education, 37:*1, pp. 15-24, 1991.
3. M. B. Gilbert, The Use of Cognitive and Affective Measures to Evaluate Early Intervention Alcohol/Drug Education Programs, *Journal of Alcohol and Drug Education, 38:*3, pp. 89-104, 1993.
4. S. Look and R. J. Rapaport, Evaluation of an Alcohol Education Discipline Program for College Students, *Journal of Alcohol and Drug Education, 36:*2, pp. 88-95, 1991.
5. H. Duran and J. Brooklyn, Inherent Problems in Substance Abuse Education on University Campuses: Student Perspectives, *Journal of College Student Psychotherapy, 2:*3-4, pp. 63-87, 1988.
6. G. M. Gonzales, The Effect of a Model Alcohol Education Module on College Students' Attitudes, Knowledge and Behavior Related to Alcohol Use, *Journal of Alcohol and Drug Education, 25:*3, pp. 1-12, 1980.
7. D. T. Hanson, Alcohol and Drug Education: An Assessment of Effectiveness, *Education, 102:*4, pp. 328-329, 1982.
8. H. W. Perkins and A. D. Berkowitz, Using Student Alcohol Surveys: Notes on Clinical and Educational Program Applications, *Journal of Alcohol and Drug Education, 31:*2, pp. 44-51, 1986.
9. W. G. Meacci, An Evaluation of the Effects of College Alcohol Education on the Prevention of Negative Consequences, *Journal of Alcohol and Drug Education, 35:*3, pp. 66-72, 1990.

10. J. S. Baer, A. Stacy, and M. Larimer, Biases in the Perception of Drinking Norms among College Students, *Journal of Studies on Alcohol, 52*:6, pp. 580-586, 1991.
11. L. F. Burrell, College Students' Recommendations to Combat Abusive Drinking Habits, *Journal of College Student Development, 31*, pp. 562-563, 1990.
12. H. W. Perkins and A. D. Berkowitz, Perceiving the Community Norms of Alcohol Use among Students: Some Research Implications for Campus Alcohol Education Programming, *The International Journal of the Addictions, 21*:9&10, pp. 961-976, 1986.
13. G. Marks, J. W. Graham, and W. B. Hansen, Social Projection and Social Conformity in Adolescent Alcohol Use: A Longitudinal Analysis, *Personality and Social Psychology Bulletin, 18*:1, pp. 96-101, 1992.
14. G. M. Barnes and J. W. Welte, Patterns and Predictors of Alcohol Use among 7-12th Grade Students in New York State, *Journal of Studies on Alcohol, 47*, pp. 53-62, 1986.
15. W. B. Hansen, J. W. Graham, J. L. Sobel, D. R. Shelton, B. R. Flay, and C. A. Johnson, The Consistency of Peer and Parent Influences on Tobacco, Alcohol and Marijuana Use among Young Adolescents, *Journal of Behavioral Medicine, 10*, pp. 559-597, 1987.
16. J. S. Baer and M. M. Carney, Biases in the Perceptions of Consequences of Alcohol Use among College Students, *Journal of Studies on Alcohol, 54*, pp. 54-60, 1993.
17. W. B. Hansen and J. W. Graham, Preventing Alcohol, Marijuana, and Cigarette Use among Adolescents: Peer Pressure Resistance Training versus Establishing Conservative Norms, *Preventive Medicine, 20*, pp. 414-430, 1991.
18. G. Agnostinelli, J. M. Brown, and W. R. Miller, Effects of Normative Feedback on Consumption among Heavy Drinking College Students, *Journal of Drug Education, 25*:1, pp. 31-40, 1995.
19. I. Ajzen and M. Fishbein, *Belief, Attitude, Intention and Behavior: An Introduction to Theory and Research,* Addison Wesley Publishing Co., Reading, Maryland, 1975.
20. D. Cahalan, *Problem Drinkers*, Jossey-Bass, San Francisco, California, 1970.
21. R. B. Huebner, Attitudes toward Alcohol as Predictors of Self-Estimated Alcohol Consumption in College Students, *International Journal of the Addictions, 11*, pp. 377-388, 1976.
22. K. M. Kilty, Attitudinal and Normative Variables as Predictors in Drinking Behavior, *Journal of Studies on Alcohol, 39*, pp. 1178-1194, 1978.
23. J. M. Havey and D. K. Dodd, Variables Associated with Alcohol Abuse among Self-Identified Collegiate COAs and their Peers, *Addictive Behaviors, 18*, pp. 567-575, 1993.
24. J. R. Stabenau, Addictive Independent Factors that Predict Risk for Alcoholism, *Journal of Studies on Alcohol, 51*, pp. 164-174, 1990.
25. R. C. Engs and D. J. Hanson, Gender Differences in Drinking Patterns and Problems among College Students: A Review of the Literature, *Journal of Alcohol and Drug Education, 35*:2, pp. 36-47, 1990.
26. E. E. Jones and H. Sigall, The Bogus Pipeline: A New Paradigm for Measuring Affect and Attitude, *Psychological Bulletin, 76*:5 pp. 349-364, 1971.

27. C. A. Presley, P. W. Meilman, and R. Lyerla, Development of the Core Alcohol and Drug Survey: Initial Findings and Future Directions, *Journal of American College Health, 42*:6, pp. 248-255, 1994.
28. C. E. Osgood, G. J. Suci, and P. H. Tannenbum, *The Measurement of Meaning,* University of Illinois Press, Urbana Illinois, 1957.

Direct reprint requests to:

George Steffian, Ph.D.
Staff Psychologist
Mental Health Services
Naval Medical Center
Bob Wilson Drive
San Diego, CA 92134-5000

J. DRUG EDUCATION, Vol. 29(2) 139-155, 1999

AN EXPLORATORY STUDY OF RECREATIONAL DRUG USE AND NUTRITION-RELATED BEHAVIORS AND ATTITUDES AMONG ADOLESCENTS*

JAMIE BENEDICT, PH.D., R.D.

WILLIAM EVANS, PH.D.

JUDY CONGER CALDER, ED.D.

University of Nevada, Reno

ABSTRACT

This study examined drug use and eating behaviors among adolescents. The data were collected by phone interviews from 401 northern Nevadan students in grades seven to twelve. Students were divided for comparison into three groups according to their involvement with drugs: Abstainers, conventional users, and high-risk users. Analyses indicated that high-risk users less frequently ate lunch, meals at home, and with their families, and ate more often at convenience stores, fast food restaurants, and with friends. In addition, female high-risk users had significantly more negative perceptions regarding their food choices than the other female groups, and were more concerned with dieting than their high-risk using male peers. Male and female high-risk users believed that their drug use affected their eating habits. Implications for prevention programming and future research are discussed.

INTRODUCTION

A growing body of clinical and empirical research suggests that recreational drug use and certain types of eating behaviors are inter-related. Much of this research, however, is based on studies that focus on the more severe and/or chronic aspect

---

*This study was supported by a grant from the Research Advisory Board of the University of Nevada, Reno.

of this relationship, such as heavy drug use or eating disorders. For example, malnutrition is known to be a common complication of alcoholism [1] and numerous studies have documented a significant percentage of adults with eating disorders also exhibit problems of alcohol/drug abuse [2-7]. Very few studies, however, have attempted to delineate the coprevalence of substance use and unhealthy eating habits among general samples, with fewer still focusing on adolescents. The present study addressed this gap in the literature by examining these behaviors and related attitudes among a general sample of adolescents.

The specific effects of many common drugs on food intake and nutrient absorption/metabolism have been well documented. Chronic and excessive alcohol use, for instance, has long been shown to have an indirect (e.g., displacement of other foods in the diet), and direct (e.g., diminished nutrient absorption, impaired glucose tolerance, increased thiamin requirement) effect on nutritional status [8-10]. Chronic nicotine use has been shown to affect nutritional status as well [11-13], and evidence has been found to suggest that some young women may use cigarette smoking as a method of weight control [14]. Cigarette smoking also has been linked to higher dietary fat intake [15, 16] and an increase in body weight after smoking cessation [17, 18]. Some widely used illicit drugs, such as cocaine and amphetamines, have been shown to suppress appetite and may result in weight loss [19, 20]. In particular, cocaine use has been associated with a lower consumption of balanced meals and low-fat foods, and an increased consumption of alcohol, coffee, and fatty foods [21].

Other investigators have attempted to understand the pattern of coprevalence between eating disorders and drug abuse. As previously stated, multiple studies have uncovered an increased tendency for individuals who are abusing food as a substance also to be abusing alcohol and drugs [7, 22, 23]. Jonas, Gold, Sweeny, and Potash found that of 259 callers to the National Cocaine Hotline who met the DSM-III diagnostic criteria for cocaine abuse, 32 percent also met the DSM-III criteria for either anorexia nervosa or bulimia nervosa [24]. Another investigation found almost half of the bulimia nervosa patients studied to be using alcohol several times a week or more [25]. High rates of amphetamine, marijuana, barbiturate, and cigarette use also have been found to be associated with individuals diagnosed with eating disorders [26, 27]. The majority of these studies have focused on females since they possess higher rates of eating disorders (although males have higher overall rates of substance use and abuse).

Filstead, Parrella, and Ebbit compared individuals who were in treatment for alcohol, drug, or polydrug abuse and who also have been diagnosed with an eating disorder [28]. Interestingly, the investigators found that 60 percent of the respondents indicated that their binge eating occurred prior to the development of alcohol-drug-related problems. Harris found that females who were not clinically diagnosed with an eating disorder, but who displayed restriction of calories and intermittent binge eating patterns, were found to exhibit a higher incidence of alcohol use, drug use, sexual promiscuity, kleptomania, and other impulsive behaviors [29].

Several studies have specifically focused on adolescents. Timmerman, Wells, and Chen found significant correlations between bulimia and alcohol abuse in a sample of secondary school students [30]. Higher rates of substance use also have been found among tenth-grade girls classified as either bingers or purgers [27]. Watts and Ellis found alcohol and (to a lesser extent) drug use to be associated with higher scores on an Eating Disorders Risk scale among seventh to twelfth grade females [31].

Although marijuana use has been linked to an increase in appetite and food intake among adults [32], a decrease in dietary quality has been found among alcohol and marijuana abusing adolescents boys [33]. Investigators discovered that the alcohol/marijuana abusers ate less fruit, vegetables, and milk, and more snack foods than marijuana abusers and nonusers. Other eating behaviors, such as frequent dieting, also have been associated with greater alcohol and tobacco use among female adolescents [34].

Unfortunately, because most studies have focused on the extremes of drug or eating behaviors, the relationship between these variables among the general adolescent population is still poorly understood. Thus, the association between drug use and nutrition-related behaviors and attitudes that may increase risk for poor health remain anecdotal and relatively unexplored. Given the continued high prevalence of drug use among adolescents, understanding this relationship is of critical importance to educators and prevention specialists who aim to insulate adolescents from the detrimental effects often associated with drug use.

METHODS

Sampling Procedures

Adolescents (n = 401) from a large urban school district were randomly selected for interview using a Computer-Assisted Telephone Interviewing (CATI) system and detailed protocol to ensure that participants met the criteria and informed consent was obtained.

First, because randomly selected households needed to contain an adolescent between the ages of thirteen and nineteen to be eligible for inclusion in the survey, verification of the ages of individuals residing in each household was required. Second, parental permission, in addition to permission from the adolescent, was required before an interview was conducted. Lastly, parents and respondents were informed that participation was voluntary and that the adolescent could refuse to answer any question or series of questions, as well as terminate the interview at any point.

The total number of eligible households remaining from the original group of 951 potential households totaled 616 (once disconnects, car phones, FAX lines, no answers, and households containing no eligible respondents were removed). Of these, parental refusals or immediate "hang-ups" totaled seventy-one; an additional twenty-seven adolescents whose parents had consented, refused to participate; and eighteen adolescents whose parents had consented, were not available for interview during the time period which the survey was conducted. The total number of completed interviews was 401. Data from two of the 401 interviews were discarded based on the reported user of "Capisol," a fictitious drug which was added to the interview as a validity check on self-reported drug use. The final total for completed interviews was therefore reduced to 399.

After approximately 300 interviews had been completed, a stratified sampling procedure was implemented to interview only substance using adolescents. This was done to ensure sufficient group sizes for comparison purposes and to parallel adolescent drug-use percentages found in previous large-scale studies [35].

Measures

Demographic Characteristics

Information on subjects' age, ethnicity, grade level and school attendance was gathered, as well as information on their family composition and parents' level of education and employment status.

Drug Use

Subjects were asked to report how often in the past six months they had used each of seventeen substances without a doctor's prescription. Subjects were divided into high-risk users (HRU), conventional users (CON), and abstainers (ABS) according to their reported drug use during the last six months. This classification is based on previous work by Skager and Frith, and Evans and Skager [35, 36]. The following criteria were adopted for participant assignment to the HRU group: 1) use of PCP, heroin, crack or cocaine; 2) weekly or more frequent use of marijuana; 3) polydrug use three or more times; 4) endorsing the most frequent use response (e.g., drinking beer more than 3 times a week or smoking more than 2 packs of cigarettes a week) of any of the following drugs: beer, wine, liquor, cigarettes, smokeless tobacco, amphetamines, or steroids; 5) an endorsement of the next to highest use category (e.g., drinking beer 1 to 3 times a week or smoking 1 to 2 packs of cigarettes a week) for three or more of the drugs listed in criteria four; 6) use of a combination of three or more of the following: LSD, other psychedelics (e.g., mushrooms, peyote or ecstasy), barbiturates, inhalants or other narcotics (e.g., codeine, morphine or percodan); and 7) some reported alcohol use in the past six months. The last criterion was added as a validity check for inclusion in the HRU group (as virtually all illicit drug-using students report some alcohol use [35]).

Assignment to the ABS group was based upon no reported alcohol or substance use. The largest group of adolescents were CON. This group was composed of adolescents who had some experience with substance use (usually alcohol), but did not engage in polydrug use, use of drugs widely regarded as dangerous (such as crack or PCP), or the high frequency of use which would place them in the HRU group. The resulting sample ($n = 399$) consisted of 21 percent ($n = 82$) ABS, 19 percent, ($n = 75$) HRU, and 60 percent ($n = 242$) CON.

Nutrition-Related Behaviors and Attitudes

A combination of open and close ended questions were included in the survey to characterize nutrition-related behaviors and attitudes. To measure the frequency of eating meals and snacks, subjects were asked four different questions (e.g., "In a typical week, how many times do you eat breakfast or something in the morning?"). Subjects' responses were collapsed into three categories; zero to two times/week, three to four times/week, and five or more times per week. Subjects also were asked questions regarding where and with whom they usually ate. Due to small cell sizes, responses were grouped into the following three categories: 1) "never" or "rarely," 2) "sometimes," and 3) "often" or "always."

In addition, participants were asked to rate themselves, using a five-point scale (with 1 = "strongly agree" and 5 = "strongly agree"), on four statements related to their food choices; if they thought their food choices were "bad," if they were concerned about eating nutritious foods, if they thought they would be healthier if they made different food choices, and if they ate certain available foods—even though they "shouldn't." Participants identified as CON or HRU were also asked to indicate their agreement with three statements on the perceived effects of drug use on food intake.

The Restrained Eating Scale was included in this survey [37] to assess the degree to which individuals exhibit behavioral and attitudinal concern about dieting and keeping their weight down. The summated-rating scale has two subscales; "Concern with Dieting" (6 items) and "Weight Fluctuation" (4 items). Results of psychometric studies of the scale suggest the scale is sound when used with a normal-weight sample [38, 39]. According to Ruderman, the greater the proportion of overweight in the sample, the lower the internal consistency and the more factors emerge in the factor analysis [40]. A recent evaluation of three measures of dietary restraint, including the Restrained Eating Scale, provided evidence of internal consistency (coefficient alpha was between .72 and .82), temporal stability (test-retest correlations = .95) and construct validity (confirmation of the two factor solution) [41]. There were, however, other findings that raised questions about the degree to which responses were related to social desirability and intentions to dissimulate [41].

A series of questions related to binge eating were also included in the survey. Participants reporting any occurrences of binge eating were asked about their behavior immediately afterward, specifically if they had purged (with diuretics, laxatives, or induced emesis), exercised excessively, or fasted.

Participants' adiposity was estimated using self-reported height and weight (used to compute body mass index = weight (kg) /height (m)^2). Lastly, each was asked to rate satisfaction with the appearance of their bodies on a scale from one (= "very dissatisfied") to five (= "very satisfied").

RESULTS

Demographic and Drug Use Group Characteristics

There were more boys (55%) than girls (45%) in the overall sample. The approximate ethnic distribution was 73 percent Caucasian/white, 12 percent Hispanic/Latino/Mexican, 4 percent Asian/Pacific Islander, 4 percent African American, and 5 percent mixed or other. The mean age of adolescents in the sample was 15.28 years (SD = 1.66). About half of the adolescents reported living with both biological parents (49%), one-third (33%) reported living in single parent families (the majority of these headed by biological mothers) and 13 percent reported living in step families. Almost 90 percent of the sample reported they were currently attending school.

No differences were noted among gender and the drug use groups, as indicated in Table 1. Ethnic differences were discovered after collapsing all minorities into one category (necessary due to the small numbers of minorities in the sample). Compared to expected values, the proportion of non-whites in the ABS group was large. Forty percent of ABS were non-whites, yet they represented only 27 percent of the total sample. Significant differences in drug use among grade levels also was noted ($p < .05$). The proportion of HRU increased from 7 percent in grades seven to eight to 39 percent among students in grades nine to ten; and 55 percent among students in grades eleven to twelve.

With regard to family structure, HRU were less likely than ABS or CON to reside with both biological parents and more likely to reside with a step family, single parent (only more likely than abstainers), or in an other family constellation ($p < .05$).

The relationship between parents' employment status and drug use was significant ($p < .05$). Among those identified as CON, more than twice as many reported their mother's worked thirty-five or more hours outside of the home each week compared to those whose mothers' were unemployed or worked part-time. With regard to fathers' employment status, the largest differences found (between expected and observed frequencies) were between the ABS and HRU. As shown in Table 1, 77 percent of participants' fathers in the ABS group were employed full-time compared to 53 percent of those in the HRU group.

No differences were noted on parents' level of education which was based on the highest level of formal education achieved by the subjects' mother or father (including step-parents if they resided in the household).

Table 1. Demographic Characteristics of Teens Surveyed by
Drug Use Groups[a]

	ABS (n = 82) %	CON (n = 242) %	HRU (n = 75) %	Total Sample N/%
Gender				
Females	45.1	45.9	40.0	178/44.6
Males	54.9	54.1	60.0	221/55.4
Ethnicity				
White	59.8	77.4	72.0	288/72.7
Non-white	40.2	22.6	28.0	108/27.3
Grade level[b]				
Grades 7-8	45.1	26.4	6.7	106/26.6
Grades 9-10	34.1	36.4	38.7	145/36.3
Grades 11-12	20.7	37.2	54.7	148/37.1
Family structure[b]				
Biological parents	68.3	47.5	34.7	197/49.4
Step-family	6.1	13.6	17.3	51/12.8
Single parent	23.2	35.1	34.7	145/32.6
Other	2.4	3.7	13.3	148/05.3
Parents' employment status				
Mother employed full-time[b]	54.9	68.6	58.7	255/63.9
Father employed full-time[b]	76.8	64.9	52.8	259/64.9
Parents' level of education				
Some high school	38.5	16.0	24.0	26/ 7.8
Some college	50.0	62.0	61.6	163/48.7
College degree or more	11.5	22.1	14.4	146/43.6

[a]Drug Use Groups: ABS = Abstainers, CON = Conventional Drug Use, HRU = High Risk Drug Use
[b]Statistically significant difference ($p < .05$) between drug use groups (ABS, CON, HRU) using a Chi-square test of independence.

Drug Use and Eating Habits

Comparisons of meal frequency and eating patterns by drug use group are presented in Table 2. Although no differences were found among the drug use groups for frequency of eating breakfast and snacking between meals, a significant difference was found for lunch. Members of the HRU group ate lunch less frequently than the other drug use groups (65% reported eating lunch 5 or

Table 2. Drug Use and Eating Habits: Results of Chi-Square Tests of Independence by Drug Use Groups[a] ($N = 394$)

	Chi-Square	df	p
Meal Frequency			
Eats breakfast	7.8	4	.09
Eats lunch	10.4	4	.03[c]
Eats dinner[b]			
Snacks between meals	4.9	4	.29
Eating Patterns (Location and Company)			
Eats alone	9.1	4	.06
Eats with family	12.3	4	.01[c]
Eats with friends	19.2	4	<.01[c]
Eats at home	2.3	4	.68
Eats at school	26.7	4	<.01[c]
Eats at friends' home	6.6	4	.15
Eats at convenience store	16.2	4	<.01[c]
Eats at fast food restaurants	14.9	4	.01[c]

[a]Drug Use Groups: ABS = Abstainers, CON = Conventional Drug Use, HRU = High Risk Drug Use.
[b]Inconclusive due to small cell sizes.
[c]Statistically significant difference ($p < .05$) between drug use groups (ABS, CON, HRU).

more times each week compared to 77% of CON and 82% of ABS). Due to the high proportion of cells with an expected frequency of less than five, the statistical analysis for dinner was inconclusive.

Several eating pattern characteristics, including location and company, were significantly different among drug use groups. Members of the HRU group ate with family members less frequently (21% reportedly never or rarely ate with family members compared to 12% of CON and 7% of ABS) and ate with friends more often (57% often or always eat with friends compared to 38 of CON and 25% of ABS). Members of the HRU group were also less likely to eat at school (15% often or always ate at school compared to 33% of CON and 51% of ABS); and more likely to eat at convenience stores (15% often or always ate at convenience stores compared to 4% of CON and 6% ABS) and fast food restaurants (45% often or always ate at fast food restaurants compared to 27% of CON and 22% of ABS).

Attitudes Regarding Food Choices

Because food intake is often gender-related, the relationships among drug use and selected variables were analyzed separately *within gender* when the sample cell sizes permitted or when the variable was continuous. The latter included attitudes regarding food choices which were analyzed using a Kruskal-Wallis One-Way ANOVA. As shown in Table 3, no differences were noted among males. Among females, however, drug use was associated with more negative perceptions about their food choices ($p < .05$). Female HRU members were much more likely to agree that ". . . almost everything I eat is bad for me," and "I eat certain foods even though I know I shouldn't."

Perceived Effects of Drug Use on Food Intake

In general, the perceived effects of drug use on food intake was greater among males (Table 4). Forty-three percent of males in the HRU group agreed/strongly agreed that they ate more, 33 percent stated that they ate less and 37 percent stated that they ate "different," when they were drunk or high (compared to 14, 19 and 16% of the CON group respectively). The only significant effect among females found was the perception that they ate more when they were drunk or

Table 3. A Comparison of Attitudes Regarding Food Choices among Drug Use Groups[a] for Male and Female Respondents

| | Mean Rank[b] | | | | | |
| | Males | | | Females | | |
	ABS (n = 45)	CON (n = 128)	HRU (n = 45)	ABS (n = 37)	CON (n = 109)	HRU (n = 30)
"It seems that almost everything I eat is bad for me."	119.2	103.1	115.4	85.2	82.7	113.6[c]
"I am very concerned about eating foods that are nutritious."	116.2	108.6	105.5	97.6	89.0	75.6
"If I changed the way I ate, I would be a much healthier person."	113.4	106.3	114.7	83.0	86.3	103.3
"I eat certain foods that are available even though I know I shouldn't."	115.6	107.9	105.5	85.7	82.5	110.9[c]

[a]Drug Use Groups: ABS = Abstainers, CON = Conventional Drug Use, HRU = High Risk Drug Use.
[b]Rank based on 5-point rating scale with 1 = strongly disagree and 5 = strongly agree.
[c]Statistically significant difference ($p < .05$) between drug use groups (ABS, CON, HRU) using a Kruskal-Wallis One-Way Analysis of Variance.

Table 4. Perceived Effects of Drug Use on Food Intake among
Male and Female Respondents[a]

	Males		Females	
	CON (n = 123)	HRU (n = 44)	CON (n = 108)	HRU (n = 30)
Percent of Respondents that Agreed/Strongly Agreed with Statement				
"I eat more when I am drunk or high."	13.8	43.2[b]	17.6	43.3[b]
"I eat less when I am drunk or high."	18.6	33.3[b]	35.0	36.7
"I eat different when I am drunk or high."	16.0	37.2[b]	17.5	31.0

[a]Drug Use Groups: CON = Conventional Drug Use, HRU = High Risk Drug Use
[b]Statistically significant difference $(p < .05)$ between drug use groups (CON and HRU) based on Chi-square test of independence.

high (43% of females in the HRU agreed/strongly agreed compared to 18% of CON members).

Restrained Eating, Binge Eating, and Drug Use

Initially, the internal consistency reliability of each of the Restrained Eating subscales was assessed. Cronbach's coefficient alpha equaled .67 for the six-item "Concern with Dieting" subscale and .59 for the four-item "Weight Fluctuation" subscale. These values are lower than what other investigators have found and may be due to the relative young age of the respondents. Because this was an exploratory study, the subscales were used to compare drug use groups. The findings do suggest, however, the need for further investigation of the psychometric properties of the instrument and its usefulness in assessing this age group.

As shown in Table 5, a two-way ANOVA was used to compare restrained eating scores by drug use and gender. In addition to the significant gender effect (females scores were higher), a significant interaction between gender and drug use was noted (see Figure 1). As drug use increased by group, scores on the "Concern with Dieting" subscale decreased among males and increased slightly among females. No differences were noted on "Weight Fluctuation" subscale scores.

With regard to the relationship between drug use and binge-eating, 61 percent of ABS, 59 percent of CON, and 45 percent of HRU reportedly never or rarely

Table 5. Restrained Eating and Drug Use: Two-Way ANOVA Results (Gender × Drug Use Groups[a]) for the "Weight Fluctuation" and "Concern with Dieting" Subscales

Source of Variation	SS	DF	MS	F	P
Concern with Dieting					
Main Effects					
Drug Use	20.39	2	10.19	0.96	0.38
Gender	293.58	1	293.58	27.75	< 0.01
Two-Way Interaction	100.07	2	50.04	4.73	< 0.01
Explained	571.88	5	114.37	10.81	< 0.01
Residual	3999.28	378	10.58		
Total	4571.16	383	11.94		
Weight Fluctuation					
Main Effects					
Drug Use	2.96	3	1.48	0.12	0.89
Gender	0.02	1	0.02	0.00	0.97
Two-Way Interaction	16.94	2	8.48	0.67	0.51
Explained	24.15	5	4.83	0.38	0.86
Residual	4939.73	389	12.70		
Total	4939.89	394	12.60		

[a]Drug Use Groups: ABS = Abstainers, CON = Conventional Drug Use, HRU = High Risk Drug Use

engaged in binge-eating. Although this did not reach statistical significance (Chi-square = 5.29), $df = 2$, $p = .07$), it does suggest that there may be a positive relationship between drug use and binge-eating. No differences were found among drug use and specific behaviors that often follow binge-eating episode, including purging, excessive exercise, or fasting.

Body Composition, Body Image, and Drug Use

Differences in adiposity (based on BMI) among the drug use groups by gender was analyzed using a two-way ANOVA. As expected, BMI was higher among males (BMI = 22.06) compared to females (BMI = 20.46) ($F = 17.42$, $df = 1$, $p < .05$). The effect of drug use, however, was not significant ($F = 1.41$, $df = 2$, $p = .245$), nor was the interaction between gender and drug use ($F = .09$, $df = 2$, $p = .91$).

The relationship between subjects' satisfaction with their bodies and drug use was analyzed using a Kruskal-Wallis One-Way ANOVA. No differences among drug use groups were noted for males or females.

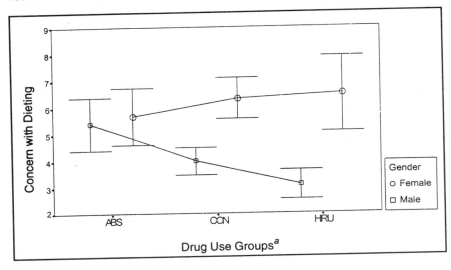

Figure 1. Interaction ($p < .05$) between gender and drug use on Restrained Eating Subscale, "Concern with Dieting."
[a]Drug Use Groups: ABS = Abstainers, CON = Conventional Drug Use, HRU = High Risk Drug Use

DISCUSSION

Several limitations of this study should be noted. First, the age differences by drug use group in this study could have influenced some of the findings. Since the HRU group was largely comprised of older teens, some of the differences found among nutrition-related behaviors and attitudes could be an artifact of age. For example, older teens may be more concerned about dating issues and thus report more dieting concern. Older teens, in general, are more independent (e.g., able to drive) which may influence where and with whom they eat. Second, our sample was not large enough to compare use of specific drugs by eating behaviors. Although it is well documented that specific drugs have differential effects on appetite and eating behaviors, in our sample it was difficult to find adolescents who used one substance at the exclusion of others (except for alcohol). Among the HRU group, multiple and even polydrug use was the norm. Third, this exploratory study examined associations only. Therefore, it was not possible to infer cause and effect relationships. These methodological limitations are issues for future research on this topic.

Given these limitations, the findings resulting from this exploratory study indicate that heavy drug use among adolescents may be associated with nutrition-related behaviors and attitudes that, over time, may compromise nutritional status and result in poor health. These findings are also consistent with previous studies demonstrating the tendency for health-compromising behaviors to co-occur [42].

Adolescents in the HRU group were less likely to eat lunch, meals at home or school, or eat with members of their family. Conversely, they were more likely to eat with friends and eat at fast food restaurants and convenience stores. Since eating has a strong social component, it should not be surprising that teens who exhibit peer-group oriented risk behaviors like heavy drug use also more often ate with peers, and patronized teen "hang-out" settings. The pattern of skipping lunch and frequenting fast food and convenience stores (as opposed to eating school meals or meals from home) may result in a diet that is high in fat and sugar, and low in nutrients. Dietary intake was not assessed here, however, previous studies of adolescent food habits that have examined these relationships have shown negative consequences of skipping meals and eating at fast food restaurants [43]. Similar to the variety of foods available at school (e.g., from the school cafeteria, food vending, snack bar, etc.), teens are presented with a wide variety of foods when they leave the school campus as well. Consequently, all teens, but most particularly those engaging in recreational drug use, will benefit from programs that teach them how to make nutritionally-sound choices in the places they prefer to eat.

Given the differences in eating habits among the drug use groups, it was interesting to find that HRU males were no more likely than male ABS or CON to have negative attitudes about their food choices. Among females, however, significantly more members of the HRU group agreed that they ate foods they knew they "shouldn't" and that their food choices, in general, were "bad." Unfortunately, due to the nature of these data, it is not known whether these beliefs are due to high-risk drug use or to the differential eating patterns noted above. Adolescent females may simply be more vigilant with regard to their food intake, hence, more likely to view their behavior as negative compared to adolescent males. The relative high prevalence of dieting and concern about body weight among adolescent females could also contribute toward these negative feelings [34].

With regard to the perceived effect of drug use on food intake, findings again varied among male and female drug use groups. Compared to CON members, significantly more female *and* male HRU agreed that drug use affected their eating habits. Although the pattern of this effect was difficult to interpret among males since each dimension was significant (eat more, eat less, and eat differently), female HRU believed that their drug use resulted in greater food intake.

The association between drug use and its perceived effect on food intake noted among females does coincide with the association that was discovered between drug use and restrained eating (as assessed by the "Concern for Dieting" subscale). According to Ruderman [40], restrained eaters worry constantly about what they eat, struggle to diet, and are more sensitive to external food cues because they are more deprived from chronic dieting [40]. Unrestrained eaters, on the other end of the continuum, eat freely as desired. According to Herman and Polivy's hypothesis, the self-control of restrained eaters may be temporarily interrupted by "disinhibitors" [44]. Alcohol has been studied as a possible disinhibitor. In experimental studies, restrained eaters who knowingly consumed alcohol, ate more compared to unrestrained eaters [45]. Thus, it is possible that because a higher proportion of HRU females in this sample were restrained eaters, drug use (including alcohol) acted as a disinhibitor for these individuals and resulted in greater food intake. This is also consistent with the trend noted between drug use and binge eating (HRU reported binge-eating more often compared to ABS and CON group members). Although the proportions did not reach statistical significance in this study ($p = .07$), the association between restrained eating and drug use may help to explain the higher incidence of binge-eating noted here and in previous research [27-29].

The results of this exploratory study also raise substantive questions for future research on the relationships among drug use and nutrition-related behaviors and attitudes—particularly among adolescent females since present results suggested that they had more negative attitudes about their eating habits and were more likely to be concerned about dieting. Assessment of dietary intake and the frequency/intensity of dieting behaviors measured over several months are clearly needed. In addition, qualitative data-gathering techniques would help verify and further elucidate the drug use and nutrition behavior findings of this study.

In summary, drug use among adolescents was associated with nutrition-related behaviors and attitudes that may further increase risk for poor nutritional status among adolescents. Previous researchers have raised concern about the nutritional well being of adolescents because of poor dietary choices and the high prevalence of dieting [34, 46, 47]. However, this study provides evidence that general trends may be amplified among heavy drug using adolescents. Longitudinal studies are needed to better understand the relationship between drug use and nutrition-related behaviors *over time* for various levels of drug use and populations. In the meantime, these findings emphasize the need for educators and prevention specialists to use a comprehensive, inter-disciplinary approach in planning health promotion programs for youth.

REFERENCES

1. L. Feinman and C. S. Leiber, Nutrition and Diet in Alcoholism, in *Modern Nutrition in Health and Disease,* M. E. Shils, J. A. Olson, and M. Shike (eds.), Lea & Febiger: Philadelphia, Pennsylvania, pp. 1081-1101, 1994.
2. J. Brisman and M. Siegal, Bulimia and Alcoholism: Two Sides of the Same Coin? *Journal of Substance Abuse Treatment, 1,* pp. 113-118, 1984.
3. D. K. Hatsukami, E. D. Eckert, and J. E. Mitchell, Affective Disorder and Substance Abuse in Women with Bulimia, *Psychological Medicine, 14,* pp. 701-704, 1984.

4. J. L. Katz, Eating Disorders: A Primer for the Substance Abuse Specialist, *Journal of Substance Abuse Treatment, 7*:3, pp. 143-149, 1990.
5. D. D. Krahn, The Relationship of Eating Disorders and Substance Abuse, *Journal of Substance Abuse, 3,* pp. 239-253, 1991.
6. G. R. Leon, K. Carroll, K. B. Cherny, and S. Finn, Binge Eating and Associated Patterns within College Student and Identified Bulimic Populations, *International Journal of Eating Disorders, 4,* pp. 43-57, 1988.
7. A. V. Taylor, R. C. Peveler, G. A. Hibbert, and C. G. Fairburn, Eating Disorders among Women Receiving Treatment for an Alcohol Problem, *International Journal of Eating Disorders, 14*:2, pp. 147-151, 1993.
8. V. Marks, Alcohol and Carbohydrate Metabolism, *Clinical in Endocrinology and Metabolism, 7,* pp. 333-349, 1978.
9. H. A. Hoyumpa, Alcohol and Thiamine Metabolism, *Alcoholism: Clinical and Experimental Research, 6,* pp. 495-505, 1983.
10. H. E. Williams, Alcoholic Hypoglycemia and Ketoacidosis, *Medical Clinical of North American, 68,* pp. 33-38, 1984.
11. R. C. Klesges and L. M. Klesges, Cigarette Smoking as a Dieting Strategy in a University Population, *International Journal of Eating Disorders, 7*:3, pp. 414-419, 1988.
12. O. Pelletier, Vitamin C and Tobacco, *International Journal of Vitamin and Nutrition Research, 16,* pp. 147-169, 1977.
13. United States Public Health Service, *The Health Consequences of Smoking-Nicotine Addiction: A Report of the Surgeon General,* 1988.
14. R. C. Klesges, A. W. Meyers, L. M. Klesges, and M. E. LaVasque, Smoking Body Weight, and Their Effects on Smoking Behavior: A Comprehensive Review of the Literature, *Psychological Bulletin, 106*:2, pp. 204-230, 1989.
15. B. M. Margetts and A. A. Jackson, Interactions Between Peoples' Diet and Their Smoking Habits: The Dietary and Nutritional Survey of British Adults, *British Medical Journal, 307,* pp. 1381-1384, 1993.
16. A. F. Subar, L. C. Harlan, and M. E. Mattson, Food and Nutrient Intake Differences between Smokers and Non-Smokers in the U.S., *American Journal of Public Health, 80*:11, pp. 1323-1329, 1990.
17. B. Caan, A. Coates, C. Schaeffer, L. Finkler, B. Sternfeld, and K. Corbett, Women Gain Weight 1 Year after Smoking Cessation While Dietary Intake Temporarily Increases, *Journal of the American Dietetic Association, 96*:11, pp. 1150-1155, 1996.
18. V. L. Ernster, Women and Smoking, *American Journal of Public Health, 83*:9, pp. 1202-1204, 1993.
19. D. A. Levitsky, Drugs, Appetite, and Body, in *Drugs and Nutrients: The Interactive Effects,* D. A. Roe and T. C. Campbell (eds.), Marcel Dekker, Inc., New York, pp. 375-408, 1984.
20. M. E. Mohs, R. R. Watson, and T. Leonard-Green, Nutritional Effects of Marijuana, Heroin, Cocaine, and Nicotine, *Journal of the American Dietetic Association, 90*:9, pp. 1261-1267, 1990.
21. F. G. Castro, M. D. Newcomb, and K. Cadish, Lifestyle Differences between Young Adult Cocaine Users and Their Nonuser Peers, *Journal of Drug Education, 17*:2, pp. 89-97, 1987.

22. C. M. Bulik, P. F. Sullivan, L. H. Epstein, M. McKee, W. H. Kaye, R. E. Dahl, and T. E. Weltzin, Drug Use in Women with Anorexia and Bulimia Nervosa, *International Journal of Eating Disorders, 11*:3, pp. 213-225, 1992.
23. M. M. Newman and M. S. Gold, Preliminary Findings of Patterns of Substance Abuse in Eating Disorder Patients, *American Journal of Drug and Alcohol Abuse, 18*:2, pp. 207-211, 1992.
24. J. M. Jonas, M. S. Gold, D. Sweeny, and A. L. C. Potash, Eating Disorders and Cocaine Abuse: A Survey of 259 Cocaine Abusers, *Journal of Clinical Psychiatry, 48*:2, pp. 47-50, 1987.
25. E. Mitchell, R. Pyle, D. Eckert, and D. Hatsukami, The Influence of Prior Alcohol and Drug Abuse Problems on Bulimia Nervosa Treatment Outcome, *Addictive Behaviors, 15,* pp. 169-173, 1990.
26. D. K. Hatsukami, J. E. Mitchell, E. D. Eckert, and R. L. Pyle, Characteristics of Patients with Bulimia Only, Bulimia with Affective Disorder, and Bulimia with Substance Abuse Problems, *Addictive Behaviors, 11,* pp. 399-406, 1986.
27. J. D. Killen, C. Barr-Taylor, M. J. Telch, T. N. Robinson, D. J. Maron, and K. E. Saylor, Depressive Symptoms and Substance Use among Adolescent Binge Eaters and Purgers: A Defined Population Study, *American Journal of Public Health, 77*:12, pp. 1539-1541, 1987.
28. W. J. Filstead, D. P. Parrella, and J. Ebbit, High Risk Situations for Engaging in Substance Abuse and Binge-Eating Behaviors, *Journal of the Study of Alcohol, 49*:2, pp. 136-141, 1988.
29. R. T. Harris, Anorexia Nervosa and Bulimia in Female Adolescents, *Nutrition Today, 26*:2, pp. 30-34, 1991.
30. G. Timmerman, A. Wells, and S. Chen, Bulimia Nervosa and Associated Alcohol Abuse among Secondary School Students, *Journal of the American Academy of Child and Adolescent Psychiatry, 29*:1, pp. 118-122, 1990.
31. W. D. Watts and A. M. Ellis, Drug Abuse and Eating Disorders: Prevention Implications, *Journal of Drug Education, 22*:3, pp. 223-240, 1992.
32. R. W. Foltin, J. V. Brady, and M. W. Fischman, Behavioral Analysis of Marijuana Effects on Food Intake in Humans, *Pharmacology, Biochemistry, Behavior, 25,* pp. 577-583, 1986.
33. J. L. Farrow, J. M. Rees, and B. S. Worthington-Roberts, Health, Developmental, and Nutritional Status of Adolescent Alcohol and Marijuana Abusers, *Pediatrics, 79,* pp. 218-230, 1987.
34. S. A. French, M. Story, B. Downes, M. D. Resnick, and R. W. Blum, Frequent Dieting among Adolescents: Psychosocial and Health Behavior Correlates, *American Journal of Public Health, 85*:5, pp. 695-701, 1995.
35. W. P. Evans and R. Skager, Academically Successful Drug Users: An Oxymoron? *Journal of Drug Education, 22*:4, pp. 353-365, 1992.
36. R. Skager and S. L. Frith, *Identifying at Risk Substance Users in Grades 9 and 11: A Report on the 1987/88 California Substance Use Survey,* Report to Attorney General John K. Van De Kamp, Office of Attorney General, Crime Prevention Center, Sacramento, California, 1989.
37. C. P. Herman and J. Polivy, Anxiety, Restraint, and Eating Behavior, *Journal of Abnormal Psychology, 91*:6, pp. 374-380, 1975.

38. W. G. Johnson, L. Lake, and J. M. Mahan, Restrained Eating: Measuring an Elusive Construct, *Addictive Behaviors, 11,* pp. 351-354, 1983.
39. A. J. Ruderman, The Restraint Scale: A Psychometric Investigation, *Behavior Research and Therapy, 21,* pp. 258-283, 1983.
40. A. J. Ruderman, Dietary Restraint: A Theoretical and Empirical Review, *Psychological Bulletin, 99*:2, pp. 247-262, 1986.
41. D. B. Alison, L. B. Kalinsky, and B. S. Gorman, A Comparison of the Psychometric Properties of Three Measures of Dietary Restraint, *Psychological Assessment, 4*:3, pp. 391-398, 1982.
42. D. Neumark-Sztainer, M. Story, S. French, N. Cassuto, D. Jacobs, and M. Resnick, Patterns of Health-Compromising Behaviors among Minnesota Adolescents: Sociodemographic Variations, *Journal of the American Public Health Association, 86*:11, pp. 1599-1606, 1996.
43. D. C. Cusatis and B. M. Shannon, Influences on Adolescent Eating Behavior, *Journal of Adolescent Health, 18,* pp. 27-34, 1996.
44. C. P. Herman and J. Polivy, Restrained Eating, in *Obesity,* A. B. Sunkard (ed.), W. B. Saunders Company, Philadelphia, Pennsylvania, pp. 208-225, 1980.
45. J. Polivy and C. P. Herman, The Effects of Alcohol on Eating Behavior: Disinhibition or Sedation? *Addictive Behaviors, 1,* pp. 121-125, 1976.
46. L. E. Cleveland, J. D. Goldman, and L. G. Borrus, *Data Tables: Results from U.S.D.A.'s 1994 Continuing Survey of Food Intakes by Individuals and 1994 Diet and Health Knowledge Survey,* Agricultural Research Service, U.S. Department of Agriculture, Riverdale, Maryland, 1996.
47. A. E. Field, A. M. Wolf, D. Herzog, L. Cheung, and G. Colditz, The Relationship of Caloric Intake to Frequency of Dieting among Preadolescent and Adolescent Girls, *Journal of the American Academy of Child and Adolescent Psychiatry, 32*:6, pp. 1246-1252, 1993.

Direct reprint requests to:

Jamie Benedict
Department of Nutrition 142
University of Nevada, Reno
Reno, NV 89557

J. DRUG EDUCATION, Vol. 29(2) 157-164, 1999

CHARACTERISTICS OF COCAINE USERS IN A PRIVATE INPATIENT TREATMENT SETTING

LON R. HAYS, M.D.

DAVID FARABEE, PH.D.

PUKUR PATEL, M.D.

University of Kentucky College of Medicine

ABSTRACT

Patient records were reviewed from an eighteen-month period of a private hospital adult addictive disease unit. Of 667 consecutive admissions, sixty-five (49 males, 16 females) were diagnosed with cocaine abuse or dependence; 38 percent were from rural areas. Although mean age of males and females was similar, males had a longer duration of use (8.2 years versus 5.8 years), however, females used an average of 14 grams per week versus 9.5 grams per week for males. African-American patients were over-represented among the cocaine using sample and also among the sample who chose smoking as their route of administration. A larger percentage of males had legal problems and admitted to "dealing," when compared to females. Those from rural areas were more likely to be married and less apt to have legal problems.

INTRODUCTION

There is a significant body of data regarding cocaine abuse and dependence. Much of our knowledge of the epidemiology of psychoactive substance abuse and dependence derives from the Epidemiologic Catchment Area Survey, the National Household Survey on Drug Abuse, and studies of clients in publicly funded treatment. The purpose of this study is to examine demographics and characteristics of cocaine abusers entering a private psychiatric hospital addictive

157

disease unit. Though located in an urban area, this particular treatment program serves a large number of patients from rural Kentucky.

The incidence of cocaine use began to increase in the late 1960s and reach a peak in the early to mid-1980s. There was then a decline in the incidence of cocaine use between 1985 and 1991 [1]. In the 1970s, cocaine users were largely employed, educated, Caucasians of the middle class. In the 1980s, there was an increase in cocaine use by minorities, youth, and lower socioeconomic groups [2]. According to the National Household Survey on Drug Abuse, the number of cocaine users dropped by 72 percent from 1985 to 1990, but there was no decline in the number of crack cocaine users [3]. According to NIDA's Drug Abuse Warning Network data, there was a five-fold increase in the number of emergency room visits by people using cocaine from 1984 to 1988 [4]. African-Americans, males, and those aged from thirty to thirty-nine were over-represented in this group. Deaths due to cocaine increased during the mid-1970s, then remained relatively stable until a marked increase in the 1980s, which correlated with the more widespread use of the crack-form of cocaine [5]. The average age of new cocaine users is about twenty-three [1].

According to the Drug Abuse Awareness Network, cocaine related emergency room visits reached their highest level in 1994 since DAWN began tracking these statistics in the early 1970s. The 142,406 cocaine related episodes reported in 1994 was a 15 percent increase over 1993 and a 40 percent increase in 1988 [6].

Increasing numbers of people seeking substance abuse treatment are users of multiple substances and the predominant drugs of choice are alcohol and cocaine. An increasing number of those are unemployed urban residents [4]. Many abusers of both alcohol and cocaine are cocaine smokers. Most crack users are younger than other groups of cocaine users; they are typically males, eighteen to twenty-nine years old, many of whom switched from intranasal use [7]. Generally accepted is the notion that cocaine smoking and injecting are more likely to lead to dependence than is snorting [8]. Both smoking and injecting cocaine are associated with higher levels of violence than is intranasal use [9].

Most studies indicate a significant degree of psychopathology among substance abusers seeking treatment. Weiss reported 50 percent of an inpatient sample of cocaine abusers had an affective disorder and subsequently found 27 percent of a larger sample to have an affective disorder, noting that affective illness may have become a less important risk factor for the development of cocaine abuse as the abuse becomes more prevalent [quoted in 4]. Other studies have demonstrated a significant number of cocaine abusers in treatment to have antisocial or borderline personality disorder [4]. One study showed elevated psychopathic deviant scales for cocaine abusers in a residential treatment program and in a hospital sample [10].

This descriptive study was undertaken to evaluate the following hypotheses developed as a result of clinical observation in this particular inpatient chemical dependency treatment program of a private psychiatric hospital.

1. African-Americans are over represented among the population of cocaine users.
2. Rural cocaine users are more likely to be Caucasian.
3. Rural cocaine users are less apt to use intravenously.
4. African-American cocaine users are more likely to smoke cocaine as their primary route of administration.
5. Males are over represented among the cocaine-using population.

METHODS

Patient records were reviewed retrospectively from an eighteen-month period of a private hospital adult addictive disease unit. This hospital is located in an urban area of 240,000, but also serves a large surrounding rural area where the predominant industry is agricultural. Sixty-five of 667 patients admitted during that time period were identified as having cocaine abuse or dependence (as per discharge diagnosis). Information was obtained regarding age, sex, race, level of education, rural versus urban environments, marital status, and employment status. Other data included amount and route of use, amount spent per week, use of other drugs, a history of previous treatment, and concurrent co-morbid diagnoses. Diagnoses in this facility are based on DSM-IV criteria. (A structured instrument is not routinely used.) Depression which cleared within the first week of treatment was generally given a diagnosis of substance-induced mood disorder.

RESULTS

The relatively small sample limits our statistical power and, to a large extent, precludes the use of significance tests. In such cases, drawing inferences based on conventional .01 or .05 alpha levels sharply increases the likelihood of making a Type II error, that is, failing to reject the null hypothesis when the alternative hypothesis is actually correct. To increase our ability to identify the hypothesized trends in these data, the alpha criteria were raised to .15, although some comparisons met more stringent alpha cutoff levels. The discussion below focuses on trends found in this clinical sample; differences meeting marginal statistical significance (i.e., $p < .15$) are indicated in Tables 1 and 2.

Sixty-five patients (49 males, 16 females) were identified as having cocaine abuse or dependence as an Axis I diagnosis. Forty were from urban areas and twenty-five from rural locales. Mean age of males and females was similar (males, 33.0 years; females 31.5 years).

A much larger percentage of males were from urban areas—67 percent versus 44 percent of females. African-Americans were over-represented among the cocaine users (55% of males and 62% of females); African-Americans comprise only 13 percent of the total patient population at this treatment facility. The vast majority of cocaine users were employed—76 percent of males and 75 percent of

Table 1.

	Males (N = 49)	Females (N = 16)
Mean age	33.0 years	31.5 years
Caucasian	22 (45%)	6 (38%)
African-American	27 (55%)	10 (62%)
Urban	33 (67%)	7 (44%)
Rural	16 (33%)	9 (56%)
Employed	37 (76%)	12 (5%)
Married	23 (47%)	6 (38%)
Mean education level	12.8 years	13.5 years
Mean duration of use	8.2 years	5.8 years
Legal problems	20 (41%)	5 (3%)
"Dealers"[a]	13 (27%)	2 (13%)
Previous treatment	23 (47%)	7 (4%)
Mood disorders	7 (14%)	4 (25%)
"Pure" cocaine users	16 (33%)	8 (50%)
Average amount used per week[a]	9.5 gm	14 gm

[a]Based on self-report

Table 2.

	Urban (N = 40)	Rural (N = 25)
Males	33	16
Mean age	33.2	32.6
Females	7	9
Mean age	32.3	30.9
Married	15 (39.5%)	13 (52%)
Legal problems	18 (45%)	6 (24%)**
African-American	27 (67.5%)	10 (40%)
Caucasian	13 (32.5%)	15 (60%)
Prior treatment	18 (45%)	12 (48%)

**$p < .01$

females; however, 10 percent of the males were disabled. Forty-seven percent of males were married, compared with 38 percent of females. Rural users were more likely than urban users to be married: 52 percent versus 40 percent. Females had a slightly higher educational level than males: 13.5 years versus 12.8 years. Males had a longer duration of use than females: 8.2 years versus 5.8 years (see Table 1).

Smoking was the predominant route of administration among the cocaine users. Forty-six of sixty-five (71%) smoked cocaine, while twenty-five (38%) used intranasally, and ten (15%) used intravenously. (Some used multiple routes of administration.) The only significant difference between urban ($N = 40$) and rural ($N = 25$) cocaine users was that 20 percent of rural users admitted to IV use versus 12 percent of urban users. Four of the sixteen (25%) females injected cocaine, while only six of the forty-nine (12%) males used IV cocaine. There were significant differences in the route of administration among African-Americans versus Caucasians: 75.7 percent of African-American users smoked cocaine versus 64.3 percent of Caucasians (chi square ($df = 1$) = 2.4, $p = .12$); 10.9 percent of African Americans used IV cocaine versus 21.4 percent of Caucasians; and only 30 percent of African-Americans used intranasally, compared to 50 percent of Caucasians (chi square ($df = 1$) = 2.8, $p = .10$.) Among those who smoked cocaine, the mean duration of use was 6.9 years, among IV users 9.6 years, and among intranasal users, 6.5 years. There were no significant differences in the mean ages based on route of administration.

Twenty of the sixty-five cocaine abusers had current legal problems. Eighteen of the twenty-four (75%) were from urban areas and twenty of the twenty-four (83.8%) were male. Urban cocaine abusers were more likely than their rural counterparts to report having current legal problems (chi square ($df = 1$) = 3.6, $p = .06$). Thirteen of the twenty-four were African-American (54.2%), compared with 57 percent of the total sample being African-American. Fifteen patients admitted to "dealing" cocaine; only two of these were female. Fifty-three percent of these were from urban areas and 47 percent were African-American.

Thirty of the sixty-five cocaine abusers (46.2%) had been in previous treatment (23 males, representing 46.9%, and seven females, representing 43.8%). Thirteen of the thirty had legal problems (43.3% compared to 36.9% of the overall sample). The mean duration of use of those having had prior inpatient treatment was 8.1 years. There was no difference between urban versus rural users in terms of a history of prior treatment (see Table 2). African-Americans were proportionately represented among those having had prior treatment (56.7% versus 56.9% overall). Almost half of the intravenous users and half of the smokers had been treated previously, whereas only 40 percent of the intranasal users had. The intravenous users spent an average of $1475 per week on cocaine, while the smokers spent an average of $1170 per week and the intranasal users spent $940 per week.

Fourteen (28.6%) of the forty-nine males were given a diagnosis of cocaine dependence (as opposed to cocaine abuse), six (37.5%) of the sixteen females received a diagnosis of cocaine dependence. However, forty-six (71%) of the sixty-five admitted to alcohol use and forty-one (63%) of the sixty-five admitted to cannabis use. Thirty-six (55.4%) received a concurrent diagnosis of cannabis abuse or dependence and seventeen (26.2%) received a concurrent diagnosis of cannabis abuse or dependence. Ten admitted to benzodiazepine abuse, while only three admitted to opioid abuse.

Diagnosis of concurrent mood disorders were made in seven males (14.3%) and four females (25%). Six of the seven males (85.7%) were from urban areas and four of the seven (57.1%) were African-American. Of the four females, two were from urban areas and two were African-American.

DISCUSSION

With regard to the five hypotheses presented: 1) African-Americans were over represented among the cocaine-using population; 2) Rural cocaine users were more likely to be Caucasian; 3) Rural cocaine users were *not* less apt to use intravenously; 4) African-American cocaine users were more likely to smoke cocaine as their primary route of administration; and 5) Males were over represented among the cocaine-using population.

Although this is meant to be a purely descriptive study, there are limitations to a retrospective chart review; obviously, only the data recorded in the chart can be used. Individual clinicians may diagnose differently based on clinical interview (both diagnoses of cocaine abuse/dependence and affective disorder). As clinicians are aware, most cocaine abusers also abuse other substances. This variable may somewhat limit the generalizability of the findings. The amount of use, dollars spent, and duration of use are all based on self-report. Although this population may not give the most reliable information, there is some evidence that substance abusers who have undergone treatment are more likely to provide valid self-report data than substance abusers who have not received treatment [12].

In spite of these limitations, the findings have implications for treatment. Little information is available regarding differences in cocaine abusers from rural areas versus urban areas. In this particular study, rural users were more likely to be married and Caucasian and were much less likely to have legal problems. There are relatively few options for rural cocaine users; a major obstacle to recovery is the rural user returning to an area without follow-up and with few, if any, AA/NA meetings. Although the number of intravenous users was small, a higher percentage of rural users and females injected cocaine and the intravenous users had a longer mean duration of use. The smokers and intravenous users were over-represented among those having had prior treatment. This is consistent with the belief that these routes of administration may contribute to more severe dependence. These users also spent more per week for their drug which concurs with the finding that financial failure is often a precipitant for seeking treatment. The risk of HIV is considered to be greater in urban areas; with significant number of rural substance abusers injecting cocaine, the risk of AIDS does have to be considered in treatment programs serving rural populations.

Concurrent mood disorders were diagnosed in 16.9 percent of this population of cocaine users. This is lower than in Weiss' study of mood disorders in cocaine addicts [quoted in 4] and much lower than reported in other studies. This seems to lend support to the notion that affective illness may have become a less important risk factor in the development of cocaine abuse. (The mood disorder diagnoses were made almost exclusively in those from urban areas.)

The number of cocaine users with legal problems in this study also has implication for treatment. There is often need for intensive social work involvement in these legal situations (i.e., postponing court dates, arranging legal assistance, communication with employers).

In summary, this study adds to the body of data regarding cocaine users and speaks specifically to differences among rural versus urban patients. Further study is needed to evaluate the implications for treatment and follow up.

REFERENCES

1. J. Gfruerer and M. Brodsky, The Incidence of Illicit Drug Use in the United States, 1962-1989, *British Journal of Addiction, 87,* pp. 1345-1351, 1992.
2. N. L. Day, C. M. Cottreau, and G. A. Richardson, The Epidemiology of Alcohol, Marijuana, and Cocaine Use Among Women of Childbearing Age and Pregnant Women, *Clinical Obstetrics and Gynecology, 36*:2, pp. 232-245, 1993.
3. National Survey Shows Continuing Decline in Use of Illicit Drugs: Cocaine Use Drops Dramatically, *Hospital and Community Psychiatry, 42*:10, p. 1078, 1991.
4. M. Closser and T. R. Kosten, Alcohol and Cocaine Abuse: A Comparison of Epidemiology and Clinical Characteristics, *Recent Development in Alcoholism, Volume 10,* M. Galanter (ed.), Plenum Press, New York, pp. 115-128, 1992.
5. L. A. Escobedo, A. J. Ruttenber, M. M. Agoes, R. F. Anda, and C. V. Wetli, Emerging Patterns of Cocaine Use and the Epidemic of Cocaine Overdose Deaths in Dade County, Florida, *Archives of Pathology Laboratory Medicine, 115,* pp. 900-905, 1991.
6. National Surveys Indicate Increase in Cocaine Use, *Substance Abuse Letter,* p. 1, November 17, 1995.
7. R. G. Smart, Crack Cocaine Use: A Review of Prevalence and Adverse Effects, *American Journal of Drug and Alcohol Abuse, 17*:1, pp. 13-26, 1991.
8. M. Gossop, P. Griffiths, B. Powis, and J. Strang, Severity of Dependence and Route of Administration of Heroin, Cocaine, and Amphetamines, *British Journal of Addiction, 87,* pp. 1527-1536, 1992.
9. A. J. Giannini, N. S. Miller, R. H. Loiselle, and C. E. Turner, Cocaine-Associated Violence and Relationship to Route of Administration, *Journal of Substance Abuse Treatment, 10,* pp. 67-69, 1993.
10. P. D. Moss and P. D. Werner, A MMPI Typology of Cocaine Abusers, *Journal of Personality Assessment, 58*:2, pp. 269-276, 1992.
11. M. Lipsey, *Design Sensitivity: Statistical Power for Experimental Research,* Sage, Newbury Park, California, 1990.

12. D. Farabee and E. Fredland, Self-Reported Drug Use Among Recently Admitted Jail Inmates: Estimating Prevalence and Treatment Needs, *International Journal of the Addictions, 31*:4, pp. 423-435, 1996.

Direct reprint requests to:

Lon R. Hays, M.D.
Associate Professor of Psychiatry
University of Kentucky Medical Center
Kentucky Clinic, Wing B
Lexington, KY 40536-0284

J. DRUG EDUCATION, Vol. 29(2) 165-174, 1999

EFFECTIVENESS OF STUDENT ASSISTANCE PROGRAMS IN NEBRASKA SCHOOLS

DAVID M. SCOTT, M.P.H., PH.D.
University of Nebraska Medical Center, Omaha

JEANNE L. SURFACE, M.A.
Wakefield Public Schools, Nebraska

DAVID FRIEDLI, B.A.
Nebraska Department of Education, Lincoln

THOMAS W. BARLOW, ED.D.
Pacific Regional Educational Laboratory, Honolulu, Hawaii

ABSTRACT

Background: This study investigated whether Nebraska schools with Student Assistance Programs (SAP) are associated with reduced adolescent alcohol use and a higher level of academic achievement than students from schools without a SAP. *Methods:* In 1992, the Toward a Drug Free Nebraska (TDFN) survey was administered to 3,454 students in grades seven to twelve at eighty-three Nebraska schools. A second survey, the TDFN "team activity report" collected from each school's team, the presence of a SAP ($n = 34$ schools) or absence of a SAP ($n = 49$ schools). Student responses for alcohol use and academic achievements were linked with the presence of a SAP through use of a school identification number on both surveys. *Results:* Students from schools with a SAP reported a lower use of alcohol in the last thirty days, compared with students from schools without a SAP program ($p < 0.05$), and they also reported a significant difference in academic achievement ($p < 0.05$). *Conclusions:* While this study used post hoc analysis of data, the results suggest lower alcohol use and higher academic achievement among students from SAP schools. Given SAPs' popularity, these trends suggest that further research should be conducted to demonstrate the effectiveness of student assistance programs.

INTRODUCTION

Student Assistance Programs (SAP) is a rapidly growing, school-based early intervention model for delivering services to adolescents with substance abuse and related problems [1, 2]. Anderson described the SAP as a comprehensive, joint school/community effort to identify, assess, refer, and support students who are affected by alcohol, tobacco, and other drug (ATOD) use problems [3]. Broad-based SAP programs were also developed to help students with problems of pregnancy, suicide, family violence, sexual abuse and drugs. ATOD use is generally a contributory factor if not a primary factor in risk behaviors by adolescents. Anderson described SAPs as programs designed to provide assistance to students who were having trouble academically and/or behaviorally, or who were at risk of ATOD use [3].

SAP DEVELOPMENT AND TRAINING

Prevention is the focus of the Toward a Drug Free Nebraska (TDFN) project that has trained school/community teams throughout Nebraska [4] since 1987. In 1990, the Nebraska TDFN Progress Report recommended that schools should establish Student Assistance Programs and directed the State Department of Education to "coordinate efforts to organize, unify and support comprehensive programs." Through TDFN, SAP training was offered to help meet the needs of students who were at risk of school-related problems and failures. SAP training was extended to any school that had completed TDFN team training and had established a comprehensive school-based prevention program. As shown in Figure 1, Student Assistance Programs are an integral component of the TDFN training model.

Student assistance is based on the philosophy that students who are identified and referred early on to a support mechanism will better be able to cope with and overcome their problems. Some identification procedures include things such as a sudden drop in grades or failing grades, change in appearance, absenteeism, or tardiness. Once the student is identified, he/she is channeled into a support group facilitated by volunteer trained persons. Student Assistance Program training is offered in two phases and are described next.

Phase 1: SAP Implementation/Core Team Training

SAP core team training provides the team with entry-level skills and protocols to begin the identification and referral process. Core team participants discuss specific school issues related to maintaining youth in school. Participants identify resources and generate an action plan that includes start-up, marketing and evaluation strategies. Policy development and incorporating SAP into school philosophy are key components. Workshop outcomes include:

Stage 1. School Community Team Training

Description: Comprehensive prevention program for all students

Components
Policy
Curriculum and Instruction
Team Maintenance
Assistance Programs
Youth Involvement
Parent Involvement
Community Involvement
Evaluation
Communication

Stage 2. Student Assistance Programs (SAP)

Description: Programs of early identification, referral, and support for students exhibiting risk behaviors

Phase
1. Implementation/Core Team Training
2. Group Facilitation Training

Stage 3. Special Populations Initiatives

Description: Programs and strategies for students who meet the federal definition of "high-risk" and high-abilities programs

Figure 1. Toward a Drug Free Nebraska training model.

- Understanding the essential features of SAP, including:
  – program components (what),
  – roles and responsibilities (who),
  – implementation and planning issues (how),
- Identifying resources;
- Raising own awareness of issues and problems relating to SAP;
- Planning for your SAP;
- Practicing skills of identification and referral of students; and
- Having examples of actual programs and practices.

Phase 2: SAP Group Facilitation Training

To qualify for this training phase, the school must have started a student assistance program. During this secondary phase, teachers and support staff develop the intervention, referral and reintegration skills necessary to lead school-based support groups. These support services are designed for children who are identified as needing assistance to be successful in school. Workshop outcomes include:

- Understanding the school-based group process and dynamics as a prevention strategy;
- Understanding the types of support groups;
- Obtaining the skills and methods for leading and facilitating support groups; and
- Understanding the importance of school-based groups.

SAPs are the unique way to reach our high-risk youth who need support to succeed in school when they are not receiving that support elsewhere. SAP provides a means of identifying children's problems early, so help can be given to them before their problems require more intensive efforts to correct them.

Several steps must be completed for a SAP to be effectively inaugurated. The first step is to gain school administration support. School administration must acknowledge that ATOD problems exist and that the school staff has the right and responsibility to intervene in problem behaviors. After administrative support is gained, the second step is the SAP Core Team training. This team provides for daily management and implementation of the SAP. To assure implementation support, the principal should be a member of the core team, although not necessarily in a leadership role. Other members should meet the following qualifications: 1) want to be involved in SAP; 2) demonstrated ability to work with students, and 3) have at least one year of school experience [5].

OVERVIEW OF SAP EVALUATION STUDIES

SAP process and outcome data are contained in local and regional evaluation studies. Most of these studies have not been published or distributed [6, 7]. Klitzner and his colleagues reviewed SAP programs and concluded, "despite the popularity of student assistance programs, the studies reviewed provide little empirical evidence of their effectiveness . . . ," and concluded that this question is "the single most pressing need in terms of evaluation research" [2]. A national survey of 900 SAPs was conducted in 1991 by the National Organization of Student Assistance Programs and Professionals (NOSAPP). Most respondents felt their SAP programs provided support to recovering students and reduced ATOD use. However, very few schools had process or outcome-based evaluation data to substantiate their beliefs [8]. While the SAP idea has been endorsed as a method to reach high-risk youth, very little has been done to evaluate the impact of SAP efforts.

Study Purpose

This study used TDFN databases [9] to assess whether Student Assistance Programs in Nebraska were effective in reducing student alcohol use and improving student academic achievement.

METHODS

Survey Administration

In 1992, the Nebraska TDFN survey was administered to 3,454 students in grades seven to twelve at TDFN Project schools. One hundred eighty-six schools, including ninety-six elementary and sixty-four secondary schools and twenty-six public schools (both elementary and secondary), participated in this evaluation. A student survey was distributed on March 1 and returned by May 15, 1992. The survey was administered to all students in the targeted core class at each school setting. Team leaders at TDFN schools acted as survey coordinators. Each coordinator was given a sheet of standardized instructions for administering the survey. Surveys were administered midweek to a core class when school attendance rates are usually highest.

At the time of this study, parental notification was not required or performed. Voluntary participation, confidentiality, and anonymity were emphasized. Students were informed by the survey coordinator at each site that they did not have to participate and that they could choose not to answer any particular question. Although the survey coordinators were not asked to measure actual response rates, this rate is believed to be similar to the mean daily school attendance rate, which is 95 percent for all Nebraska schools. Student responses were recorded on a standard computer response form. To ensure confidentiality and anonymity, only a school identification (ID) number was placed on the response form. Upon completion, all surveys were placed in an envelope, sealed and returned to the project investigators for scoring and tabulation.

Student Survey Design

For grades seven through twelve, the TDFN survey was a battery of 110 questions including demographic data, ATOD use, and related risky behaviors. The student survey was developed based on a review and adaptation of existing instruments, such as the University of Michigan's Monitoring the Future Survey and the Search Institute Survey. This survey uses measurement instruments from other investigators in the field that have already been shown to be reliable and valid measures. We included an honesty-control item in the survey. When a student reported that he or she had given a dishonest response, that student's entire survey was deleted.

Team Activity Report Design and Administration

The "Team Activity Report" was administered to each school's TDFN team. Each team leader was instructed to administer the survey during a team meeting. The survey was distributed and due on the same date as the student survey. This sixty-seven-item Team Activity Report [9] included the number of completed team projects, frequency of team meetings, and the presence of a student assistance program. A school I.D. number identifying that team was included on the computer response sheet. Consequently, linking the presence of a student assistance program, and reported alcohol use on the student surveys was possible. By linking these databases, the investigators could assess impact on student academic achievement, alcohol use, and the presence of a SAP.

Certain questions were tabulated with the question, "Does your school have a student assistance team?" While the initial responses to this question were in a Likert scale, for this report, Student Assistance Program activity levels were combined into a dichotomous yes/no response for analysis purposes. Of the eighty-three secondary schools answering this question, 41 percent ($n = 34$) of schools reported the presence of a SAP and 59 percent ($n = 49$) of schools reported the absence of a SAP.

Data Analysis

All data were entered into a SAS database at the University of Nebraska Medical Center's Computing Center, then analyzed using the SAS (Version 6) program with the FREQ procedure [10]. A tabular analysis involved both frequency counts and percentages. Chi-square analysis using an alpha level of 0.05 was used to test for significant differences between SAP participant schools and non-SAP participant schools. This study used a post hoc analysis of TDFN data.

RESULTS

Alcohol Use

When the 3,454 student responses were totaled from the secondary survey, 971 secondary students reported alcohol use in the last 30 days as reported in Table 1, and 30.7 percent of the students were from schools without a SAP. Of schools with a Student Assistance Program, 24.3 percent of the students reported alcohol use. This difference was statistically significant (chi-square = 16.49, $DF = 1$, $p = 0.0001$). Thus, most secondary students from schools with a SAP reported a lower use of alcohol, compared with those from schools without a SAP program.

Table 1. Alcohol Use by Secondary Students

| | Alcohol Users | | | | | |
| | Last Thirty Days[a] | | Last Year[b] | | Total Students | |
	n	(%)	n	(%)	n	(%)
Without SAP	635	(30.7)	1,025	(49.5)	2,070	(59.9)
With SAP	336	(24.3)	568	(41.0)	1,384	(40.1)
Total	971	(28.1)	1,593	(46.1)	3,454	(100.0)

[a]Significant difference between schools with SAP and without SAP for users and nonusers in the last thirty days (chi-square = 16.49, $DF = 1$, $p = 0.0001$).

[b]Non-significant difference between schools with SAP and without SAP for users and nonusers in last year (chi-square = 2.29, $DF = 1$, $p = 0.13$).

Alcohol Use Frequency

As reported in Table 2, 2,075 secondary students (60.1%) reported abstaining from alcohol use. Of those, 58.9 percent of the students were from schools without a SAP, while 61.8 percent were from schools with a SAP. Another 1,379 students (39.9%) reported consuming one or more drinks. In comparing the number of drinks for the two groups, the percentage of students in each group (except five or more drinks) was similar. While the alcohol use frequencies were lower for SAP schools in comparison to schools without a SAP, they were not statistically significant.

Average Reported Grades

Table 3 summarizes the average academic achievement (grades A-F) reported by secondary students. Of students with a SAP were statistically significantly different compared with those from non-SAP schools (chi-square = 12.12, $DF = 4$, $p = 0.0165$). For students reporting their average grade as "C" or above, 93.6 percent of students were in the SAP schools, compared with 92.9 percent in the non-SAP schools. For students with "D" or below, SAP schools had a 6.4 percent rate compared with 7.1 percent of students for non-SAP schools. Overall, SAP school students average grades were at a slightly higher level than non-SAP schools.

DISCUSSION

This study used post hoc analysis of data and was exploratory in nature. While lower alcohol use rates were associated with schools with SAP programs, causality cannot be concluded based on this type of study. The data for this study were analyzed retrospectively and confounding variables should be considered.

Table 2. Alcohol Drink Frequency by Secondary Students

	Number of Alcoholic Drinks					
	None n (%)	1 n (%)	2-4 n (%)	5-10 n (%)	11+ n (%)	Total Students n (%)
Without SAP	1,220 (58.9)	258 (12.5)	203 (9.8)	161 (7.8)	228 (11.0)	2,070 (59.9)
With SAP	855 (61.8)	179 (12.9)	127 (9.2)	89 (6.4)	134 (9.7)	1,384 (40.1)
Total	2,075 (60.1)	437 (12.7)	330 (9.6)	250 (7.2)	362 (10.5)	3,454 (100.0)

Table 3. Average Grades by Secondary Students[a]

	Number of Students					
	A n (%)	B n (%)	C n (%)	D n (%)	F n (%)	Total n (%)
Without SAP	637 (30.8)	785 (37.9)	501 (24.2)	111 (5.4)	36 (1.8)	2,070 (59.9)
With SAP	366 (26.5)	593 (42.9)	337 (24.4)	61 (4.4)	27 (2.0)	1,384 (40.1)
Total	1,003 (29.0)	1,378 (39.9)	838 (24.3)	172 (5.0)	63 (1.8)	3,454 (100.0)

[a]Significant difference between schools with SAP and without SAP for average grade (chi-square = 12.12, $DF = 4$, $p = 0.0165$).

For instance, are the findings due to more intensive prevention efforts in SAP schools than non-SAP schools? Schools that support a SAP usually have a higher level of ATOD prevention activities than in non-SAP schools. In Nebraska, to quality for SAP phase two training, the school must have started a student assistance program. During this phase, teachers and support staff develop skills to help at-risk children who need assistance in school. As SAP programs are carried out, other school policies, procedures, and programs are changed to make school a more successful environment. The team activity report did not differentiate SAP phase one trained schools from SAP phase two trained schools, so this confounding variable cannot be statistically tested. Since data was analyzed retrospectively, the investigators cannot conclude that the findings were caused by the SAP program. However, this study does suggest important trends and suggests that experimental studies should be conducted to demonstrate the effectiveness of student assistance programs.

The findings of this study show that secondary school students report a lower alcohol use rate in the last thirty days in those schools with a SAP when compared with those schools without one. These students also reported a significant difference in academic achievement. In the State of Washington, Gabriel noted a slight increase in grade point averages (GPA) after student assistance program services were provided at the middle and high school level [11]. Dr. Gabriel also found that ATOD use was lower among students from SAP schools. Pollard and Houle results also showed that alcohol and other drug use for schools without a SAP were increasing at a faster rate than at the student assistance program sites [12]. These studies [11, 12] provide convergent support to this study's results.

CONCLUSION

These findings support the 1990 report of the National Commission on Drug Free Schools that recommended that every school should establish a student assistance program. According to the report, implementation of a SAP will specifically help students who have alcohol, tobacco or other drug problems. These problems ultimately will affect the student's ability to remain in school and succeed at academic endeavors [13]. While this study used post hoc analysis of data, the results suggest lower alcohol use and slightly higher academic achievement among students from SAP schools. Given SAPs' popularity, these trends suggest that further research should be conducted to demonstrate the effectiveness of student assistance programs.

ACKNOWLEDGMENTS

The Toward a Drug Free Nebraska staff especially Barbara Fisher and Tom Reardon at the UNMC Academic Computing Services for database design are acknowledged.

REFERENCES

1. D. D. Moore and J. R. Forster, Student Assistance Programs: New Approaches for Reducing Adolescent Substance Abuse, *Journal of Counseling and Development, 71,* pp. 326-329, 1993.
2. M. Klitzner, D. Fisher, K. Stewart, and S. Gilbert, *Early Intervention for Adolescents,* Pacific Institute for Research and Evaluation, Bethesda, Maryland, 1992.
3. G. Anderson, *When Chemicals Come to School.* Clinical Recovery, The Student Assistance Program Model, Milwaukee, Wisconsin, 1987.
4. D. M. Scott, P. A. Merkel, and T. W. Barlow, Process Evaluation of Nebraska's Team Training Project, *Journal of Drug Education, 24*:3, pp. 269-279, 1994.
5. Mid-Continent Regional Education Lab (McREL), *Student Assistance Program Implementation Training,* Midwest Regional Center for Drug Free Schools, Oakbrook, Illinois, 1989.
6. K. A. Carlson, J. D. Hughes, J. K. LaChapelle, M. C. Holayter, and F. M. Deebach, Student Assistance Programs: Do They Make a Difference? *Journal of Child and Adolescent Substance Abuse, 4*:1, 1994.

7. National Organization of Student Assistance Program and Professionals, *National Survey of Student Assistance Programs 1991: Selected Results,* NOSAPP, Boulder, Colorado, 1991.

8. K. A. Carlson, *Student Assistance Programs: A Summary of Recent Research,* Olympic Educational Service District #114, Bremerton, Washington, July 1993.

9. D. M. Scott, *Evaluation of the Toward a Drug Free Nebraska School/Community Team Training Project: 1990-91 Year in Review,* University of Nebraska Medical Center, College of Pharmacy, Department of Pharmacy Practice, Omaha, Nebraska, 1992.

10. *SAS/STAT User's Guide,* Release 6.03 Edition, SAS Institute, Cary, North Carolina, 1988.

11. R. M. Gabriel, D. W. Weaver, E. L. Einspruch, and K. O. Yap, *Assessment of the Effectiveness of the Washington State Omnibus Alcohol and Controlled Substance Abuse Act: Drug and Alcohol Abuse Prevention and Early Intervention in Schools Program,* Evaluation Findings and Recommendations, Northwest Regional Educational Laboratory, Portland, Oregon, 1992.

12. J. A. Pollard and D. M. Houle, *Student Assistance Program Demonstration Project Evaluation: Final Report,* Southwest Regional Educational Laboratory, Los Alamitos, California, 1993.

13. National Commission on Drug-Free Schools, *Toward a Drug Free Generation: A Nation's Responsibility, Final Report,* 1990.

Direct reprint requests to:

David M. Scott, M.P.H., Ph.D.
College of Pharmacy
University of Nebraska Medical Center
600 South 42nd St.
Box 986045
Omaha, NE 68198-6045

J. DRUG EDUCATION, Vol. 29(2) 175-185, 1999

A COMPARISON OF MEMORY FOR AND ATTITUDES ABOUT ALCOHOL, CIGARETTE, AND OTHER PRODUCT ADVERTISEMENTS IN COLLEGE STUDENTS*

OTTO ZINSER

JAMES E. FREEMAN

DAVID K. GINNINGS

East Tennessee State University

ABSTRACT

The purpose of this study was to compare the attitude ratings and recall scores of cigarette, alcohol, automobile, deodorant, jeans, soft drink, athletic shoe, breakfast cereal, and fast food restaurant advertisements. Male and female college students rated the advertisements of these product groups on a number of traits—adventurous, eye-catching, appealing, informative, believable, good times, recreational, effectiveness, romantic, athletic, buy product, and honesty. Drawing on their everyday experience, the students also were asked to recall as much about the advertisements from these product groups as they could. The results revealed that the rating and recall scores of the alcohol advertisements were significantly higher than those for the cigarette advertisements and among the highest of all of the advertisement groups. The female recall scores generally were significantly higher than the male recall scores. In contrast to the cigarette advertisements, the high scores of the alcohol advertisements were interpreted to be due in part to the wider distribution alcohol advertising has had. That alcohol advertising ranked among the highest of all of the advertising groups indicates that college students view alcohol advertising very favorably.

*The authors wish to thank Ms. Alicia Williams and Ms. Melissa Barnes for scoring the memory data.

The extent to which advertising influences young people to begin and continue consuming cigarette and alcohol products has been studied extensively in recent years. Of major concern has been the extent to which advertising contributes to the health problems people eventually incur in the consumption of these products.

CIGARETTE ADVERTISING

A number of investigators have reported evidence which suggests that cigarette advertising is related to cigarette consumption. Chapman and Fitzgerald investigated brand preference and advertising recall in 1,195 Australian secondary school children and reported that four of the 130 available brands—three of which were the most heavily advertised brands—accounted for 78.7 percent of the cigarettes smoked [1]. Moreover, they found that smokers correctly identified edited cigarette advertisements and slogans almost twice as well as nonsmokers did. They concluded that advertising serves as a cue to smoking behavior, whether it is already established or something that could develop in the future, and that the focus on four brands suggests that cigarette advertising plays an important cultural role in the lives of adolescent smokers.

A number of investigators made a study of the content of cigarette advertising. Altman, Slater, Albright, and Maccoby performed a content analysis of youth magazine cigarette advertisements and found that they frequently contained images of risk and adventure which have been interpreted to appeal to youth [2]. Albright, Altman, Slater, and Maccoby examined advertisements in eight popular magazines from 1960-1985 and not only found a substantial increase in the frequency of cigarette advertisements in popular magazines, but also a substantial increase from 1972-1985 in the frequency of cigarette advertisements in youth- and female-oriented magazines [3]. McCarthy and Gritz analyzed the content of 5,800 magazines cigarette advertisements of brands known to be popular among urban teenagers and found independence and self-reliance themes being used in the cigarette advertisements of the most popular brands [4]. Evaluations of selected advertisements by 1,034 sixth, ninth, and twelfth graders and assessment of their attitudes toward future smoking revealed that identification with a same-sex model in the selected advertisements occurred most frequently in the adolescents who were most likely to smoke in the future.

Another approach has been to study the attitudes young persons have formed toward cigarette advertisements. Potts, Gillies, and Herbert surveyed 258 English fifteen-year olds concerning their smoking behavior and opinions of cigarette advertisements [5]. They found that smokers rated cigarette advertisements favorably on exciting, interesting, witty, persuasive, glamorous, eye-catching, and attractive and concluded that cigarette advertisements may help maintain smoking in adolescents by reinforcing a favorable attitude toward smoking. In a similar way, Zinser, Kloosterman, and Williams investigated college student smokers, former smokers, and nonsmokers' attitudes toward five magazines cigarette advertisements interspersed among ten noncigarette advertisements on the following scales: action, adventurous, liking, relaxing, enjoyment, glamorous, romantic, product quality, ad effectiveness, and fun [6]. They found 1) that smokers rated the cigarette advertisements more favorably than the nonsmokers and former smokers did; 2) that the smokers and nonsmokers did not vary in their perception of the noncigarette advertisements; and 3) that the nonsmokers and former smokers were in greater agreement than the smokers were with the idea that the cigarette advertisements are a cause of the onset and maintenance of smoking. The results suggested that cigarette smoking leads to more favorable perceptions of cigarette advertisements, but, paradoxically, also to the view in smokers that cigarette advertisements have little to do with causing smoking, possibly out of a desire to be self-determining [7].

ALCOHOL ADVERTISING

Similarly, some researchers also have reported a relationship between alcohol advertising and drinking behavior. For example, Atkin, Hocking, and Block found that seventh to twelfth graders who reported greater exposure to alcohol advertisements also reported drinking more, or expected to begin drinking more, than classmates who reported less exposure to alcohol advertisements [8]. Likewise, underage drinkers (10 to 17 years old) identified and recognized brand images more often in alcohol advertisement photographs and expressed greater liking for humorous alcohol advertisements, than nondrinking classmates [9]. Finally, for a group of fifth-sixth graders, Grube and Wallack reported that knowledge about alcohol advertising was related to a more favorable attitude toward drinking and expected drinking as an adult [10].

Altman, Schooler, and Basil examined demographic data relative to the locations of 901 billboards in San Francisco [11]. They found that tobacco and alcohol were the most heavily advertised products, that billboards in Afro-American and Hispanic neighborhoods carried a disproportionately higher number of tobacco and alcohol advertisements than those in Caucasian and Asian neighborhoods, that billboards advertising menthol cigarettes and malt liquor were more frequent in black neighborhoods, and that billboards advertising beer and wine were more frequent in Hispanic neighborhoods.

In contrast, other researchers have found no relationship between alcohol advertisement exposure and drinking. The continued utilization of television as an alcohol advertisement medium in the United States has afforded researchers an opportunity to assess their effects upon consumption. Kohn and Smart presented subjects viewing a videotaped soccer game with various numbers of beer advertisements and assessed consumption during and following viewing [12]. They concluded their results did not support current concern about the effect of televised alcohol advertisements on alcohol consumption. Sobell, Sobell, Riley, Klajner, Leo, Pavan, and Cancilla found no differences between type of advertisements (food, beer, and nonalcohol drink) and program type (with or without alcohol scenes) in terms of subsequent drinking behavior [13]. Sobell, Sobell, Toneatto, and Leo found that although abstinence ratings were significantly lower for alcohol abusers exposed to alcohol-cued programming segments, compared to abusers not exposed to this material, the subjects reported a higher level of confidence in their ability to abstain when these segments were paired with alcohol commercials [14]. Finally, Lipsitz, Brake, Vincent and Winters failed to find a difference on a alcohol-drinking expectancy measure in fifth to eighth graders who had viewed beer, soft drink, or beer advertisements in combination with counter-alcohol-drinking-messages [15].

Another set of studies examined the effect of alcohol advertising bans. Smart and Cutler assessed the effects of a fourteen-month alcohol advertisement ban in British Columbia and concluded that the ban had no effect on the consumption of beer, wine, and liquor [16]. In a similar study, Ogborne and Smart analyzed alcoholic beverage sales data from Manitoba prior to and following restriction of advertising [17]. Their results indicated that the advertising restriction was unrelated to type of alcoholic product consumed, per capita consumption or alcoholism rate. Personal income emerged as the best predictor of consumption, and total consumption emerged as the best predictor of alcoholism rate. Makowsky and Whitehead studied the effect of the abolition of a fifty-eight-year ban on alcoholic beverage advertising in Saskatchewan [18]. They found that there was no absolute increase in the sale of alcoholic beverages. There was only a shift in sales: an increase in the sale of beer and a decrease in the sale of spirits. Smart reviewed the results of econometric, exposure, experimental, and advertisement restriction/ban studies and concluded that advertising of alcohol has little effect upon consumption [19]. Young, Oei, and Crook's [20] assessment of the relationship between American college students' perceptions of televised alcohol advertisements and drinking patterns supports Smart's [19] conclusions.

Objectives

The general purpose of this investigation was to measure and compare attitude ratings of cigarette and beer and alcohol advertisements as product groups in the context of the advertisement ratings of other product groups in college students. It was expected, given the absence of cigarette advertising in the electronic media and the considerable negative publicity the cigarette industry has incurred in recent years, that college students would perceive cigarette advertisements less favorably than advertisements from other product groups, including alcohol advertisements. A second objective was to determine how students perceive alcohol advertising relative also to other, noncigarette product groups. A third purpose was to measure and compare the recall of the brands and content of cigarette, alcohol, and other product advertisement groups. It was expected that the recall of the cigarette advertisements would be among the lowest of the product classes and that the recall of the alcohol advertisements would be higher than that of the cigarette advertisements. The fourth purpose was to test for gender differences.

METHOD

Participants

One hundred and thirty-one male and 184 female undergraduates—seventeen to sixty-two years of age with a mean of twenty-two years and median of twenty years—from a southeastern university served as participants. All subjects received extra credit points toward their course grade for participating. One hundred and fifty-two reported having smoked—49.4 months on the average and 9.7 cigarettes per day. One hundred and sixty-four reported having never smoked. Two hundred and sixty-five reported having consumed alcohol—4.1 drinks per week on the average. Fifty-one reported having abstained totally. One hundred and eighty-nine reported that they currently drink.

Materials

One booklet was prepared to obtain advertisement recall data, a second to obtain advertisement ratings, a third and a fourth to obtain demographic information and to assess personal variables, and the last to present closing instructions. The instructions accompanying the first booklet requested that the subjects list general information, general impressions, specific content, and product names they could recall from all of the following advertisement classes: cigarettes, beer and other alcoholic beverages, automobiles, deodorants, jeans, soft drinks, athletic shoes, breakfast cereals, and fast food restaurants. The subjects were instructed to strive for accuracy and to leave the space provided blank for any product class that they confidently could not recall anything about. The subjects were also informed that they would be limited to two minutes to respond to each product class.

The instructions preceding the second booklet requested that the subjects rate, on a scale of 1 to 10 (Lo to Hi), each of the product classes on the following characteristics: adventurous, eye-catching, appealing, informative, believable, good times, recreational, effectiveness of ads, romantic, athletic, buy product, and honest. The subjects were informed that they would be limited to 30 seconds to respond to each product class.

The third, the demographic questionnaire, requested the subjects provide information about their gender, age, academic classification, and consumption habits of all of the product classes. The fourth booklet assessed advertisement medium exposure. The final instructions directed the subjects on the compilation of their response sheets and requested that they refrain from discussing the research with anyone to avoid influencing the responses of future participants.

Procedure

Upon obtaining written informed consent from the subjects, each group was presented with the first booklet; the subjects were tested in groups varying from three to thirty-one in number. The instructions were read aloud. The experimenter announced each product class and the time to "begin." Upon the passage of two minutes, the experimenter announced "stop." The order of the presentation of the product classes was randomized from group to group.

Upon completion of the first booklet, the subjects were asked to turn the booklet over, lay it aside, and not to return to it. Then the experimenter read the instructions aloud for the ratings booklet. For each product class, the experimenter announced the product class and when the subject was to "begin" providing ratings. Upon the passage of thirty seconds, the experimenter announced "stop." The order of product class presentation for recall was retained for the ratings.

Upon completion of the second booklet, the subjects were again requested to turn it over, lay it aside, and not to return to it. The demographic questionnaire was then distributed; the subjects were instructed to complete it, then to turn over, and not to return it. The product use questionnaire followed. Upon completion of these questionnaires, the closing instructions were distributed and read aloud. All testing materials were then collected.

RESULTS

Two female graduate students, naive to the purposes of the experiment, scored the recall data. Each student was asked to use their best judgment in assigning a point for each valid specific and general content element recalled by the subjects and two points for each valid product recalled. The average of the two scores generated by the raters served as the recall measure for each subjects' recollections of each product category. The correlation between the recall scores generated by the two raters was +.39 for the alcohol advertisements and +.49 for the cigarette advertisements. The mean recall scores and rating scores across all subjects for each advertisement class are presented in Table 1. The mean recall and rating scores broken down by gender are presented in Tables 2 and 3.

A median split of consumption rates of current alcoholic beverage drinkers and cigarette smokers into low alcohol (LAC) and high alcohol consumption (HAC) and low cigarette (LCC) and high cigarette consumption (HCC) subgroups was performed. The recall scores were subjected to a four-factor MANOVA (smoking versus alcohol advertisements x gender x LAC/HAC x LCC/HCC) with repeated measures across advertisements. Only the advertisements ($F(1,180) = 23.46$, $p > .05$), and the gender ($F(1,181) = 4.75$, $p < .05$) effects were statistically significant. The subjects recalled more from the alcohol advertisements than from

Table 1. Recall Means and Attitude Rating Means of
Classes of Advertisements

Classes of Advertisements	Recall Means	Classes of Advertisements	Rating Means
Beer & Alcohol	14.98	Athletic Shoes	6.50
Automobiles	14.97	Automobiles	6.12
Soft Drinks	14.93	Jeans	6.00
Fast Food Restaurants	14.81	Beer & Alcohol	5.90
Breakfast Cereals	14.34	Soft Drinks	5.71
Jeans	12.81	Fast Food Restaurants	5.06
Athletic Shoes	12.73	Deodorants	4.70
Cigarettes	12.32	Breakfast Cereals	4.63
Deodorants	12.26	Cigarettes	3.82

Table 2. Recall Means by Classes of Advertisements and Gender

Classes of Advertisements	Males	Classes of Advertisements	Females
Automobiles	14.71	Soft Drinks	15.74
Beer & Alcohol	14.46	Fast Food Restaurant	15.59
Soft Drinks	13.80	Breakfast Cereals	15.45
Fast Food Restaurants	13.72	Beer & Alcohol	15.35
Breakfast Cereals	12.76	Automobiles	15.15
Athletic Shoes	12.31	Jeans	13.75
Jeans	11.50	Deodorants	13.16
Cigarettes	11.38	Athletic Shoes	13.04
Deodorants	10.98	Cigarettes	12.99

the cigarette advertisements and the females recalled more of the advertisements than the males did. The same analysis performed on the rating data yielded only an advertisements main effect, $F(1,186) = 197.18, p > .05$. The subjects rated the alcohol advertisements significantly higher than the cigarette advertisements.

DISCUSSION

Cigarette and Alcohol Advertising

As expected, the results of this study revealed that recall scores and ratings were significantly higher for the alcohol advertisements than for the cigarette

Table 3. Rating Means by Classes of Advertisements and Gender

Classes of Advertisements	Males	Classes of Advertisements	Females
Athletic Shoes	6.65	Athletic Shoes	6.39
Beer & Alcohol	6.06	Automobiles	6.20
Automobiles	6.00	Jeans	6.10
Jeans	5.85	Soft Drinks	5.91
Soft Drinks	5.43	Beer & Alcohol	5.78
Fast Food Restaurants	4.78	Fast Food Restaurants	5.25
Deodorants	4.40	Deodorants	4.95
Breakfast Cereals	4.39	Breakfast Cereals	4.80
Cigarettes	3.64	Cigarettes	3.95

advertisements in males and females. These results suggested that cigarette advertisements are viewed less favorably by college students than alcohol advertisements and that alcohol advertisements are in the company of the most favorable of advertisement groups—fast food restaurants, automobiles, and soft drinks.

Previous research has demonstrated that alcohol and cigarette advertisements are preferentially oriented toward certain themes and target populations [2, 21]. It has also been demonstrated that themes conveyed in magazine cigarette advertisements preferentially target youthful readers [2-4]. Furthermore, investigations conducted by Chapman and Fitzgerald [1], Potts et al. [5], Zinser et al. [6] and others have reported results suggesting that adolescents choose brands from among the most widely advertised and are more cognizant of and favorable toward advertisements of products they use.

That beer and alcohol advertisements attempt to put alcohol products in a favorable light seems obvious [22]. The results of this study suggest they have been successful in this regard. That college students perceive and recall them comparatively better than cigarette advertisements may be partly due to the beer industry having access and the cigarette industry not having access to the electronic media as an advertisement medium. It is possible that the cigarette advertisement recall and rating scores of this study are a function of the negative publicity that cigarette smoking has received in recent years. Moreover, it is also possible that the cessation of televised cigarette advertisement in 1971 affected the smoking advertisement data. Madden and Grube's finding that from 1990-1992, 77 percent of all of the beverage advertising at sporting events was alcohol advertising is also worthy of note [23]. Social factors, such as parental and peer influence not withstanding, the very extensive use the alcohol industry makes of advertising may contribute to the very favorable view college students have of alcohol advertising and their associated products.

Gender

Across all types of advertisements, the recall scores of females were significantly higher than those of males. Other researchers have reported females recalling more information than males [6].

Although there was no interaction between advertising classes and gender, the differences between alcohol and cigarette advertisements in the recall and rating scores was smaller for the female subjects than for the male subjects. It also will be noted that compared to the other advertisement classes males recalled the alcohol advertisements nearly the best and that females, despite not having recalled the most about alcohol advertisements when compared with the other product classes, recalled more about them than males did.

Limitations and Conclusions

That the correlations between the raters' scores were not higher suggests that the raters were somewhat inconsistent in their evaluation of the memory data, perhaps because they were not equally knowledgeable about the advertisement groupings presented. Substantial differences in knowledge and in the evaluation method and criteria used could have accounted for much of the inconsistency in the recall scores between the two raters. In addition to this problem, the recall methodology of this study may be criticized on the use of female raters. Inclusion of a male rater might have altered the results and made the evaluations more representatives of both sexes; however, it is not likely that the recall results would have been markedly different since the pattern of results in the recall data were basically similar to those in the rating data.

The results of this study suggest that the cumulative effect of many years of multi-media advertising has provided alcohol products with a comparatively favorable standing, roughly equal to that of many other nonalcoholic products, despite publicity about the negative consequences of the abuse of these products by young and old alike. What weakens this assertion is that studies like the present do not provide a clear indication of a causal relationship between alcohol advertising and the status of alcohol products because the evidence is retrospective and circumstantial. Moreover, this guarded conclusions is presented in the context of continued conflicting reports about the influence of advertising on alcohol consumption [24, 25].

REFERENCES

1. S. Chapman and B. Fitzgerald, Brand Preference and Advertising Recall in Adolescent Smokers: Some Implications for Health Promotion, *American Journal of Public Health,* 72:5, pp. 491-494, 1982.

2. D. Altman, M. Slater, C. Albright, and N. Maccoby, How an Unhealthy Product is Sold: Advertising in Magazines, 1960-1985, *Journal of Communication, 37*:4, pp. 95-106, 1987.
3. C. Albright, D. Altman, M. Slater, and N. Maccoby, Cigarette Advertisements in Magazines: Evidence for a Differential Focus on Women's and Youth Magazines, *Health Education Quarterly, 15,*:2, pp. 335-344, 1988.
4. W. J. McCarthy and E. R. Gritz, *Madison Avenue as the Pied Piper: Cigarette Advertising and Teenage Smoking,* paper presented at the American Psychological Association Convention, New York, 1987.
5. H. Potts, P. Gillies, and M. Herbert, Adolescent Smoking and Opinion of Cigarette Advertisements, *Health Education Research: Theory and Practice, 1*:13, pp. 195-201, 1986.
6. O. Zinser, R. Kloosterman, and A. Williams, Perceptions of Cigarette Advertisements by College Student Smokers, Former Smokers, and Nonsmokers, *Journal of Social Behavior and Personality, 6*:2, pp. 354-366, 1991.
7. E. L. Deci and R. M. Ryan, *Intrinsic Motivation and Self-Determination in Human Behavior,* Plenum Press, New York, 1985.
8. C. K. Atkin, J. Hocking, and M. Block, Teenage Drinking: Does Advertising Make a Difference? *Journal of Communication, 34,* pp. 157-167, 1984.
9. P. P. Aitken, D. R. Eadie, D. S. Leathar, and R. E. McNeill, Television Advertisements for Alcoholic Drinks Do Reinforce Under-Age Drinking, *British Journal of Addiction, 83*:12, pp. 1399-1419, 1988.
10. J. W. Grube and L. Wallack, Television Beer Advertising and Drinking Knowledge, Beliefs, and Intentions among Schoolchildren, *The American Journal of Public Health, 84*:2, pp. 254-259, 1994.
11. D. Altman, C. Schooler, and M. Basil, Alcohol and Cigarette Advertising on Billboards, *Health Education Research: Theory and Practice, 6*:4, pp. 487-490, 1991.
12. P. Kohn and R. Smart, The Impact of Television Advertising on Alcohol Consumption: An Experiment, *Journal of Studies on Alcohol, 46*:4, pp. 295-301, 1984.
13. L. Sobell, M. Sobell, D. Riley, F. Klajner, G. Leo, D. Pavan, and A. Cancilla, Effect of Television Programming and Advertising on Alcohol Consumption in Normal Drinkers, *Journal of Studies on Alcohol, 47*:4, pp. 333-340, 1986.
14. L. C. Sobell, M. B. Sobell, T. Toneatto, and G. I. Leo, Severely Dependent Alcohol Abusers May be Vulnerable to Alcohol Cues in Television Programs, *Journal of Studies on Alcohol, 54,* pp. 85-91, 1993.
15. A. Lipsitz, G. Brake, E. J. Vincent, and M. Winters, Another Round for the Brewers: Television Ads and Children's Alcohol Expectancies, *Journal of Applied Social Psychology, 23*:6, pp. 439-450, 1993.
16. R. Smart and R. Cutler, The Alcohol Advertising Ban in British Columbia: Problems and Effects on Beverage Consumptions, *British Journal of Addiction, 71,* pp. 13-21, 1976.
17. A. Ogborne and R. Smart, Will Restrictions on Alcohol Advertising Reduce Alcohol Consumptions? *British Journal of Addiction, 75,* pp. 293-296, 1980.
18. C. Makowsky and P. Whitehead, Advertising and Alcohol Sales: A Legal Impact Study, *Journal of Studies on Alcohol, 52*:6, pp. 555-567, 1991.

19. R. Smart, Does Alcohol Advertising Affect Overall Consumption: A Review of Empirical Studies, *Journal of Studies on Alcohol, 49*:4, pp. 314-323, 1988.

20. R. Young, T. Oei, and G. Crook, Differences in the Perception of Alcoholic and Nonalcoholic Beverage Advertisements, *Psychologia, 34,* pp. 241-247, 1991.

21. J. Matarazzo, Behavioral Health's Challenge to Academic, Scientific, and Professional Psychology, *American Psychologist, 37*:1, pp. 1-14, 1982.

22. A. Wyllie, F. Holibar, S. Casswell, N. Fuamatu, K. Aiolupatea, H. M. Barnes, and A. Panapa, A Qualitative Investigation of Respondents to Televised Alcohol Advertisements, *Contemporary Drug Problems, 24*:1, pp. 103-132, 1997.

23. P. A. Madden and J. W. Grube, The Frequency and Nature of Alcohol and Tobacco Advertising in Televised Sports, 1990 through 1992, *The American Journal of Public Health, 84*:2, pp. 297-299, 1994.

24. H. Saffer, Studying the Effects of Alcohol Advertising on Consumption, *Alcohol Health and Research World, 20*:4, pp. 266-273, 1996.

25. J. E. Calfee and C. Scheraga, The Influence of Advertising on Alcohol Consumption: A Literature Review and an Econometric Analysis of Four European Nations, *International Journal of Advertising, 13*:4, pp. 287-301, 1994.

Direct reprint requests to:

Otto Zinser, Ph.D.
Psychology Department
East Tennessee State University
Johnson City, TN 37614

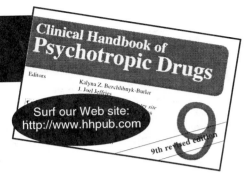

FOCUS ON ALCOHOL

Edited by SEYMOUR EISEMAN

PRIMARY ORIENTATION: prevention of drug misuse
A must for the drug educator

To adequately address and deal with the detrimental effects of alcohol, attempts must be made to learn and understand the motivations and attitudes which contribute to its use and misuse.

This essential collection represents a psychosocial perspective of the effects of alcohol while providing relatively unknown—but central research needed for a comprehensive understanding of the behaviors associated with alcohol use.

Table of Contents

Part I — Theory ● Behavioral Intention as an Indicator of Drug and Alcohol Use ● Pre-Service Teachers Use of and Attitudes Toward Alcohol and Other Drugs ● Relationship Between Alcohol Consumption and Alcohol Problems in Young Adults ● The Private Sector: Taking a Role in the Prevention of Drug and Alcohol Abuse for Young People Part 2 — Research ● Early Onset of Drinking as a Predictor of Alcohol Consumption and Alcohol Related Problems in College ● A Short- and Long-Term Evaluation of Here's Looking at You Alcohol Education Program ● Evaluating the Effectiveness of a School Drug and Alcohol Prevention Curriculum: A New Look at "Here's Looking at You, Two" ● Alcohol Education Research and Practice: A Logical Analysis of the Two Realities Long-Term ● Evaluation of a Life Skills Approach for Alcohol and Drug Abuse Prevention ● Does Drug and Alcohol Use Lead to Failure to Graduate from High School? Children's ● Changing Attitudes Regarding Alcohol: A Cross-Sectional Study ● Increased Exposure to Alcohol and Cannabis Education and Changes in Use Patterns Part 3 — Practice ● Are Drinkers Interested in Inexpensive Approaches to Reduce their Alcohol Use? ● Alcohol and Soap Operas: Drinking in the Light of Day ● Effects of a Preventive Alcohol Education Program after Three Years ● Public Attitudes to and Awareness of Fetal Alcohol Syndrome in Young Adults ● College Students' Definitions of Social and Problem Drinking ● Teaching Adolescents about Alcohol and Driving: A Two Year Follow-up ● Alcohol and Drug Education Programs

Format: 6' x 9", 272 pages, Paper, ISBN: 0-89503-083-7

Price: $35.95 + $4.00 postage and handling

Baywood Publishing Company, Inc.
26 Austin Avenue, Amityville, NY 11701
call (516) 691-1270 fax (516) 691-1770 orderline (800) 638-7819
e-mail: baywood@baywood.com ● web site: http://baywood.com

DECISIONS:
A CALL TO ACTION

Seymour Eiseman, Dr. P.H.
Professor Emeritus
Department of Health Science
California State University, Northridge

&

Robert A. Eiseman, B.A.
Instructor, Biology
University High School
Los Angeles, California

about the book

    This book represents a method by which students are assisted to make wise decisions about the use of alcohol and other drugs. Situations which are essential to effective daily living are employed to reach effective decisions. The role of parents in assisting the children toward a better understanding of the nature of drug use is also explored. Specifically, the use of alcohol and other drugs in the workplace places the drug situation directly in the light of the job market. The current problem of HIV and drugs is also discussed, along with drugs and pregnancy.

intended audience

- College freshman classes
- Teacher preparation classes at college and university levels
- Community colleges
- Parents, high school seniors
- Senior Citizens groups
- Lodges and fraternal groups

what people are saying

"A no-nonsense, easy-to-use guide to alcohol and other drug prevention in schools."

James Robinson III
Texas A&M University, College Station, Texas

Format Information: 6" x 9", 92 pgs., ISBN: 0-89503-148-5, Paper, $19.95, $3.50p/h

Baywood Publishing Company, Inc.
26 Austin Avenue, Amityville, NY 11701
call (516) 691-1270 **fax** (516) 691-1770 **orderline** (800) 638-7819
e-mail: baywood@baywood.com • **web site:** http://baywood.com

SUBSTANCE ABUSE PREVENTION:

A Multicultural Perspective

Edited by Snehendu B. Kar

Alcohol, tobacco, and other drugs (ATOD) abuse is a major threat to our health and quality of life. In this volume, nationally recognized substance abuse specialists, public health researchers, and community-based practitioners undertake an in-depth state-of-the-art review of substance abuse prevention intervention from a multicultural perspective.

Special emphasis is on the application of the lessons learned from fields of substance abuse and the new public health paradigm as a modus operandi for ATOD prevention in multicultural communities. The book further makes specific recommendations for prevention policy, research, professional preparation, and effective intervention strategies.

In thirteen chapters, twenty-four authors share their analyses, concerns, and conclusions in several domains including the: meaning and dynamics of multiculturalism affecting prevention intervention, relative risks and knowledge gaps across ethnic groups, social trends affecting health risks and substance abuse, lessons learned from substance abuse research and prevention, role of the media, promises and limits of the new public health paradigm for assessment, policy development, assurance of preventive services, and social action and empowerment for prevention in partnership with the public.

This pioneering volume will serve as a valuable resource to researchers, policy makers, educators, professionals and organizations interested in the health and quality of life of our communities as we approach the 21st century.

Format Information: 6" x 9", 336 pages, ISBN: 0-89503-194-9, $42.00 plus $4.00 postage and handling

Baywood Publishing Company, Inc. 26 Austin Avenue, Amityville, NY 11701
Call (516) 691-1270 Fax (516) 691-1770 **Orderline** (800) 638-7819
e-mail: baywood@baywood.com ● **web site:** http://baywood.com

Journal of DRUG EDUCATION

INSTRUCTIONS TO AUTHORS

Submit manuscript to: Dr. Seymour Eiseman, Editor
Department of Health Science
California State University, Northridge
Northridge, CA 91330

Manuscripts are to be submitted in triplicate. Retain one copy, as manuscript will not be returned. Manuscript must be typewritten on 8-1/2" × 11" white paper, one side only, double-spaced, with wide margins. Paginate consecutively starting with the title page. The organization of the paper should be indicated by appropriate headings and subheadings.

Originality Authors should note that only original articles are accepted for publication. Submission of a manuscript represents certification on the part of the author(s) that neither the article submitted, nor a version of it has been published, or is being considered for publication elsewhere.

Abstracts of 100 to 150 words are required to introduce each article.

References should relate only to material cited within text and be listed in numerical order according to their appearance within text. State author's name, title of referenced work, editor's name, title of book or periodical, volume, issue, pages cited, and year of publication. Do not abbreviate titles. Please do not use ibid., op. cit., loc. cit., etc. In case of multiple citations, simply repeat the original numeral. Detailed specifications available from the editor upon request.

Footnotes are placed at the bottom of page where referenced. They should be numbered with superior arabic numbers without parentheses or brackets. Footnotes should be brief with an average length of three lines.

Figures should be referenced in text and appear in numerical sequence starting with Figure 1. Line art must be original drawings in black ink proportionate to our page size, and suitable for photographing. Indicate top and bottom of figure where confusion may exist. Labeling should be 8 point type. Clearly identify all figures. Figures should be drawn on separate pages and their placement within the text indicated by inserting: —Insert Figure 1 here—.

Tables must be cited in text in numerical sequence starting with Table 1. Each table must have a descriptive title. Any footnotes to tables are indicated by superior lower case letters. Tables should be typed on separate pages and their approximate placement indicated within text by inserting: —Insert Table 1 here—.

*Authors will receive twenty complimentary reprints of their published article.
Additional reprints may be ordered.*

Volume 29, Number 3 — 1999

JOURNAL OF

DRUG

EDUCATION

CONTENTS

Executive Editor:

SEYMOUR EISEMAN, DR.P.H.

Baywood Publishing Company, Inc.

ISSN 0047-2379

Journal of DRUG EDUCATION

EXECUTIVE EDITOR
SEYMOUR EISEMAN, DR. P.H.
Department of Health Sciences
California State University, Northridge

The *Journal of Drug Education* is a peer-refereed journal.

Journal of Drug Education is noted in: *Abstracts on Criminology and Penology; Academic Abstracts; Adolescent Mental Health Abstracts AGRICOLA; ALCONARC: ASSIA: All-Russian Institute of Scientific and Technical Information; Applied Social Sciences Index & Abstracts; Cambridge Scientific Abstracts; Cancer Prevention and Control Database; Counseling and Personnel Services Information Center; Criminal Justice Abstracts; Criminology, Penology and Police Service Abstracts; Cumulative Index to Nursing & Allied Health Literature (CINAHL); Current Contents; Current Index to Journals in Education; Dokumentation Gefahrdung durch Alkohol, Rauchen, Drogen, Arzneimittel; Drug Abuse and Alcoholism Review; EMBASE/Excerpta Medica; Health Promotion and Education Database; H.W.Wilson; International Bibliography of Periodical Literature; International Bibliography of Book Reviews; International Pharmaceutical Abstracts; Kindex Medicus; MEDLINE; NCJRS Catalog; National Institute on Alcohol Abuse and Alcoholism's Alcohol and Alcohol Problems Science Database, ETOH; Psychological Abstracts; Smoking and Health Database; Safety and Health at Work ILO-CIS Bulletin;* and *Sociological Abstracts*

The *Journal of Drug Education* is published by the Baywood Publishing Company, Inc., 26 Austin Ave., P.O. Box 337, Amityville, NY 11701. Subscription rate per Volume (four issues): Institutional—$175.00 Individual—$48.00 (prepaid by personal check or credit card). Add $7.00 per volume for postage inside the U.S. and Canada and $12.50 elsewhere. Back list volumes are available at $192.50. Subscription is on a volume basis only and must be prepaid. Copies of single issues are not available. No part of this journal may be reproduced in any form without written permission from the publisher.

J. DRUG EDUCATION, Vol. 29(3) 187-188, 1999

EDITORIAL: CONSENSUS STATEMENT, 14th JULY 1997 OF THE FARMINGTON CONFERENCES

The purpose of *this statement* is to define the basis for shared identity, commitment, and purpose, among journals publishing in the field of psychoactive substance use and associated problems. Our aim has enhanced the quality of our endeavors in this multidisciplinary field. We share common concerns and believe that we do well to join together in their solution. To that end we accede to this document as a statement of our consensus and as basis for future collaboration.

1. Commitment to the peer review process

1.1 We are committed to peer review and would expect research reports and scientific reviews to go through this process. As regards the extent to which other material will be so reviewed, we see that as a matter for editorial discretion, but policies should be declared.

1.2 Referees *should be told* that their access to the articles on which they have been requested to comment is in strict confidence. Confidentiality should not be broken by pre-publication statements on the content of the submission. Manuscripts sent to reviewers should be returned to the editor or destroyed.

1.3 Referees *should be asked to* declare to the editor if they have a conflict of interest in relation to the material which they are invited to review, and if in doubt they should consult the editor. We define "conflict of interest" as a situation in which professional, personal, or financial considerations, could be seen by a fair-minded person as potentially in conflict with independence of judgment. Conflict of interest is not in itself wrong-doing.

2. Expectations of authors

2.1 **Authorship:** All listed authors on an article should have been personally and substantially involved in the work leading to the article.

2.2 **Avoidance of double publication:** Authors are *expected to ensure* that no significant part of the submitted material has been published previously and that it is not concurrently being considered by another journal. An exception to this general position may be made when previous publication has been limited to another language, to local publication in report, or publication of a conference abstract. All such instances, we would expect authors should consult the editor. Editors are encouraged to develop policies concerning electronic publication. Authors are asked to provide the editor at the time of submission with copies of published or submitted reports that *are related to that submission.*

2.3 Sources of funding for the submitted paper must be declared *and will be published.*

2.4 Conflicts of interest experienced by authors: *Authors should* declare to the editor if their relationship with any type of funding source might fairly be construed as exposing them to potential conflict of interest.

2.5 Protection of human and animal rights: *Where applicable* authors *should* give an assurance that ethical safeguards have been met.

2.6 Technical preparation of articles: We will publish guidance for authors on the technical preparation of articles with the form of instruction at the discretion of individual journals.

3. Formal response to breach of expectations be an author

3.1 Working in collaboration with our authors, we have a responsibility to support the expectations of good scientific publishing practice. To that end each journal will have defined policies for response to attempted or actual instances of *duplicate* publicatplagiarismarism, or scientific fraud.

4. Maintaining editorial independence

4.1 *We are committed to independence in the editorial process. To the extent the owner or another body may influence the editorial process, this should be declared, and in that case any sources of support from the alcohol, tobacco, pharmaceutical, or other relevant interests should be published in the journal.*

4.2 *We will publish declarations on any sources of support received by a journal, and will maintain openness in regard to connections which a journal or its editorial staff may have established which could reasonably be construed as conflict of interest.*

4.3 Funding for journal supplements: When we publish journal supplements, an indication will be given of any sources of support for their production.

4.4 Refereeing journal supplements: An editorial note will be published to indicate whether it has or has not been peer reviewed.

4.5 Advertising: Acceptance of advertising will be determined by, or in consultation with, the editor of each journal.

Seymour Eiseman

J. DRUG EDUCATION, Vol. 29(3) 189-203, 1999

MODIFIED STAGES OF ACQUISITION OF GATEWAY DRUG USE: A PRIMARY PREVENTION APPLICATION OF THE STAGES OF CHANGE MODEL

R. MARK KELLEY, PH.D.
University of Wisconsin–LaCrosse

GEORGE DENNY, PH.D.

MICHAEL YOUNG, PH.D.
University of Arkansas

ABSTRACT

The purpose of the study was to identify the stages of acquisition of gateway drugs in fourth, fifth, and sixth graders. The Stages of Acquisition model is a primary prevention application of the Stages of Change model. The subjects in the study were 811 students from seventeen elementary schools in Arkansas and Missouri. The instrument elicited information regarding the stages of acquisition and individual self-reported drug use. The data were analyzed using frequency, distribution, discriminant analysis, and correlation analyses. Stage placement was confirmed using a series of drug use measures. Results confirmed the existence of discrete stages of acquisition. Results supported the concept of gateway drugs in that subjects indicated they had progressed further through the stages of acquisition of alcohol use than through the stages of acquisition of cigarettes use, smokeless tobacco use, or marijuana use.

INTRODUCTION

National survey data indicate that drug use among American youth is the highest in the industrialized world [1]. Data also indicate that after a decade of decline, drug use among American youth is increasing [2]. Such sobering news should prompt researchers and educators to search for more effective prevention models.

189

Two models that seem to explain the acquisition of behavior, such as drug use, and behavior change are the Stages of Change model [3, 4] and the Multi-Component Motivational Stages (McMOS) model [5]. These models have been used to examine the "Stages of Acquisition" and the "Stages of Habit Change" within a variety of populations [6, 7]. This study examines the Stages of Acquisition in upper elementary school students.

DiClemente and Prochaska [8] developed the Stages of Change Model to describe the cognitive stages through which individuals progress during the process of cessation of habitual action [8-13]. The model was first applied to smoking cessation. Some applications of this model have been made to the study of the acquisition of health-related behaviors such as alcoholism, mammography screening, exercise, and the use of sunscreens [14, 15].

Werch and DiClemente developed the McMOS model to explain the process by which a person acquires a habit (drug use) and/or changes a habit (drug use) [5]. The McMOS model contains five stages of habit acquisition and five stages of habit change: precontemplation, contemplation, preparation, action, and maintenance [6, 7, 16]. For habit acquisition the stages are: precontemplation—those who are not thinking about starting use; contemplation—those who are seriously considering initiating use; preparation—those who are intending to use in the near future; action—who are initiating actual use; and maintenance—those who are continuing use. For habit change the stages are as follows: precontemplation—those who are not considering stopping use; contemplation—those who are seriously considering stopping use; preparation—those who are intending to stop in the near future; action—those who are making attempts to stop use; and maintenance—those continuing nonuse. The McMOS model also includes a drug specific prevention hierarchy, which is supported by previous research [17, 18]. Their research indicates that there is a progression in drug use from the use of alcohol (beer or wine) to the use of cigarettes or hard liquor to the use of marijuana and then to the use of other illicit drugs.

This study proposes a modification of the Stages of Habit Acquisition as theorized in the McMOS model. The modification is the inclusion of a new stage which is named the Recontemplation stage. The Recontemplation stage includes those individuals who have tried the substance, but after trying the substance decide not to try the substance again. This new model, The Modified Stages of Acquisition model, includes six discrete cognitive stages: 1) Precontemplation—those who *have not* tried the substance and are *not planning* to try the substance; 2) Contemplation—those who *have not tried* the substance but *are* thinking about trying it sometime; 3) Recontemplation—those who *have* tried the substance but are *not* planning to try it again; 4) Initiation—those who have tried the substance and are planning to try/use it again soon, 5) Action—those who have been using the substance for a short period of time (6 months or less); 6) Maintenance—those who have been using the substance for a long period of time (more than 6 months). The present study is part of the ongoing effort to identify the Modified Stages of Acquisition of gateway drug use in elementary school students.

METHODS

Subjects

The data in the study were collected as part of the evaluation of an elementary school drug education program. The subjects were 811 students from seventeen different elementary schools in Arkansas and Missouri. Of the responding subjects, 402 (49.8%) of the subjects were females and 409 (50.2%) were males. By grade, 477 (58.5%) of the subjects who participated in the study were in the fourth grade, 261 (32.2%) were in the fifth grade and sixty-two (7.6%) were in the sixth grade. Eleven subjects (1.7%) did not respond to the grade variable. By ethnicity, 563 (96.4%) of the subjects who responded to this question were White, three (0.3%) subjects were African American, five (0.6%) were Hispanic or Mexican American, four (0.5%) were Asian, one (0.1%) was Native American, and three (0.3%) reported their race as "other." There were 232 (28.6%) subjects who did not respond to this question. An examination of the data revealed that none of the subjects from three different schools responded to the race question. Follow-up contact with those schools provided no explanation of the missing data.

Instrument Development

The instrument used in the study was a forty-item questionnaire which was administered in the classroom by the classroom teacher. The instrument elicited information about the Modified Stages of Acquisition of alcohol, smokeless tobacco, cigarettes, and marijuana, demographic information and the subjects' usage of alcohol, smokeless tobacco, cigarettes, and marijuana. All of the items of the instrument were obtained from a variety of previously published instruments. These items were modified for readability and age appropriateness of questions.

The questions which placed students into one of the stages of the Modified Stages of Acquisition model were adapted and modified from the instrument described by Werch, Meers, and Farrell [7]. These authors found the items selected "to produce robust and replicable categorical classification" [7]. A Modified Stages of Acquisition question for each substance was included in the instrument. For example, the alcohol stages question read "Pick the one answer that is most true for you about alcohol." Each response to these questions represents a stage in the Modified Stages of Acquisition model. The seventh response was used to identify any subject in any of the Stages of Change. These questions were used to establish stage placement.

1. "I have not tried alcohol and am not planning to try it." (Precontemplation)
2. "I have not tried alcohol but am planning to try it sometime soon." (Contemplation)

3. "I have tried alcohol but am not planning to try it again." (Recontemplation)
4. "I have tried alcohol and plan to try it again." (Initiation)
5. "I have been using alcohol for a short time (less than 6 months)." (Action)
6. "I have used alcohol for a long time (more than 6 months)." (Maintenance)
7. "I used alcohol for a long time (more than 6 months) but quit using it." (Habit Change)

A variety of procedures were used to confirm the validity and reliability of the instrument. These procedures included analysis of readability, stability, content validity, and concurrent validity. Result of these procedures are presented in the results portion of the article.

Procedures

Participation in the evaluation of the program required the active consent by the parents. Students voluntarily and in a regular classroom setting completed the forty-item questionnaire using an optical scan answer sheet. Teachers used transparencies to display questionnaire items and read all items aloud to the students. The protocol followed by the teachers called for them to emphasize the voluntary nature of the study, the confidentiality of the study, the right to pass on any item and the importance of providing honest responses for all items that were answered. At the conclusion of the test, the completed answer sheets were placed into an envelope provided by the researchers. The teacher sealed the envelope and placed it into the school mail in the presence of a student. This procedure ensured the confidentiality of the subjects.

RESULTS

Readability

Four methods were used to confirm the clarity, ease-of-use, and readability: 1) the instrument was reviewed by a focus group consisting of teachers of the target population; 2) the instrument was reviewed by an elementary reading specialist; 3) a computerized readability analysis was performed; and 4) the instrument was reviewed by the developer of the McMOS model. The computerized reading level assessment test yielded a Flesch Reading Ease Grade Level of 6.3 and a Flesch-Kincaid Score of 3.1. The results indicated the reading level of the instrument was appropriate for the subjects in the study (fourth, fifth, and sixth graders). All of the above methods confirmed the clarity, ease-of-use, readability of the instrument.

Reliability

The stability of the Stages of Acquisition questions was assessed by calculating the percentage of responses which were equal at both test times. For the Stages of Alcohol Acquisition, twenty-one (72%) of the twenty-nine subjects' responses on the initial test matched their responses on the retest. For the Stages of Cigarette Acquisition, twenty-seven (93%) of the twenty-nine subjects' responses on the initial test matched their responses on the retest. For the Stages of Smokeless Tobacco Acquisition, twenty-eight of the twenty-nine subjects' responses on the initial test matched their responses on the retest. For the Stages of Marijuana Acquisition, all twenty-nine of the subjects' responses on the initial test matched their responses on the retest. The percentage of subjects whose responses matched was treated as a measure of stability yielding stability coefficients ranging from $r = .72$ for the Stages of Alcohol Acquisition to $r = 1.0$ for the Stages of Marijuana Acquisition.

The stability of the usage measures was assessed by combining all of the items measuring the subjects' usage of each substance into a summated rating scale. This created an alcohol profile variable, a cigarette profile variable, a smokeless tobacco profile variable, and a marijuana profile variable at the initial test and the retest. The correlation coefficient between each of the profile variables at the initial test and the retest was treated as a measure of the stability of the substance usage measures. These analyses yielded the following reliability coefficients for each substance profile: Alcohol profile ($r = .77$); Cigarette profile ($r = .98$); and Smokeless Tobacco ($r = .88$). There was no variability for the Marijuana profile at the initial test time, therefore, no correlation coefficient could be calculated for the Marijuana profile.

Validity

The content validity of the instrument to measure the Stages of Acquisition was assessed by a panel of experts including the developer of the original instrument, a nationally known drug education specialist, the researchers of the study and a measurement expert. The panel concluded the instrument correctly identified the Modified Stages of Acquisition.

Evidence for concurrent validity was sought by using each students' responses to the use items to validate their placement into the Modified Stages of Acquisition. The questionnaire contained a series of usage questions for each substance (alcohol, cigarettes, smokeless tobacco, and marijuana). These questions were used to confirm the validity of each student's own placement into the Modified Stages of Acquisition. For each stage placement, the researchers determined which responses to each of the usage questions were consistent with each stage placement. For example, for the Precontemplation stage of alcohol use the subjects should respond in the following manner: "Have you ever drunk alcohol on at least one occasion?" = No; "During the last six months, how often have you used alcohol?" = None; "Have you had a drink of alcohol in the last year?" = No; "Have you had a drink of alcohol in the last month?" = No; "Have you had a drink of alcohol in the last week?" = No; "During the last month, how much did you usually drink at one time?" = Did not drink; and "During the last thirty days, how often have you used alcohol?" = None. Of the 811 total subjects, 63 percent (511) responded consistently to all of the alcohol usage questions with regard to their Stage of Alcohol Acquisition. With regard to their Stage of Cigarette Acquisition, 82 percent (667) of the subjects responded consistently to all of the cigarette usage questions. With regard to their Stage of Smokeless Tobacco Acquisition, 85 percent (687) of the subjects responded consistently to the smokeless tobacco usage questions. With regard to their Stage of Marijuana Acquisition, 92 percent (746) of the subjects responded consistently to the marijuana usage questions. The percent of consistent responses was treated as a measure of construct and concurrent validity.

Discriminant Function Analysis

Additional evidence of concurrent validity was sought through discriminant analysis. Several discriminant function analyses were performed to further confirm that the student responses to the stage placement question for a substance were consistent with the responses to the usage questions for that substance. Thus, the discriminant analyses served as measures of both internal consistency and concurrent validity. These analyses are described in the following section.

Stages of Alcohol Acquisition

A discriminant function analysis was performed on the Stages of Alcohol Acquisition using seven usage items as predictors of membership in four groups. Predictor variables were whether subjects had tried alcohol at least one time, how often they had used alcohol in the last six months, whether they had drunk alcohol in the last year, whether they had drunk alcohol in the last month, whether they had drunk alcohol in the last week, how much alcohol they had consumed at one time in the last month, and how often they had consumed alcohol in the last thirty days. Groups were the Precontemplation, Contemplation, Recontemplation, and Initiation Stages of Alcohol Acquisition. The Action, Maintenance, and Habit Change stages were omitted because each stage contained fewer than seven subjects.

Of the original 811 cases, forty-seven were excluded from the analysis. The reasons for exclusion were missing or out-of-range group codes ($n = 13$), at least one missing discriminating variable ($n = 26$), or both problems ($n = 8$).

Two significant discriminant functions were calculated, with a combined χ^2 ($df = 18$) = 447.40 ($p = 0.0001$). When these discriminant functions were used to classify the subjects, 73 percent of the subjects were correctly classified. After removal of the first function, there was still significant discriminating power, χ^2 ($df = 10$) = 63.40 ($p = 0.0001$). The third discriminant function did not have a significant χ^2 value (see Table 1). The first and second functions accounted for 88.36 and 11.15 percent of the variance respectively. Based on the loading matrix, function one seemed to be related to having drunk alcohol at least once while function two seemed to be related to having drunk alcohol at least once but not having drunk alcohol in the last thirty days. Table 2 contains loading matrix for the Stages of Alcohol discriminant analysis.

Stages of Cigarette Acquisition

A discriminant function analysis was performed on the Stages of Cigarette Acquisition using six usage items as predictors of membership in four groups. Predictor variables were whether subjects had tried cigarettes at least one time, how often they had used cigarettes in the last six months, whether they had used cigarettes in the last year, whether they had used cigarettes in the last month, whether they had used cigarettes in the last week, and how many cigarettes they had consumed at one time in the last month. Groups were the Precontemplation, Contemplation, Recontemplation, and Initiation Stages of Cigarette Acquisition. Again, the Action, Maintenance, and Habit Change Stages of Cigarette Acquisition were omitted because they contained fewer than six subjects.

Of the original 811 cases, thirty-nine were excluded from the analysis. The reasons for exclusion were missing or out-of-range group codes ($n = 17$), at least one missing discriminating variable ($n = 16$), or both problems ($n = 6$).

Table 1. Discriminant Function Analyses for the Modified Stages of Acquisition for Alcohol, Cigarettes, Smokeless Tobacco, and Marijuana

Analysis of Combined Stages of Alcohol Acquisition	χ^2	df	χ^2 Probability	Predictor Items	Percent Correctly Classified
Stages of Alcohol Acquisition (Combined)	447.4	18	<0.01	17, 21, 25, 26, 27, 40	72.88
Stages of Cigarette Acquisition (Combined)	609.66	18	<0.01	18, 22, 30, 28, 29, 39	90.03
Stages of Acquisition (Combined)	653.27	18	<0.01	19, 31, 32, 23, 33	89.81
Stages of Marijuana Acquisition (Combined)	54.05	3	<0.01	24, 34, 36	95.81

Table 2. Loading Matrix for Stages of Alcohol Discriminant Analysis

Item Number	Function 1	Function 2
Q17	0.67	0.52
Q21	-0.25	1
Q25	0.25	0.2
Q26	0.3	-0.37
Q27	-0.19	0.16
Q40	-0.02	-0.41

Q17 — Have you drunk alcohol on at least one occasion?
Q21 — During the last six months, how often have you used alcohol?
Q25 — Have you had a drink of alcohol in the last year?
Q26 — Have you had a drink of alcohol in the last month?
Q27 — Have you had a drink of alcohol in the last week?
Q40 — During the last thirty days, how often have you used alcohol?

A stepwise discriminant function analysis using the Stages of Cigarette Acquisition as the grouping variable found that all six of the predictor variables (significantly ($p = 0.0001$) contributed to the prediction equation. Three significant discriminant functions were calculated, with a combined χ^2 ($df = 18$) = 609.66 ($p = 0.0001$) (see Table 1). When these discriminant functions were used to classify the subjects, 90 percent of the subjects were correctly classified. After removal of the first function, there was still significant discriminating power, χ^2 ($df = 10$) = 122.28 ($p = 0.0001$). After also removing the second function, there was still significant discriminating power, χ^2 ($df = 4$) = 13.51 ($p = 0.009$). Functions one, two, and three accounted for 84 percent, 14.4 percent, and 1.6 percent, respectively. Based on the loading matrix, function one seemed to be related to having tried cigarettes one time which functions two and three seemed to be related to having smoked a cigarette in the last six months and in the last year respectively. Table 3 contains loading matrix for the Stages of Cigarette discriminant analysis.

Stages of Smokeless Tobacco Acquisition

A discriminant function analysis was performed on the Stages of Smokeless Tobacco Acquisition using five usage items as predictors of membership in four groups. Predictor variables were whether subjects had tried smokeless tobacco at least one time, how often they had used smokeless tobacco in the last six months, whether they had used smokeless tobacco in the last year, whether they had used smokeless tobacco in the last month, and whether they had used smokeless

Table 3. Loading Matrix for Stages of Cigarette Discriminant Analysis

Item Number	Function 1	Function 2	Function 3
Q18	0.98	0.13	−0.22
Q22	−0.53	0.63	0.22
Q29	0.17	−0.6	0.11
Q30	0.07	−0.58	−0.12
Q39	−0.37	0.53	0.27
Q28	−0.44	−0.58	0.62

Q18 — Have you smoked your first cigarette?
Q22 — During the last six months, how often have you smoked cigarettes?
Q28 — Have you smoked a cigarette in the last year?
Q29 — Have you smoked a cigarette in the last month?
Q30 — Have you smoked a cigarette in the last week?
Q39 — During the last thirty days, how many cigarettes did you usually smoke?

tobacco in the last week. Groups were the Precontemplation, Contemplation, Recontemplation, and Initiation Stages of Smokeless Tobacco Acquisition. The Action, Maintenance, and Habit Change Stages of Smokeless Tobacco Acquisition were omitted because each stage contained fewer than five subjects.

Of the original 811 cases, twenty-two were excluded from the analysis. The reasons for exclusion were missing or out-of-range group codes ($n = 10$), at least one missing discriminating variable ($n = 9$), or both problems ($n = 3$).

A stepwise discriminant function analysis using the Stages of Smokeless Tobacco Acquisition as the grouping variable found that all five of the predictor variables significantly ($p = 0.0001$) contributed to the prediction equation. Three significant discriminant functions were calculated, with a combined χ^2 ($df = 15$) = 653.27 ($p = 0.0001$) (see Table 1). When significant discriminant functions were used to classify the subjects, 90 percent of the grouped cases were correctly classified. After removal of the first function, there was still significant discriminating power, χ^2 ($df = 8$) = 30.28 ($p = 0.0002$). After also removing the second function, there was still significant discriminating power, χ^2 ($df = 3$) = 13.30 ($p = 0.004$). Function one accounted for 96.9 percent of the variance while functions two and three accounted for 1.7 percent and 1.4 percent of the variance respectively. Based on the loading matrix, function one seemed to be related to having ever tried smokeless tobacco while functions two and three seemed to be related to having used smokeless tobacco in the last week and in the last six months respectively. Table 4 contains loading matrix for the Stages of Smokeless Tobacco discriminant analysis.

Table 4. Loading Matrix for Stages of Smokeless Tobacco Discriminant Analysis

Item Number	Function 1	Function 2	Function 3
Q19	0.8	0.04	0.44
Q23	-0.21	0.04	1.02
Q31	0.43	-0.35	0.08
Q32	-0.32	-0.28	-0.63
Q33	-0.05	0.92	-0.34

Q19 — Have you ever tasted smokeless tobacco (dip or snuff)?
Q23 — During the last six months, how often have you used smokeless tobacco?
Q31 — Have you used smokeless tobacco (dip or snuff) in the last year?
Q32 — Have you used smokeless tobacco (dip or snuff) in the last month?
Q33 — Have you used smokeless tobacco (dip or snuff) in the last week?

Stages of Marijuana Acquisition

A discriminant function analysis was performed on the Stages of Marijuana Acquisition using five usage items as predictors of membership in four groups. Predictor variables were whether subjects had tried marijuana at least one time, how often they had used marijuana in the last six months, whether they had used marijuana in the last year, whether they had used marijuana in the last month, and whether they had used marijuana in the last week. Groups were the Precontemplation and Contemplation Stages of Marijuana Acquisition. The Recontemplation, Initiation, Action, Maintenance, and Habit Change Stages of Marijuana Acquisition were omitted because each stage did not contain at least five subjects.

Of the original 811 cases, twenty-eight were excluded from the analysis. The reasons for exclusion were missing or out-of-range group codes ($n = 7$), at least one missing discriminating variable ($n = 18$), or both problems ($n = 3$). One significant discriminant function was calculated, with a combined χ^2 ($df = 3$) = 54.05 ($p = 0.0001$) (see Table 1). When the significant discriminant function was used to classify the subjects, 96 percent of the grouped cases were correctly classified. This function accounted for 100 percent of the variance. Based on the loading matrix, function one seemed to be related to having ever tried marijuana. Table 5 contains loading matrix for the Modified Stages of Marijuana discriminant analysis.

Stage Placement

A summary of the stage placement for each substance is contained in Table 6. For all substances (alcohol, cigarettes, smokeless tobacco, and marijuana), the

Table 5. Loading Matrix for Stages of Marijuana Discriminant Analysis

Item Number	Function 1
Q24	0.85
Q34	−0.52
Q36	0.38

Q20 — Have you ever smoked marijuana?
Q24 — During the last six months, how often have you used marijuana?
Q34 — Have you used any marijuana in the last year?
Q35 — Have you used any marijuana in the last month?
Q36 — Have you used marijuana in the last week?

Table 6. Stages of Acquisition Frequencies

Stages	Alcohol	Smokeless Tobacco	Cigarettes	Marijuana
Precontemplation 1	283 (61.0%)	332 (71.6%)	375 (80.8%)	434 (93.5%)
Contemplation	9 (1.9%)	11 (2.4%)	6 (1.3%)	2 (0.4%)
Recontemplation	112 (24.1%)	74 (15.9%)	42 (9.1%)	4 (0.9%)
Initiation	38 (8.2%)	24 (5.2%)	18 (3.9%)	2 (0.4%)
Action	2 (0.4%)	2 (0.4%)	1 (0.2%)	0
Maintenance	1 (0.2%)	2 (0.4%)	4 (0.9%)	1 (0.2%)
Habit Change	4 (0.9%)	1 (0.2%)	1 (0.2%)	0
Missing	14 (3.0%)	16 (3.4%)	15 (3.2%)	20 (4.3%)

majority of the subjects were in either the Precontemplation or Recontemplation stage. The limited number of subjects who placed themselves into one of the latter stages of the MoSoA model confounds the analysis and interpretation of the results.

DISCUSSION

There are several issues that need to be addressed that relate to the study. First, there are several limitations of the study. All of the data used in the study are subject to the limitations that are common to all self-report data. The sample used in the study is a convenience sample made up of intact classrooms.

There are several points of discussion related to the instrumentation. First, the evidence of validity for the MoSoA items is better for Cigarettes, Smokeless Tobacco, and Marijuana than it is for Alcohol. For example, one evidence of concurrent validity was sought by using each student's responses to the use items to validate their placement into the MoSoA items. For alcohol, 63 percent of the respondents stage placement was consistent with their responses to the usage items while 82 percent, 85 percent, and 92 percent of the respondents stage placement was consistent with the usage items for cigarettes, smokeless tobacco, and marijuana respectively. This finding was consistent with the percentage of correct reclassification computed as part of the discriminant function analyses for alcohol (73%), cigarettes (90%), smokeless tobacco (90%), and marijuana (96%). This lower reclassification rate for alcohol may indicate a need to further refine the MoSoA alcohol item and/or the alcohol usage items. It is also possible that this finding may be due to greater variance in the responses to the MoSoA alcohol item. However, the responses to the MoSoA smokeless tobacco item are more similar to the MoSoA alcohol item than to the responses to the MoSoA cigarette or marijuana items.

Second, the overwhelming majority of the respondents placed themselves into one of the early stages of the MoSoA model (Precontemplation, Contemplation, Recontemplation). This lack of variance in responses to the MoSoA items substantially limited the ability of any statistical analysis to discriminate between the responses. During the examination of the data, one of the researchers commented that, with this sample, a reclassification percentage similar to that achieved with the discriminant analyses would have been possible by assuming that every respondent was in the Precontemplation stage. This alternative reclassification method would have resulted in reclassification rates of 75 percent for alcohol, 86 percent for cigarettes, 89 percent for smokeless tobacco, and 98 percent for marijuana. This finding appears to be a result of the grade level/age of the subjects and is not likely to be repeated with sample with more variance in their responses to the MoSoA items.

One of the purposes of the study was to explore the viability of the inclusion of a new stage called the Recontemplation stage into the McMOS model proposed by Werch and DiClemente [5]. This stage includes those students who have tried the substance but who do not intend to try it again. In this study, the Recontemplation stage was the second most commonly selected stage for all substances and the majority of subjects who indicated they had tried each substance indicated they did not intend to continue use. For example, 24 percent of the respondents placed themselves into the Recontemplation stage for alcohol. Seventy-one percent of the respondents who indicated they had tried alcohol placed themselves into this stage indicating they did not intend to continue use. This finding indicates there may be a "sub-sample" of adolescents who are in an experimental stage of usage which have not previously been identified and do not have prevention messages targeted to their current decision-making stage. The authors are not familiar with drug education programs which have identified this "sub-sample" and have developed specific prevention messages which reinforce the decision to not continue use of alcohol, cigarettes, smokeless tobacco, or marijuana. If future studies involving the Modified Stages of Acquisition model continue to confirm the existence of such a large percentage of students in the Recontemplation stage, it may indicate a "gap" in the current drug education prevention programming. Students who have tried a particular drug but are not planning to try it again may require a different drug use prevention message than students who may or may not have tried the substance but are planning to initiate use of the drug.

The results of the study indicate that the Modified Stages of Acquisition model may be a useful tool in the planning and implementation of primary prevention drug education programs. The study provides support for the McMOS Model as theorized by Werch and his colleagues [5, 7] and may indicate the need to include an additional stage. When the Precontemplation and Recontemplation stages of the present study are combined, the proportion of students in each of the stages of acquisition for each substance are quite similar to those found by Werch et al. [6] in an earlier study of sixth, seventh, and eighth grade students. Further research with elementary, junior high, and high school aged subjects is needed to examine the differences and similarities of these groups with respect to the Modified Stages of Acquisition model.

Further studies are needed to confirm the findings of the study. These studies should attempt to include subjects who are more varied in their Modified Stages of Acquisition placement and a broader representation of minorities.

REFERENCES

1. L. D. Johnston, P. M. O'Malley, and J. G. Bachman, *Illicit Drug Use, Smoking and Drinking by American High School Student, College Students, and Young Adults: 1975-1987*, U.S. Government Printing Office, Washington, D.C., 1988.

2. L. D. Johnston, P. M. O'Malley, and J. G. Bachman, *National Survey Results on Drug Use from the Monitoring the Future Study, 1975-1993: Volume I, Secondary School Students*, U.S. Government Printing Office, Washington, D.C., 1994.
3. J. O. Prochaska and C. C. DiClemente, Transtheoretical Therapy: Toward a More Integrative Model of Change, *Psychotherapy: Theory, Research and Practice, 20*, pp. 161-173, 1983.
4. J. O. Prochaska and C. C. DiClemente, Stages and Processes of Self-Change of Smoking: Toward an Integrative Model of Change, *Journal of Consulting and Clinical Psychology, 51*, pp. 390-395, 1983.
5. C. E. Werch and C. C. DiClemente, A Multi-Component Stage Model for Matching Drug Prevention Strategies and Messages to Youth Stage of Use, *Health Education Research: Theory and Practice, 9*:1, pp. 37-46, 1994.
6. C. E. Werch, D. Anzalone, E. Castellon-Vogel et al., Factors Associated with Stages of Alcohol Use Among Inner City School Youth, *Journal of School Health, 65*:7, pp. 255-259, 1995.
7. C. E. Werch, B. W. Meers, and J. Farrell, Stages of Drug Use Acquisition among College Students: Implications for the Prevention of Drug Abuse, *Journal of Drug Education, 23*:4, pp. 375-386, 1993.
8. C. C. DiClemente and J. O. Prochaska, Self-Change and Therapy Change of Smoking Behavior: A Comparison of Processes of change in Cessation and Maintenance, *Addictive Behaviors, 7*, pp. 133-142, 1982.
9. J. O. Prochaska, C. C. DiClemente, W. F. Velicer et al., Predicting Change in Smoking Status for Self-Changers, *Addictive Behavior, 10*, pp. 395-406, 1985.
10. C. C. DiClemente and J. O. Prochaska, Processes and Stages of Change: Coping and Competence in Smoking Behavior Change, in *Coping and Substance Abuse*, S. Shiffman and T. A. Willis (eds.), Academic Press, New York, pp. 319-343, 1985.
11. C. C. DiClemente, J. O. Prochaska, and M. Gilbertini, Self-Efficacy and the Stages of Self-Change of Smoking, *Cognitive Therapy and Research, 9*, pp. 181-200, 1985.
12. C. C. DiClemente, J. O. Prochaska, W. F. Velicer et al., The Process of Smoking Cessation: An Analysis of Precontemplation, Contemplation and Preparation Stages of Change, *Journal of Consulting and Clinical Psychology, 59*, pp. 295-304, 1991.
13. J. O. Prochaska and C. C. DiClemente, Stages of Change in the Modification of Problem Behaviors, *Progress in Behavior Modification, 28*, pp. 183-218, 1992.
14. C. C. DiClemente and S. O. Hughes, Stages of Change Profiles in Alcoholism Treatment, *Journal of Substance Abuse, 2*, pp. 217-235, 1990.
15. J. O. Prochaska and C. C. DiClemente, Toward a Comprehensive Model for Change, in *Treating Addictive Behaviors*, W. R. Miller and N. Heather (eds.), Plenum Press, New York, 1986.
16. C. E. Werch and D. Anzalone, Stage Theory and Research on Tobacco, Alcohol, and Other Drug Use, *Journal of Drug Education, 25*:2, pp. 81-98, 1995.
17. J. S. Brook, M. Whiteman, and A. S. Gordon, Stages of Drug Use in Adolescence: Personality, Peer, and Family Correlates, *Developmental Psychology, 19*, pp. 269-277, 1983.

18. D. Kandel, Stages in Adolescent Involvement in Drug Use, *Science, 190,* pp. 912-914, 1975.

Direct reprint requests to:

R. Mark Kelley, Ph.D.
Assistant Professor and
Director of School Health Education Graduate Program
209 Mitchell Hall
University of Wisconsin–LaCrosse
LaCrosse, WI 54601

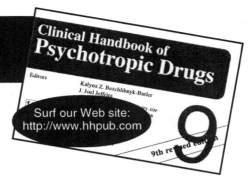

J. DRUG EDUCATION, Vol. 29(3) 205-215, 1999

PEER CLUSTER THEORY AND ADOLESCENT ALCOHOL USE: AN EXPLANATION OF ALCOHOL USE AND A COMPARATIVE ANALYSIS BETWEEN TWO CAUSAL MODELS

CHRISTOPHER D. ROSE, M.A.
Western Kentucky University

ABSTRACT

This study tests the premise of peer cluster theory as it applies to individual alcohol use, and makes a comparative analysis between its ability to explain alcohol use and marijuana use. Using the results of a 1996 drug and alcohol survey of 1312 Western Kentucky University students, path analysis was used to measure the influence of six of peer cluster theory's psychosocial characteristics on the percentage of the respondent's college friends who use alcohol. All of these variables were then regressed on the respondent's alcohol use. The results of the causal models did show some support for peer cluster theory. The direct effect of the student's association with alcohol-using peers on individual alcohol use was shown to have the strongest direct influence on this outcome variable. However, a few limitations of this theoretical perspective were identified. The causal model for alcohol use showed that the indirect influence of two of these psychosocial characteristics (parental attitudes on alcohol use and success in school) was weaker than their direct influence on individual alcohol use. And, the comparative analysis showed that peer cluster theory is better suited to explain the use of marijuana than the use of alcohol.

INTRODUCTION

The following study entailed two objectives. The first objective was to determine if peer cluster theory could explain individual alcohol use. Peer cluster theory proposes that each variable antecedent to an individual's association with alcohol users should only influence individual alcohol use indirectly. In addition, the

205

theory proposes that an individual's association with alcohol users should have not only the strongest direct influence over individual alcohol use, but also the only direct influence [1].

To achieve this first objective, a causal model of alcohol use was established to measure the unique influence of six of Beauvais and Oetting's psychosocial characteristics on an individual's decision to associate with peers who use alcohol and, in turn, the unique influence of each antecedent variable on individual alcohol use. To determine the significance of the findings, path analysis was used as the measure of assessment.

The second objective was to determine if peer cluster theory was better suited to explain the use of illicit drugs (such as marijuana), or the use of licit drugs (such as alcohol). To achieve this second objective, the causal model of alcohol use was compared to a causal model of marijuana use.

METHODS

Sample

A sample of Western Kentucky University's undergraduate student population was established by randomly selecting seventy classes from the total number of undergraduate classes offered during the fall semester of 1996. Of the seventy classes that were selected, a scheduling date for the administration of the survey was set for sixty-three of the classes. Of the seven missed classes, two were no longer meeting as a class and five could not be reached in time to schedule a survey time during the two weeks allowed for data collection.

The researcher administered the surveys to each selected class at the scheduled time of the class meeting, requesting the participation of only those students who had not previously completed a survey. Respondents were guaranteed anonymity and asked to voluntarily fill out a survey concerning several demographics, alcohol and marijuana use among their college friends and family, and their own recent levels of alcohol and marijuana use.

Based on class enrollment, 1838 students were originally selected to participate, but only 1312 of these students actually completed the survey (a completion rate of 71%). Five hundred and twenty-six subjects did not fill out the survey because of absences from class or tardiness to class on the day of data collection. Because of the possibility that some of these students may have missed as a consequence of alcohol or drug abuse, it is possible that the sample underestimates the true levels of drug use on this particular campus. However, it should be recognized that such an underestimation does not necessarily alter the bivariate or partial correlations between variables. To the extent that this is true, an underestimation does not pose a problem for the multivariate analysis.

Independent Measures: Antecedent Variables

The first exogenous variable, *gender,* was operationally defined simply as the respondent's gender: male or female. Because path analysis requires that all variables in the model are measured on either an interval or ratio scale of measurement, a dichotomous variable was created to represent gender. If a respondent reported that he was male, the response was coded as a zero. If a respondent reported that she was a female, her response was coded as a one.

The second exogenous variable, *importance of religion to the family,* was defined with the use of an attitude question. Each respondent was asked, on a scale of 0 to 9, to rate how important religion was to his or her family. A rating of 0 suggested that religion was not important to their family, and a rating of 9 suggested that religion was very important to their family.

The third exogenous variable, *parental attitudes about alcohol use,* was also defined with the use of an attitude question. Each respondent was asked, on a scale of 0 to 9, to rate his or her parents' attitudes concerning the use of alcohol. A rating of 0 suggested that the respondent's parents were strongly opposed to the use of alcohol, and a rating of 9 suggested that the respondent's parents strongly favored the use of alcohol.

The fourth exogenous variable, *number of family members with drug-related problems,* was operationalized as the total number of members within the respondent's family that had drug-related problems. This variable had a potential range from 0 to 10. The fifth exogenous variable, *success in school,* was defined as the approximate cumulative grade average that the respondent reported. The variable included both (+) and (–) letter grades and ranged from a low of F (value of 1) to A+ (value of 13).

The Measures of the First Endogenous Variables: The Intervening Variables

The first endogenous variable to enter the causal model for alcohol use was *peer alcohol use.* In the first model, this endogenous variable was measured according to the percentage of the respondent's college friends who use alcohol at least weekly. To measure this variable, each respondent was asked to report the percentage of his or her college friends that use alcohol at least weekly. The possible responses ranged from 0 percent to 90 percent or more. The coding for the responses to each of these questions was as follows: a code of 0 indicated 0 percent; a code of 1 indicated 10 percent; a code of 2 indicated 20 percent; a code of 3 indicated 30 percent; a code of 4 indicated 40 percent; a code of 5 indicated 50 percent; a code of 6 indicated 60 percent; a code of 7 indicated 70 percent; a code of 8 indicated 80 percent; a code of 9 indicated 90 percent or more.

In the second model, the endogenous variable, *peer marijuana use,* was defined by asking the respondents to report the percentage of his or her college friends that use marijuana at least weekly. The possible responses and codings for this variable were the same as described above.

Dependent Measures: The Outcome Variables

The outcome variable for each model also varied. In the first model, the dependent variable, *subject alcohol use,* was defined as the respondent's reported frequency of alcohol use, ranging from no use in the past year to weekly (or more frequent) use.[1] An index was created to rate alcohol use for each respondent. If a respondent reported that he or she had never used alcohol, a score of 0 was recorded for that respondent's level of alcohol use. If a respondent indicated that he or she had used alcohol once in the last year, a score of 1 was recorded for that respondent's level of alcohol use. For those respondents who indicated that they used alcohol six times within the last year, a score of 6 was recorded for the level of alcohol use. If he or she used alcohol once a month within the last year, the respondent received a score of 12. If a respondent reported that he or she used alcohol twice a month within the last year, a score of 24 was assigned. For those respondents who reported that they had used alcohol either once a week, three times a week, five times a week, or every day within the last year, a score of 52 was assigned.

In the second model, the outcome variable, *subject marijuana use,* was defined as the respondent's reported frequency of marijuana use within the last year. The same scaling weights and recodes used for the causal model of alcohol use were applied to the causal model for marijuana use. For a graphic depiction of the two causal models, see Figures 1 and 2.

RESULTS

Path Analysis: The Alcohol Model

Figure 3 shows the results of the path analysis for the causal model for alcohol use with those path coefficients that were significant at the .01 level of alpha. In this analysis, the outcome variable, *subject alcohol use,* was regressed on the endogenous variable and the five exogenous variables. Table 1 shows the direct, indirect, and total effects of each variable in the first model that were significantly related to *subject alcohol use* ($p < .01$).

Summary of the Causal Model for Alcohol Use

Of all the variables within this causal model for alcohol use, the strongest predictors of individual alcohol use were *peer alcohol use* ($\beta = .52$) and *parental*

---

[1] Although respondents were given the option of indicating whether they used marijuana once a week, three times a week, five times a week, or everyday, these three categories were recoded into one category because of the infrequent responses that fell into the latter three categories.

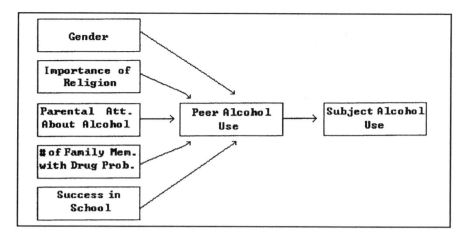

Figure 1. A causal model for alcohol use.

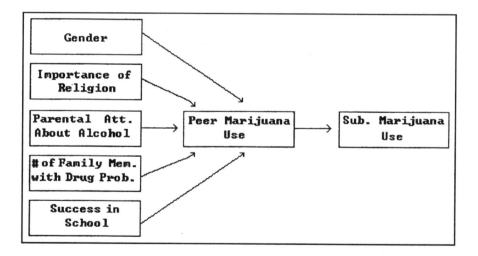

Figure 2. A causal model for marijuana use.

attitudes about alcohol use (total effect = .30). Forty-one percent of the variation in *subject alcohol use* was explained by five of the independent variables (*number of family members with drug-related problems* did not significantly relate), but the majority of this explanation was the result of peer influence. In addition, two exogenous variables were found to not only indirectly affect individual alcohol use but to directly affect it as well. In fact, the direct effects of these

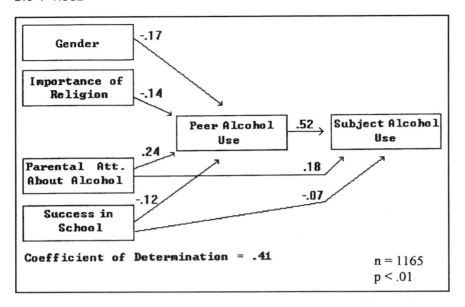

Figure 3. A causal model for alcohol use (analyzed).

Table 1. Direct, Indirect, and Total Effects of Exogenous and
Endogenous Variables on Subject Alcohol Use
(*N* = 1165)

Variables Effect	Direct Effect	Indirect Effect	Total
Gender	—	−.09	−.09
Importance of religion to family	—	−.07	−.07
Parental attitudes about alcohol use	.18	.12	.30
Success in school	−.07	−.06	−.13
Peer alcohol use	.52	—	.52

p < .01

variables were found to have a stronger influence on *subject alcohol use* than the indirect effects of these two exogenous variables.

These results indicate that, in the case of *parental attitudes about alcohol use* and *success in school,* the majority of influence on individual alcohol use was not the result of influence on *peer alcohol use* which is, undoubtably, inconsistent with the perspective of peer cluster theory.

The Comparative Analysis

Figure 4 shows the results of the causal model of marijuana use. The comparison between the causal model of alcohol use and the causal model for marijuana use does indicate that peer cluster theory is better suited to explain individual marijuana use. The causal model for alcohol use shows that two exogenous variables (*parental attitudes about alcohol use* and *success in school*) directly influenced subject alcohol use. In fact, the direct effect of these variables on the outcome variable was stronger than their indirect effect (see Table 2).

On the contrary, the causal model of marijuana use only shows that one exogenous variable (*importance of religion to the family*) has a direct influence on *subject marijuana use.* In addition, it was determined that the direct effect of *importance of religion to the family* on *subject marijuana use* was weaker than its indirect effect.

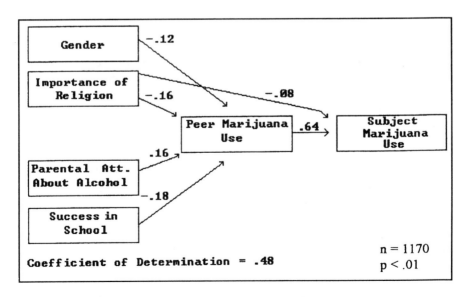

Figure 4. A causal model for marijuana use (analyzed).

Table 2. Direct, Indirect, and Total Effects of Exogenous and
Endogenous Variables on Subject Marijuana Use
($N = 1170$)

Variables Effect	Direct Effect	Indirect Effect	Total
Gender	—	–.08	–.08
Importance of religion to family	–.08	–.10	–.18
Parental attitudes about alcohol use	—	.10	.10
Success in school	—	–.12	–.12
Peer marijuana use	.64	—	.64

$p < .01$

DISCUSSION

The Causal Model for Alcohol Use

Although the analysis of the causal model for alcohol use did show some inconsistencies with the perspective of peer cluster theory, it did provide some support for the proposed theoretical model. The model clearly showed that gender influenced peer associations, with males associating with a higher percentage of frequent alcohol users than females and that gender only influenced individual alcohol use indirectly. The results also indicated that those respondents coming from religious families associated with a smaller number of frequent alcohol users than those respondents coming from a family where religion is of less importance. The model also indicated that religious importance only influenced individual alcohol use indirectly.

However, *parental attitudes about alcohol use* was shown to have a direct impact on the subject's alcohol use, a finding that is contrary to the perspective of peer cluster theory. Even more contradictory, *parental attitudes about alcohol use* was shown to have a stronger direct influence on individual alcohol use than its indirect influence on individual alcohol use, a finding that is inconsistent with the perspective of peer cluster theory [1].

Success in school was also shown to influence peer associations. It was found that those respondents reporting a low grade point average associated with a higher number of frequent alcohol users than those respondents reporting a high grade average, a finding that is consistent with the perspective of peer cluster theory and previous research [2-5]. However, it was also discovered that success in school produced a direct impact on drug use and, in fact, this direct impact was stronger than its indirect impact—a finding that is inconsistent with peer cluster theory.

In Beauvais and Oetting's model a similar finding is also reported [3]. Within their model the indirect effect of *school adjustment* (success in school and liking for school) has a direct influence on individual drug use ($\beta = -.11$). However, within this earlier model the indirect effect of *school adjustment* ($\beta = -.24$) on *drug use* is stronger than its direct effect on this outcome variable. The previous finding may suggest that a broader definition of school adjustment, a definition that includes a precise measurement of "liking for school," may result in findings that are more congruent with the premise of peer cluster theory. The addition of a precise measurement of "liking for school" should be considered if a future model is to be established.

The causal model for alcohol use also showed that *peer alcohol use* was by far the strongest predictor of a respondent's alcohol use, a finding supportive of the perspective of peer cluster theory. In fact, peer use accounts for more than half of the explained variation in individual alcohol use.

Implications of This Study

This study does suggest that peer cluster theory does have the ability to explain individual alcohol use. However, the study also indicates that peer cluster theory may be better suited to explain the use of illicit drugs rather than the use of licit drugs like alcohol. In Beauvais and Oetting's model a much more supportive model of peer cluster theory was produced, but the operational definition of the outcome variable in this earlier model must be considered [3]. In Beauvais and Oetting's model, the outcome variable was defined as one's involvement with the use of alcohol *and* ten other drugs.

Within this study, the outcome variable for the causal model for alcohol use was defined solely on the individual's alcohol use within the last year. The difference in the support provided by Beauvais and Oetting's model and the causal model of alcohol use presented in this study may suggest that peer cluster theory's ability to explain individual drug use may be limited when drug use is defined to include only alcohol use. For peer cluster theory to effectively predict drug use, it may be necessary when defining drug use to include in conjunction with alcohol use those drugs that are defined as illegal substances or illicit forms of drug-related behavior. Support for this suggestion was shown with the analysis of the causal model for marijuana use, which showed that within this study the premise of peer cluster theory was more effective when predicting individual marijuana use.

Based on the differences between these two models, it is suggested that the premise of peer cluster theory may be better suited to explain the use of illicit drugs such as marijuana, cocaine, heroin, d-Lysergic acid diethylamide (LSD), and other drugs that society classifies as excessively deviant. It is likely that if these drug behaviors were regressed on these same psychosocial characteristics, the exogenous variables would only influence these drug behaviors through peer use.

The limitation in peer cluster theory's ability to explain individual alcohol use, as opposed to its more adequate ability to explain illicit drug use, lies in the many different ways that an individual can be exposed to alcohol use and related behaviors. Not all members of American society see the use of alcohol as a deviant act and, therefore, those who use alcohol in moderation are not necessarily seen as deviants. As a result, a child can often be introduced to the use of alcohol by one's parents who participate in a behavior that is defined as socially acceptable. Apart from this introduction, the use of alcohol can also be initially introduced to the individual by the media and advertisement agencies hoping to sell their client's product to the next generation. These advertisements and parental use can often hit the child with the thrills and glories of alcohol use. A possible result may be that an adolescent is not as dependent on peers to introduce and teach the use of a drug to which they have already been introduced and provided with a large variety of diverse teachers.

Marijuana and other illicit forms of drugs (cocaine, heroin, d-Lysergic acid diethylamide, etc.), however, are the drugs that the majority of American society does deem as unacceptable. Because these drugs are deemed as unacceptable, an adolescent is not bombarded with advertisements of and about the use of marijuana use. In fact, these adolescents are bombarded with just the opposite. The media tends to portray these substances as the evils of society, governmental programs declare war on these subscales, and punishments and labels are placed on those who participate in such deviant behaviors. These deviant labels and, sometimes, exaggerations about these substances may force an individual to rely more heavily on his or her peers to introduce the aspects of these deviant drugs and teach them the appropriate behaviors and norms that are associated with its use.

REFERENCES

1. F. Beauvais and E. R. Oetting, Peer Cluster Theory: Drugs and the Adolescent, *Journal of Counseling and Development, 65,* pp. 17-22, 1986.
2. D. Elandt and R. Saltz, College Student Drinking Studies 1976-1985, *Contemporary Drug Problems, 13,* pp. 117-159, 1986.
3. F. Beauvais and E. R. Oetting, Peer Cluster Theory, Socialization Characteristics, and Adolescent Drug Use: A Path Analysis, *Journal of Counseling Psychology, 34,* pp. 205-213, 1987.

4. J. G. Bachman, L. D. Johnston, P. M. O'Malley, and J. Schulenberg, High School Educational Success and Subsequent Substance Use: A Panel Analysis Following Adolescents into Young Adulthood, *Journal of Health and Social Behavior, 35,* pp. 45-62, 1994.
5. C. E. Grenier, A Substance Abuse Survey Analysis of LSU Students: Profiles and Correlates, Spring 1991, *Journal of Adolescent Chemical Dependency, 2,* pp. 93-129, 1993.

Direct reprint requests to:

Christopher D. Rose, M.A.
Department of Sociology
Western Kentucky University
1 Big Red Way
Bowling Green, KY 42101-3576

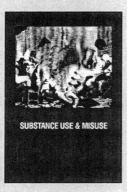

J. DRUG EDUCATION, Vol. 29(3) 217-233, 1999

A QUALITATIVE EXPLORATORY STUDY OF SUBSTANCE ABUSE PREVENTION OUTCOMES IN A HETEROGENEOUS PREVENTION SYSTEM*

JOHN D. CLAPP, PH.D.
San Diego State University

THERESA J. EARLY, PH.D.
The Ohio State University

ABSTRACT

The prevention of abuse of alcohol and other drugs is a concern for parents, policy-makers, educators, and social service professionals. Prevention programs are sponsored by many different types of social and educational agencies using a variety of intervention strategies. This article reports a study of a sample of such programs in the state of Nevada. The overall prevention system in the state espouses a "risk and resiliency" approach to prevention. Focus group methodology was used to study perception of outcomes of these programs from the viewpoints of various program stakeholders (youth participating in the programs, parents of participants and program staff). Analysis of the qualitative data yielded findings about potential outcomes as well as implicit program theories. Implications for future planning efforts as well as further evaluation efforts are discussed.

Problems associated with alcohol, tobacco, and other drugs (ATOD) are among the most serious public health threats in the United States. Current social indicators suggest Nevada residents are in the upper 10 percent nationally for high-risk drinking and smoking behaviors [1]. To address such problems in Nevada, the Nevada Bureau of Alcohol and Drug Abuse (BADA) funds a variety of prevention programs ($N = 62$). Figure 1 presents the BADA-funded programs by

---

*Each author contributed equally to this article.

program type. Approximately 72 percent of these programs target school-aged youth. Programs are funded for one year and receive between $1,600 and $126,000 with the average program receiving $27,585.

To date, the BADA ATOD prevention system has not been evaluated as a whole. Similarly, evaluation of individual programs is rare, and such evaluations vary greatly in their rigor and utility. This situation is compounded by a heterogeneous prevention system. BADA prevention strategy embraces a "risk and resiliency" approach to ATOD prevention that seeks to reduce individual and community risk factors while enhancing factors that protect against ATOD problems. Programs within this system are given great flexibility to develop interventions consistent with this framework. Given this, BADA-funded programs are diverse, using interventions ranging from golf instruction programs to academic tutorials. Additionally, programs within BADA's ATOD prevention system vary greatly in target populations, geographic setting, organizational context, size, duration, and the like. Thus, neither programmatic interventions (independent variables) nor outcomes (dependent variables) are adequately specified for use of traditional summative evaluation methods.

This study sought to identify potential prevention outcomes and activities common to diverse programs within the Nevada ATOD prevention system. In addition, the study hoped to better articulate the types of risk and protective factors targeted within the Nevada ATOD prevention system. Beyond description, the investigators hoped to inform the literature on risk and resiliency programs by identifying a cross-section of prevention activities that may enhance protective factors and/or reduce risk factors related to ATOD problems.

ALCOHOL, TOBACCO, AND OTHER DRUG PREVENTION TARGETING YOUTH

For over a decade, the primary prevention of ATOD problems among youth has received attention from politicians, the public, and health and behavioral

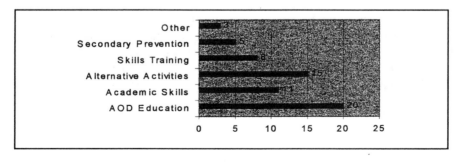

Figure 1. BADA prevention programs by program type.

researchers. Despite this, to date there is inconclusive evidence concerning which approaches to ATOD prevention work. In a critical review of a wide array of ATOD prevention efforts, Moskowitz concluded that, "there is currently little evidence to support the efficacy of primary prevention programs. Although such programs may influence knowledge, beliefs, or attitudes, they generally do not affect behaviors or problems" [2, p. 79]. In contrast, Tobler using meta analytic techniques, found that peer-led programs were successful in reducing alcohol, tobacco, and marijuana use [3]. In addition, Tobler reported that programs using "alternative activity" approaches were effective in changing non-ATOD behaviors like academic performance [3]. When looking solely at ATOD use (self-reported or observed), peer-led programs had the greatest effect size (.42) followed by alternative activity programs (.20). However, Botvin and Botvin reported that alternative activity programs have generally failed to demonstrate efficacy in reducing ATOD use [4]. Further, Botvin and Botvin reported that no prevention approach has demonstrated long lasting effects on ATOD use.

RISK AND RESILIENCY

As noted above, the effectiveness of ATOD prevention efforts is uncertain. A major limitation of many programs is a simplistic conceptualization of the etiology of ATOD problems [5]. Mauss et al. suggested that the risk and resiliency approach to prevention is a promising deviation from more simplistic models [5].

Hawkins, Catalano, and Miller reviewed 140 research articles to identify risk and protective factors associated with ATOD use [6]. Based on their review, the following common risk factors were identified: 1) individual factors including alienation and rebellion; 2) peer factors including peer ATOD use; 3) family factors like cohesion; 4) school factors like academic achievement; 5) community factors including economics and crime; and 6) alcohol and other drug use factors including availability. Factors that protect against ATOD use include: 1) coping skills; 2) parenting skills; 3) school achievement; 4) positive social influences; 5) social skills; and 6) health-related social norms. Thus, both risk and protective factors occur at the individual and environmental levels.

In their book *Communities that Care,* J. David Hawkins and his associates detail the "social development model" that serves as the theoretical foundation for the risk and resiliency approach [7]. Based on social learning theory and control theory, the social development model employs the concept of social bonding to maximize ATOD-related protective factors while reducing risk factors. As Hawkins et al. note, "strong positive bonds have three important components: 1) *attachment*—positive relationships with others; 2) *commitment*—an investment in the future; and 3) *belief* about what is right and wrong, and an orientation to positive, moral behavior and action" [7, p. 14, emphasis in original]. In turn, bonding is a function of opportunities to bond, skills to maintain relationships, and positive reinforcement. Reinforcement occurs both at the individual level by recognizing pro-social behavior and at the community level through norms opposing ATOD use. Thus, intervention must focus on these factors and target multiple levels (i.e., individual, group, and community). As such, strategies include community mobilization, voluntarism, and educational strategies [7].

METHODS

Design and Purpose

The purpose of this exploratory study was to identify potential outcomes of Nevada Bureau of Alcohol and Drug Abuse-sponsored prevention programs as part of an effort to implement evaluation of the prevention system. Further, the investigators hoped to identify programmatic characteristics that may contribute to client outcomes. Thus, the intent was to shed light on both the interventions programs employed (independent variables), and the outcomes programs might produce (dependent variables).

We selected focus group methodology for two reasons. First, focus groups allowed us to interview several programmatic stakeholders in a relatively short period of time. Second, we hoped to ground future quantitative measures in qualitative observations to enhance the validity of future research on this population.

Sample and Respondents

BADA staff purposively selected programs to obtain a cross-section of the types of programs funded as well as regional and urban/rural variation. The strategy resulted in inclusion of five programs: three urban programs in southern Nevada, one urban program in northern Nevada, and one rural program in northern Nevada.

We suggested that BADA staff help programs identify six to ten respondents for each focus group. Staff at each program used purposive or convenience sampling strategies at each selected site. We hoped to interview program staff, clients (aged 12 to 18 years), and parents of clients at each selected site. Unfortunately, we were only able to interview respondents from all these groups at two of the five selected sites. At one site, a snowstorm precluded holding a client or parent focus group. At another site, no parents elected to participate in the focus group or grant consent for their children to participate. Program staff at this site suggested that the parents' reluctance to participate was a function of their residency status; apparently, several of the parents were Mexican nationals living and working in the United States illegally. At a third site, no parents showed up for their scheduled focus group. The staff at this site indicated that the parents were too busy working to attend the focus group. Thus, client, staff, and parent focus groups were held at two sites; client and staff focus groups were held at one site; and staff focus groups were held at two sites. Groups varied in size from three to ten respondents, with an average of five respondents in each group. Subjects participated in the study voluntarily and received no payments for their participation. For four programs, the focus groups were held at the respective program sites. Groups for the fifth program, whose activities took place in a number of different elementary schools, were held at the sponsoring agency.

The focus group interview schedule included an introduction to the project and the following three broad areas: 1) perceived program effects; 2) important aspects of the program; and 3) suggested changes for the program. In addition, in each focus group we asked respondents to briefly describe their programs. The investigators and BADA staff facilitated the focus groups.

We tape recorded and transcribed each focus group. In addition, we took detailed field notes during the focus groups. Field notes were transcribed to word processor files immediately following focus groups and were augmented based on the investigators' recall of the session [8, 9].

Analysis

The analysis plan was designed to maximize consistency and trustworthiness. To this end, one investigator analyzed and coded the transcripts and field notes. Coding focused on emergent themes in the transcripts. The second investigator checked the coding and helped clarify themes. We used journal entries as "audit trails" to document the development of coding procedures.

We used a three phase coding process to analyze the data. First we read the transcripts and took notes on recurrent themes in the data. Based on recurrent themes in the data and the literature concerning risk and resiliency [6, 7], we developed twenty-one codes. We then coded all transcripts and field notes. After the initial coding of the data, we examined our codes and combined conceptually similar or redundant codes. This process yielded seventeen codes. The data were then coded a second time using these refined codes. During the second coding pass, we also examined responses for their analytic meaning.

The first level of analysis of the focus group data was an attempt to detect outcomes that program stakeholders believe are being produced. The logic of most of the interventions was unclear at the start, but as we explored what the participants said, it became clear that there were implicit intervention theories guiding the programs. Thus, the second level of analysis sought to uncover the implicit intervention theories. Both levels of analysis, in theory, could produce testable propositions for future evaluations. A final step in our analysis was to compare the outcome and intervention theory information with writings on risk and resiliency, including the theory of social bonding. This last step is an attempt to determine the extent to which the programs are consistent with the risk and resiliency approach intended by the funding agency.

To ensure trustworthiness, a limited member checking strategy was employed. A report of preliminary findings was generated and distributed to BADA staff for comments. This report contained descriptive analysis using quotes from respondents to illustrate the coding categories. There were no additions or alterations to the preliminary findings.

FINDINGS

The findings of the project to date include descriptions of the programs, descriptions of program outcomes from the various perspectives, and interpretation of the data, which will be presented as mini-"grounded theories."

Program Descriptions

Two of the five programs focused on academic skill building as a means of prevention. One of the programs was an after-school tutoring program administered by a local community center and held in several neighborhood elementary schools. Program recipients were elementary students from low socioeconomic, ethnic minority neighborhoods in Las Vegas. Through this program, students were able to stay after school four days per week to get help with homework, have snacks, and have adult supervision. The other program with a formal academic skills element was at a minimum security juvenile detention camp in rural northern Nevada. BADA funded three components of the comprehensive program. The academic portion of this program focused on enhancing reading and writing skills. Writing assignments added to the therapeutic aspect of the overall rehabilitation program. This program also had two other foci: a family relations intervention and a vocational skills intervention. The family relations portion consisted of working separately with the youth and their parents on understanding each other better, to prepare parents and youth for the youths' return home. Students in the vocational skills portion are able to earn academic credits and learn building trades through a 200-hour vocational course held several afternoons and Saturdays at the camp.

One program used an "alternative activity" intervention of teaching golf skills to adolescents one day per week. This program was administered by an alcohol and drug prevention program in an urban Native American colony in Reno. The target population for this program was not limited to colony members; several participants were Caucasian males and the balance of participants were Native American males and females. Participants contracted not to use alcohol or other drugs, to try to perform well in school, and to not be involved in violence while they were in the golf program.

Another "alternative activity" program in Las Vegas was an educational theater troupe for adolescents. Participants in the theater troupe were ethnically diverse but seemed to be primarily from middle socioeconomic status families. The adolescents participated in writing and performing plays dealing with topics such as substance abuse issues, child abuse, AIDS, and teen suicide. Educational sessions focused on knowledge, attitudes, and behaviors related to similar social problem themes. The plays are performed in a variety of contexts, from schools to youth group homes and detention facilities. The troupe is reformed about every four months with some members continuing and others coming and going. While in the troupe, the youth contract to participate in the educational programs, rehearsals and performances, to avoid alcohol and drugs, and to maintain a C average in school. The youths' parents also contract to allow their teens to participate in the program without preventing participation as a behavioral consequence.

One program, in an elementary school in a predominantly lower income Hispanic area in Las Vegas, used a traditional ATOD prevention curriculum in classroom settings. The curriculum was taught under contract by a community mental health center staff member. Instruction was primarily in English with Spanish as a supplement.

Perceptions of Outcomes

Examining the outcomes that focus group participants described for program participants reveals perceived outcomes that are consistent with enhancing protective factors and reducing risk factors. Overall, the programs had a focus on academic skills and/or achievement. Several of the programs directly targeted academic skills (e.g., helping with writing or English as a second language) and others required maintaining minimum standards of academic achievement as a condition for continued participation in the activity. Two of the programs were directly related to school—the after-school tutoring program staffed by school teachers and the residential juvenile justice facility that included instruction in reading and writing as part of its overall intervention. Even programs with no obvious connection to school, however, such as the program in golf instruction, had the minimum grade average expectation, and respondents reported participants' bringing grades up to meet the expectation.

Several different aspects of school achievement were described as improving for program participants: grades, getting work done, and knowing how to do work. Focus groups from the tutoring program, for instance, reported that children were getting their homework done at the program. Both teachers and parents attributed this outcome to the structure provided and to the presence of teachers The following comments from teachers illustrate this point:

> It's just an availability of time that adults can provide for the children. A lot of the kids, they don't have any adults to go to. Nobody's home, nobody helps them with their homework. And like he was saying, *completion* of homework, feeling better about myself because I actually have someone there to help.

> I think it's the way they feel about themselves, you know, getting that homework done, and they know it's right because if you're there, you're going to check it, and they feel good when they go back to school the next day because everything is all right. So they feel good about themselves and they come back in the next day, they show you exactly what they got on their papers, and they say, "I'm catching on. I know this stuff."

A teacher translated for Spanish-speaking parents who described similarly how their children benefited from the program:

> This parent says that her child is able to come home and is free from homework. She feels relaxed, whereas before she would come home and be pressured when she didn't understand something in the homework and the parent's not able to help them . . . In our school, I'm taking all the newcomers from out of the country, so they don't know any English at all, and since I'm basically the only Spanish teacher in the school, I take these children and I teach them English. [referring to another parent] She's happy because the child has accelerated in the language and has been able to feel more comfortable because the program helps them learn English.

Another important aspect of the changes in academic skills and achievement, evident in the comments above, is that not only were children doing better, they also felt better about themselves both because they got their homework done and because they were learning. The emotional aspect of the changes attributed to the programs was described as improved self-esteem, increased confidence, and pride.

Emotional changes in program participants were described in several focus groups, ranging from the perceived increase in self-esteem described above to learning that anger is okay and feeling increased tolerance of differences among people. Respondents from the tutoring program described children getting along better because the program broke down barriers of grade levels and other groupings. One teacher described the change she saw:

> Many of the students that I'm dealing with are obviously being cognitively stimulated, but more so they're better affectively stimulated, because they're relating with other students and not only at their grade level, and not only necessarily from the same background or experience, so some of their decisions are more informed with respect to dealing with those other students during the normal course of the day. A lot of stereotype barriers have been broken.

Parent, staff, and youth theater troupe respondents also described increased tolerance as an outcome of that program. In the words of the youth:

I've become more sensitive to feelings. I won't openly say something because I think, oh, maybe this has happened to them or maybe their home life is different. You know, we really see another side of the world that we don't see in our own homes or with our friends or something.

There's a lot of education involved. I mean, everybody attacks certain issues with certain preconceived notions and this just dispels them all. It gives you the hard-core facts so you leave here with a certain positive energy, I guess would be a way to describe it, just knowing what you know. And you can use that to help others.

Just being in this group can definitely change any kind of view—you can't look at someone, you can't judge a book by its cover, and everyone always says that, but this group really brings that home, when you go and perform for groups . . . you'll always have one or two of the audience members come up to you and say, "That's exactly what I went through" and they'll be crying or they'll be happy—and you'll feel it, you'll feel what they're feeling, and it's a very good feeling—it empowers you and them.

Parents of theater troupe participants described other aspects of moral development and increased social responsibility as well:

She was very much wanting to get involved in something that had to do with drama and she wanted something to give her some social responsibility, so this was kind of a nice match . . . She looks at situations, she makes her decisions, she makes her choices, she can give you extremely valid reasons for them and she can live with them. She does have a very strong sense of social responsibility.

. . . it's important to have the group to experience things with. It's important to do the presentations as well, the best way to learn is to teach and this has given her the opportunity to provide this information and really open her eyes and raise her potential consciousness and others' consciousness.

Teenagers have so much emotion they don't know what to do with anyway. They can go crazy with it and the group gives them a purpose, you know. You know I heard her talking one-day in her room . . . She was playing this girl that was in a gang and she had a black dress. She had worn this black dress, and she had worn this black dress about twelve times in the last four months. She bought the dress for one girl's funeral and ended up wearing it to like all her friends' funerals that had died in the gang. When I heard her talking, I didn't know it was her. I really thought it was someone else in her room saying this, and I'm standing there listening to her and her voice was cracking. You know, like she was really into it and when she came out she says, "You know, mom, I really thought I'd like to be in a gang but I never thought about people dying." . . . they don't worry about the consequences, but the consequences are there and the group actually brought that out to her.

The affective and behavioral changes regarding increased tolerance are related to social skills. When people are more tolerant of others, they are more likely not only to get along but to have meaningful relationships with others. Strong bonds with others theoretically contribute to a variety of protective factors.

Implicit Program Theories

The preceding section outlined some of the outcomes that stakeholders believe the programs are producing. In this section, we will describe observations based on the focus group data about the mechanisms through which these outcomes may be produced, which Chambers, Wedel, and Rodwell described as program theory: ". . . a rough account of the logic of a social program" [10, p. 107]. What follows is an attempt to glean the implicit intervention theories of the various prevention programs studied. As Chambers et al. noted, specifying program theory is a necessary step in evaluation of social programs, in order to obtain implementation data and interpret evaluation findings. Emergent program theories are presented below for each program.

School-Based Program (Urban)

Conceptually, this program followed a model in which learning English and dealing with emotions lead to acculturation (see Figure 2). Coupled with knowledge about the social and physical dangers of AOD use, this program postulates increased acculturation leads to reduced AOD risk. As one teacher suggested concerning the relationship between acculturation and emotions:

all of them (her students) are of Mexican descent. I don't know if it's part of their culture or their unsureness about sharing . . . But (since the program started) they have come a long way.

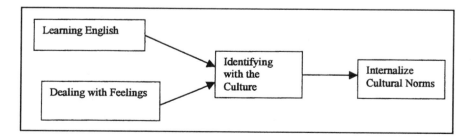

Figure 2. School-based conceptual model.

Further, the prevention staff person for the program noted the children have made a conceptual link between AOD use and emotions:

> The question today was, "If we are suppose to be talking about drugs, why are we talking about feelings?" . . . she raised her hand and said "because when you're feeling sad, people that are sad, there's a bigger chance that they will go into drugs and gangs.

Urban Teen Theater Program

This program tacitly embraced a more complex program model (see Figure 3). Focus group participants indicated that the program has two primary outcomes that are protective factors concerning AOD use—social responsibility and self-esteem/personal confidence. This dual path model is represented in Figure 3. The social responsibility pathway was a very common theme in the focus group interviews:

> We try to make them activists . . . We try to make sure that they leave the group with a real sense of who they are, how they feel about the world and what's going on around them, how they can make a difference. (Staff member)

> I think (child's name) realizes that she has a real responsibility in the community and that she can make a difference. (Parent)

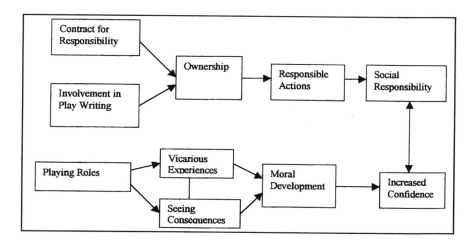

Figure 3. Theater program conceptual model.

> Just being this group can definitely change any type of view—you can't look
> at someone, you can't judge a book by its cover, and everyone always says
> that, but this group really brings that home. (Teen participant)

Role playing is also an important aspect of the program which is conceptually
linked with moral development and increased confidence.

> every night after a performance, you'll always have one or two of the
> audience members come up and say, "that's exactly what I went through" and
> they'll be crying or they'll be happy or—and you feel it, you feel what they
> are feeling, and it's a very good feeling—it empowers you and them. (Teen
> participant)

> But when it comes to alcohol and drugs they get to act it out. They get to act
> out their emotions and get more information about the subject. (Parent)

> I think with the drama, they get to an opportunity to act out, they get to play
> the other side of it, the drug abuser. So they get some insight into that
> experience, um and I think that helps them with their own development. They
> get to pretend the consequences. (Parent)

> This may be a substitute for the titillation of experimentation. (Parent)

After School Tutorial Program (Urban)

This program implicitly hoped to help participants develop stronger bonds with
their school. As Figure 4 illustrates, academic skill building, in concert with
quality time with adults, contribute to greater school bonding in this program
theory. As one teacher suggested:

> The students are willing to try, whereas before they might have felt they
> couldn't do it . . . They feel like you're not just a teacher, you're their friend.

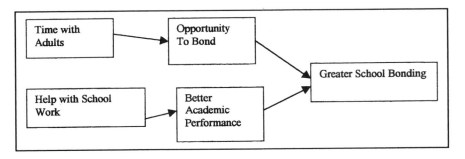

Figure 4. After school program conceptual model.

Similarly, parents stated:

> (translated by teacher) The most positive thing was that they were able to learn English and progress and understand their homeroom teacher a little better and that way they don't feel so left out.

> . . . there is lesser kids so there is more time for the teacher to be one-on-one basis as far as helping them with homework and that kind of stuff. And I work two jobs, so when I get off work, I don't have a lot of time to sit there and say, "Okay, two plus two is whatever" when she already knows that, she gets that at the after-school program.

Golf Instruction Program (Urban)

Of all the programs we studied, the golf instruction program had the least articulated program theory. However, this program did have an implicit theory that suggested that contracting not use AOD combined with athletic skills would result in increased academic performance and social attachment. Figure 5 graphically presents this theory.

> Supporting this tacit conceptual approach, focus group respondents indicated: They are really trying hard (referring to school work), they are really proud of how good they are doing.

> (referring to AOD) It has a lot more motivation for them now than it did because they have grown to love it and look forward to it (golf).

> I think what makes me so excited about the program [is] because I've gotten to know the kids. I'm going to hire a few of them in the spring time. There's a good possibility, I'd say four or five of them have a good chance to play high school golf in the spring, they've come far enough ability-wise.

When asked what the program participants get out of the program besides golf skills, the respondents indicated:

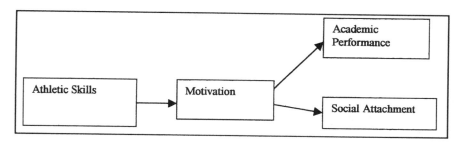

Figure 5. Urban golf program conceptual model.

Responsibility

Commitment

Better grades

I think maturity-wise, too, they've come a long ways. Because out on the course, you do have to behave, it's not a kids' environment, being around adults all the time. They *are* well behaved—their language is good, they're not rowdy. They've come a long way even from the first few times out.

Concentrating, more now than when they started.

Rural Detention Center

This program had a fairly well-articulated program theory that postulated family skills, vocational skills, and academic skills would lead to reduced criminal behavior including AOD use (see Figure 6). As the program staff indicated:

The more successful in writing and comprehension, the more successful they are going to be when they get out there on there own.

The other thing that (staff person's name) presents to the parents is the fact that when Johnny came in, he was like this, and when Johnny leaves he's going to be like this, so that Johnny has a chance, at least allowing to prove himself again as opposed to getting hassled as soon as he walks in the door.

Like I said earlier, these kids are so far behind in credits they need all the schooling they can get. Most of the kids that come here are not college bound,

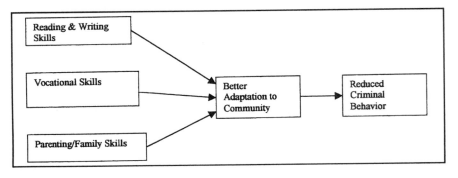

Figure 6. Rural detention center conceptual model.

we know that, we understand that, not that they are not capable of it, it's just somewhere in their life they've never lived up to the expectations and can never get caught up, no matter how long it will take. . . . So that's why we look at vocational technology or the building trades.

We hope we're giving them enough tools that they can get out and, go out and earn the money or go out and *buy* the stereo rather than ripping it out of your car.

DISCUSSION

This study examined the perceived program outcomes of five AOD prevention programs in a heterogeneous prevention system. The prevention system founding these programs embraces a risk and resiliency model based on the work of Hawkins and associates [7]. Data from the present study indicates that, in general, the perceived or potential program outcomes and mini-grounded theories associated with the programs we examined are consistent with this approach. The programs we studied focused on several factors relevant to the risk and resiliency approach—academic skills and bonding, social responsibility, etc.

Despite this, none of the programs we examined implemented a comprehensive risk and resiliency program similar to the one detailed by Hawkins et al. [7]. In fact, one of the key assumptions made by Hawkins and associates is that prevention efforts must be comprehensive and community-based to work. The prevention system in Nevada was broad in scope, but all the elements presented in the risk and resiliency literature are not systematically represented in the Nevada system. Allowing disparate grantees to address single aspects of the risk and resiliency model is probably insufficient to bring about the desired effect. Moreover, the geographic and social diversity of a state, make such an approach suspect.

Beyond the lack of conceptual coherence at the state level, our analysis suggests that most programs cannot clearly articulate their own programmatic theories. When we asked each program to describe their efforts, no program clearly identified a theory of prevention, nor did any program specifically mention "risk and resiliency." The mini-ground theories present earlier emerged from the data and were not clearly specified by program staff or recipients. However, all of the programs could clearly articulate their programmatic activities. Logic models or similar planning models might help program see the link between their interventions and their desired goals more clearly [11].

Our analysis identified selection issues that should be highlighted. Some of the prevention programs studied have target populations that are not high risk, based on risk factors identified in the literature. While it may have broad political appeal to target programs more generally, a risk and resiliency approach is based on identified risk factors determining target populations and identified resiliency factors guiding program interventions. The urban theater troupe, for example, involves primarily youth from middle to upper socioeconomic backgrounds, who are not at particularly high risk for ATOD abuse. Secondarily, the program targets youth who are at greater risk, through the performances in settings such as group homes and detention centers. However, recent shifts in drug use patterns (e.g., heroin use among affluent teens) may indicate a new or previously-undetected at-risk population related to the anomie of higher SES youth. The activities and reported outcomes of this program could be conceptualized as appropriate prevention strategies for this type of ATOD abuse through the groups' meeting the needs of youth for belonging and emotional outlet. This type of role-playing, vicarious experience intervention also is being used in prevention efforts on college campuses across the country.

Wear links also seem to exist between the prevention intervention chosen and the population risk factors. For instance, participants in the golf program are at-risk of ATOD use because of low SES and because of race (for the Native American participants). The resiliency the program intends to build is a positive physical outlet. However, the particular physical outlet chosen may not be available to the participants outside of their participation in this program. Golf is an expensive pastime. Once the youth encounter barriers to continued participation in the sport, gains made in areas of protective factors may be erased or worse yet, the youth may experience greater frustration and loss of self-esteem, leading to increased risk of ATOD abuse.

From a political standpoint, the approach adopted by Nevada may also be problematic. Focusing on risk and protective factors for AOD use and problems is often somewhat removed from actual AOD-related problems. As such, it is often difficult to demonstrate the efficacy or relevance of programs that do not seek to reduce AOD use directly. For instance, a policy maker may be hard pressed to see the relevance of an instructional golf program to AOD prevention. More traditional programs like DARE may be more intuitively appealing to policy makers (regardless of effectiveness) simply because they have face validity. In contrast, risk and resiliency approaches require more conceptual understanding on the part of policy makers and program staff alike.

Finally, we want to reiterate that this study was exploratory in many ways, using focus group methodology in order to obtain wide perspectives on prevention program outcomes. A next step that is needed is using this information to inform more rigorous evaluation of the system to determine the extent to which the programs are producing these outcomes. A more formal evaluation would likely involve taking more direct measures of behavioral, attitudinal, and knowledge changes of participants, using more structured research designs to be able to appropriately attribute observed changes to program activities.

REFERENCES

1. J. Calder, Unpublished data, University of Nevada, Reno, 1996.
2. J. M. Moskowitz, The Primary Prevention of Alcohol Problems: A Critical Review of the Research Literature, *Journal of Studies on Alcohol, 50*:1, pp. 54-88, 1989.
3. N. S. Tobler, Drug Prevention Programs Can Work: Research Findings, *Journal of Addictive Diseases, 11,* pp. 1-28, 1992.
4. G. J. Botvin and E. M. Botvin, School-Based and Community-Based Prevention Approaches, in *Substance Abuse: A Comprehensive Textbook,* J. H. Lowinson, P. Ruiz, R. B. Millman, and J. G. Langrod (eds.), Williams & Wilkins, Baltimore, pp. 910-927, 1992.
5. A. L. Mauss, R. H. Hopkins, R. A. Weisheit, and K. A. Kearney, The Problematic Prospects for Prevention in the Classroom: Should Alcohol Education Programs Be Expected to Reduce Drinking by Youth? *Journal of Studies on Alcohol, 49*:1, pp. 51-60, 1989.
6. J. Hawkins, R. Catalano, and J. Miller, Risk and Protective Factors for Alcohol and Other Drug Problems in Adolescence and Early Adulthood: Implications for Substance Abuse Prevention, *Psychological Bulletin, 112*:1, pp. 64-105, 1992.
7. J. D. Hawkins, R. F. Catalano, and Associates, *Communities That Care,* Jossey-Bass, San Francisco, 1992.
8. R. B. Warren and D. I. Warren, How to Diagnose a Neighborhood, in *Strategies of Community Organization,* F. M. Cox, J. L. Erlich, J. Rothman, and J. Tropman (eds.), F. E. Peacock and Publishers, Itasca, Illinois, pp. 27-40, 1987.
9. H. R. Bernard, *Research Methods in Anthropology: Qualitative and Quantitative Approaches,* Sage, Thousand Oaks, California, pp. 224-229, 1994.
10. D. Chambers, K. Wedel, and M. Rodwell, *Evaluating Social Programs,* Allyn and Bacon, Boston, 1992.
11. R. M. Goodman and A. Wandersman, FORECAST: A Formative Approach to Evaluating Community Coalitions and Community-Based Initiatives, *Journal of Community Psychology,* Special Issue CSAP Monograph Series, pp. 6-25, 1994.

Direct reprint requests to:

Dr. John D. Clapp, Ph.D.
San Diego State University
School of Social Work
San Diego, CA 92182-4119

Progress in Preventing AIDS?
Dogma, Dissent and Innovation
Global Perspectives
Editors: David Buchanan and George Cernada

An exciting new reader highlights recent pivotal articles on global AIDS prevention. This state-of-the-art volume is must reading for social scientists and health and development professionals; and an appropriate text for college students.

Current scientific approaches to assessing preventive needs are examined in its first section. Social and behavioral approaches useful for large-scale field programs are presented in terms of meeting public needs, particularly those of youth and the disenfranchised.

Second, the dissident view: skeptics and dissenters call attention to the politics of AIDS, question the commitment of governments, even the whole idea of progress in AIDS prevention.

A third section highlights innovative community approaches to AIDS education and prevention: involving traditional healers; using drama and songs; community controlled planning.

This work includes many informative and readable contributions by experts from Africa, Asia, Latin America, and North America!

368 pages, Paper, ISBN: 0-89503-176-0
$46.95 + $4.00 postage and handling

Baywood Publishing Company, Inc.
26 Austin Avenue, Amityville, NY 11701
Call (631) 691-1270 • **e-mail:** baywood @baywood.com
Fax (631) 691-1770 • **toll-free Orderline (800) 638-7819**
web site: http://baywood.com

J. DRUG EDUCATION, Vol. 29(3) 235-249, 1999

EXAMINING THE RELATIONSHIP BETWEEN GENDER AND DRUG-USING BEHAVIORS IN ADOLESCENTS: THE USE OF DIAGNOSTIC ASSESSMENTS AND BIOCHEMICAL ANALYSES OF URINE SAMPLES

WILLIAM H. JAMES, PH.D.
University of Washington, Seattle

DAVID D. MOORE, PH.D.
University of Puget Sound

ABSTRACT

The present study examined the relationship between gender and drug-use among adolescents using diagnostic assessments and biochemical analyses of urine samples. The data were collected in the context of a referral and assessment program for adolescents suspected of using drugs, using the Adolescent Substance Battery [1]. A six-month random sample of 20 percent of adolescents assessed for drug use were targeted for biochemical assay. Compliance for urine delivery was relatively high at 91 percent. Urine samples were quantitatively screened for pharmaceuticals using a standard thin-layer chromatography (TLC) technique [2]. Statistical significance was found in the relationship between gender and marijuana use ($p < .05$). This study confirms that gender and drug-using behaviors among adolescents need additional research and evaluation.

INTRODUCTION

There are two major national databases and sources of long-term data on adolescent drug use, the National High School Seniors Survey (NHS) and the National Household Survey on Drug Abuse (NHS), both funded by the National Institute on Drug Abuse. These surveys focus on prevalence—whether or not the adolescents have used or do use alcohol or other drugs—as compared to patterns of use (e.g., experimentation, regular use, bingeing, heavy use, polydrug use). Two

235

measures that can contribute significant information toward understanding the patterns of drug use among adolescents are: 1) self-reported assessments of drug use and 2) urine screening. These two measures are accurate and beneficial clinical procedures that have increased in utilization over the past decade with at-risk adolescent populations [3-17].

The increase in the amount and frequency of overall drug use by adolescents in the past ten years [18, 19] has facilitated the use of self-report assessments and urine screening for school-based prevention and intervention programs. School-communities are now more knowledgeable about the use of self-report assessments and urine testing for diagnosing drug use and informing clinical decisions. This knowledge has led to increasing numbers of adolescent treatment programs using or considering self-report assessments and urine screening for adolescent populations [20]. This study was conducted to examine the relationship between gender and drug-use in adolescents through the use of diagnostic (self-report) assessments and biochemical analyses of urine samples.

The utilization of urine drug screening for assessment purposes has been used for over a decade with adolescent populations [3, 5-12, 14, 15-17, 21-24]. Although there has been an increase in the use of urine screening with adolescents for clinical purposes, there are limited gender-specific findings in the research literature. Gender-specific findings are critical to assisting prevention, intervention, and treatment programs in addressing developmental difference between males and females [25-27]. Dawson analyzed gender differences in the probability of alcohol treatment and utilized interview data from 7,359 adults eighteen years of age and older who met the criteria for alcohol abuse or dependency as specified by the DSM-IV [28]. Gender differences were found as the median interval from onset of disorder to first treatment was between two and three years longer for men than women. Although Dawson's study was not focused exclusively on an adolescent population and the use of drug screening, it did provide comparative data that underscore many of the differences between males and females in treatment. For example, men and women have different median intervals to the initiation of treatment. Other gender differences include factors such as social, work, and legal consequences being less important in influencing the entry of females into treatment. More significant factors for females in structuring treatment programs to meet the disparate gender needs include marital disruption, more alcoholic partners among females, a higher level of emotional distress and comorbid psychiatric symptoms among females, and a greater level of violence and sexual abuse among females [29-33].

The following studies focused on the adolescent population and examined gender-specific differences, and some used urinalysis as a measurement or monitoring tool for drug use. Dembo et al., [4, 34] in a longitudinal study of juvenile detainees, found statistically significant relationships between the youth's demographic characteristics (age, race, and gender), referral history, reason for placement in the detention center, cocaine use (as measured by urinalysis), and recidivism during the twenty-four and thirty months following their initial interviews. The magnitude of these relationships increased with the length of the follow-up period. Thomas describes an adolescent drug treatment program that has attempted to use urinalysis in ways that move beyond the issues of substance use and nonuse [16]. The program is based on the premise that drug use by an adolescent can be adaptive and purposeful in the family system. The program reports that adolescent substance abuse can be a family developmental issue, highlighting issues of separation and individuation. The program advances a treatment condition of systemic change rather than alleviation of the symptoms only and involves members of the family in the treatment process. The neuropsychological effects of chronic marijuana abuse on intelligence and memory of adolescents was examined by Millsaps et al. [35]. Fifteen marijuana-dependent abusers (mean age 16.9 years) were administered the full Wechsler Memory Scale—Revised and the Wechsler Adult Intelligence Scale—Revised (WAIS-R). The subjects had no history of other substance or alcohol abuse or dependence, cerebral trauma, or psychiatric or neurological disorders. They had been abstinent from marijuana for an average of twenty-seven days, verified by urinalysis. Comparisons among intelligence and memory indices revealed significant findings consistent with the pattern produced by cerebral dysfunctioning. Specifically, memory indices were significantly reduced in relation to both intellectual functioning and attentional ability, while intelligence was in the normal range and unchanged relative to the estimated premorbid level. The conclusions were that this profile is a characteristic finding in patients who are recovering from chronic impairment of memory function. Tennant evaluated whether a urine screening technique facilitated the entry of adolescents into treatment [15]. The study analyzed urine samples from 100 consecutive adolescent outpatients (aged 11 to 19 years). A total of 43 percent of the adolescents tested positive for one or more drugs of abuse, 6 percent had two or more drugs in their urine, and 25 percent of those who tested positive entered treatment. Eight percent proved dependent on drugs to the point of requiring medical detoxification or inpatient treatment. Azrin and colleagues evaluated a new behavioral method of treating drug abuse by randomly assigning twenty-six youth (age 13 to 18 years) to either a supportive counseling program or to a newly designed behavioral treatment for six months [36]. The behavioral program was designed to restructure family and peer relations and to control drug use urges. Drug use was measured by urinalysis, supplemented by family report and self-report. During the last month of the program, 9 percent of youth receiving support counseling were abstinent versus 73 percent of youth receiving behavioral treatment. A greater reduction of drug use was confirmed by urinalysis data alone, days per month of drug use, or overall number of months of abstinence. Improved functioning of youths in the behavioral program was shown by greater school/work attendance, youth and parent relationship satisfaction ratings, conduct ratings, decreased depression, and decreased frequency of alcohol use compared with that of youth in the counseling program. Kelleher, Rickert, Hardin, Pope, and Farmer evaluated the effects of early adolescent alcohol use on rural adolescents and found that adolescents from the delta area, especially girls, reported drinking less frequently and in less abusive patterns than did adolescents from other areas, while adolescents from the highland area reported rates and patterns of drinking similar to those of urban adolescents [37]. The purpose of a study by Deykin, Buka, and Zeena was to examine depressive illness among chemically dependent adolescents [38]. Using the National Institute of Mental Health Diagnostic Interview Schedule, the researchers interviewed 223 adolescents who were in residential treatment for alcohol or drug dependence. The results of the study indicated that only female gender, paternal psychopathology, and victimization (physical abuse, sexual abuse) emerged as important variables associated with depression.

METHOD

Subjects

A census district sample framework for randomly selected schools was supplied by Olympic Counseling Services. Group homes and juvenile detention facilities were not included in the sample. A school was defined as grades six through twelve. Adolescents were regarded as ineligible for the study if they were not able to complete the survey. A total of thirty-seven urban, suburban, and rural schools were included in the census. Of these, thirteen were high schools and twenty-four were middle schools. The thirty-seven schools enrolled 32,747 students aged eleven to nineteen years old. Of these, 16,804 (51%) were high school students. The remaining 15,943 (49%) students were middle school students. Census data showed the study sample to be approximately representative of students living in the Pacific Northwest. Of these, 1,637 were assessed for suspected drug use, including 654 middle school students (40%) and 983 high school students (60%). A random 20 percent of the assessed adolescents were targeted for urine sample collection. A total of 296 urine samples were collected, representing 18 percent of the total sample and 90 percent of participants targeted for urine collection. Urine sample results were deleted from the analysis where matching assessment data could not be found, leaving a final sample size of 296.

Measurement: The Adolescent Substance Battery

Chemical dependency specialists interviewed the adolescents referred for an evaluation and provided a diagnostic assessment for each individual using the Adolescent Substance Battery [1]. Each participant was administered the Adolescent Substance Battery developed to quantify the level of drug impairment experienced by the adolescent and the level of treatment needed. This battery included a structured interview that was designed to provide additional diagnostic information on substance use problems. Substance abuse and chemical dependency diagnoses were based on criteria in the Diagnostic and Statistical Manual, Fourth Edition (DSM-IV) published by the American Psychiatric Association [39]. Two psychometric instruments were used as part of the battery to evaluate defensiveness. The battery took approximately ninety minutes to administer based on a reading level of grade six or higher. The battery sequence was: Confidentiality of Records Agreement, Confidential Intake Questionnaire, Client Substance Index, Psychological Screening Inventory, and a Student Assistance Evaluation form where the diagnosis is noted. The components described below were used in a sequential manner with each participant.

Confidentiality of Student Records

The confidentiality of the adolescent's records is protected by Federal laws and regulations (42 C.F.R., Part 2) and the information may not be disclosed unless; the patient consents in writing, the disclosure is allowed by court order, the disclosure is made to medical personnel in a medical emergency, the disclosure is to qualified personnel for research, audit, or program evaluation, or the adolescent commits or threatens to commit a crime either at the program or against any person who works for the program. Violation of the Federal laws and regulations governing confidentiality is a crime and suspected violations may be reported to the United States Attorney in the district where the violation occurs. Federal laws and regulations do not protect any information about suspected child abuse or neglect from being reported under Washington State law to appropriate state or local authorities. This information was reviewed with each participant to insure that they understood the confidentiality requirements.

Confidential Intake Questionnaire

The Confidential Intake Questionnaire described the confidentiality of the adolescent's record and the procedure for appeal and review. After this review, the specialist asked each participant to read and sign a confidentiality statement. The structured interview began with the Confidential Intake Questionnaire. The specialist reviewed the answers on this instrument for approximately fifteen minutes and used an active listening question-answer modality. If the adolescent indicates that others are to blame for their problem, they are not confronted about discrepancies in attitudes, or drug-using behaviors. This allows for the development of trust and empathy so that the adolescent can safely ventilate fear, frustration, and other emotions. The specialist makes clarifying notations directly on the Questionnaire and fills in questions that the adolescent left blank. The specialist also notes the types of denial throughout the interview that may include basic denial (discrepancies and contradictions), minimizing (quantities of drug use or other experiences vary), and rationalizing (using excuses and blaming others). The adolescent completes the paper-and-pencil Confidential Intake Questionnaire that is designed to provide basic descriptive information on gender, race/nationality, age, school attendance, source of referral, reason for taking evaluation, and insurance or payment plan. The questionnaire also gathers information on counseling needs, educational background and status, employment history, medical condition and family history with alcohol and other drugs, residential status, legal issues such as arrests and probation, family relationships and support, thoughts and feelings such as anger, withdrawal, attitudes and habits, and a confidential section on sexually transmitted diseases.

Psychological Screening Inventory

The psychological screening inventory is administered to the adolescent and it is an instrument designed to measure alienation, social nonconformity, discomfort, expression, and defensiveness. High scores in any of these areas results in an increased awareness of factors in the adolescent's life that are related to the area of concern.

Client Substance Index

The specialist then moves to the thirty-minute Client Substance Index (CSI), a paper-and-pencil instrument that measures substance use history. The CSI is completed by the adolescent. A blank page is used as a note-taking page for the specialist to fill in the school grade where significant substance use began. The specialist places the CSI next to the blank page and notes on the page the type of substance used and the amount of use for each grade and summer period. For each section of the CSI, the specialist reflectively listens to the answer and notes responses on the history page. The questions on the Client Substance Index are designed to measure attitudes and activities concerning drug use. The adolescent is asked about each drug they have used or tried, their age when they tried the drug, and frequency of use. At the end of this substance history, two potential evaluations may result. One is a specific diagnosis: (no significant problem, misuse, abuse, or chemical dependency), and the other is a deferred diagnosis due to client defensiveness.

Specific diagnosis—No significant problem: This is a diagnostic evaluation where there are no signs and symptoms of alcohol or other drug use. Experimentation with alcohol and other drugs may be a part of this category. *Misuse:* A diagnostic evaluation where intoxication and impairment occurs because of the use of alcohol or other drugs. *Abuse:* A diagnostic evaluation where use of alcohol and other drugs may be continuous, episodic/binges, or disease in remission. *Chemical dependency:* A diagnostic evaluation where dependency on alcohol or other drugs is continuous, episodic/binges, or disease in remission.

*Deferred diagnosis—*A diagnostic evaluation where defenses do not allow a diagnosis. Defensiveness may indicate misuse, abuse, chemical dependency, or other issues which place the adolescent at risk. An extended evaluation period is used to monitor individuals with this diagnosis as they are placed in an ongoing abstinence monitoring, counseling, and reassessment program.

Measurement: Biochemical Analyses of Urine Samples

The utilization of urine drug screening for adolescents provides information that is beneficial for diagnostic purposes. Urine screening has an important purpose as a diagnostic tool to assist in evaluating drug use. In the case of adolescents who are using illicit drugs, urine screening reveals the levels of use of drugs such as marijuana, cocaine, amphetamines, opiates, phencyclidines, and over-the-counter drugs that include cough medicines with codeine, morphine, and other narcotics. Urine screens are also extremely valuable as a clinical treatment tool. The optimal use of urine screens and self-report measures provide an understanding of the amount and frequency of drug use. All urine samples were screened for pharmaceuticals using a standard thin-layer chromatography (TLC) technique. Positive findings were confirmed by two-dimensional TLC and gas-liquid chromatography (GLC). These procedures facilitated the detection of the metabolites or unchanged forms of a large number of drugs including barbiturates, opiates, benzodiazepines, and cocaine.

The use of urine drug screening technology is efficient, timely, and costs between \$15 and \$25 per individual depending on the number of drugs screened and the need for confirmation testing. Urine screening is conducted according to the manufacturer's instruction for the type of screening assays. The screening is designed to detect and quantify a drug's primary metabolite with some cross reactivity to its minor metabolites, in a range between its 95 percent sensitivity level and upper limits chosen for the drug. Ranges for drug metabolites are as follows: amphetamines, 50 ng/ml to 3000 ng/ml; cannabinoids (THC), 50 ng/ml to 750 ng/ml; cocaine, 300 ng/ml to 5000 ng/ml; phencyclidine (PCP), 5 to 500 ng/ml; opioids, 40 to 1000 ng/ml; and ethanol concentrations range from 10 to 300 ng/ml. Quantitative values provide some indication of the level and timing of marijuana use when urine samples are collected. The quantitative values are influenced by many factors, such as frequency and duration of use, purity of the drug, and individual metabolism. The higher the value, the more likely that the use of the drug has been heavy and/or recent. Low values correlate with light use or heavy use prior to the urine collection. Levels that are moderate are best interpreted in relationship to previous results or reliable data on usage history. Urine concentrations above the upper thresholds are indicative of marijuana dependency or binge use while lower concentrations normally suggest low use or an attempt to cut down or withdraw. Urine screens are done for diagnostic and clinical purposes in treatment programs and are not typically confirmed by other screening technology unless requested by the parents, the school, or the program.

Analysis of Data

For the purpose of statistical analyses, a Mann-Whitney U-Test was conducted using the urinalysis level of marijuana use as the ordinal variable and gender as the nominal or independent (female, male) variable. The criteria used for deciding on marijuana to be used in the data analysis was that it was detected in the urine samples of 84 percent of subjects testing positive for drug use. For cannabinoids, three levels of marijuana use were examined: low use, below 100 ng/ml; moderate use, between 100 and 250 ng/ml; and high use, above 250 and up to 750 ng/ml. The independent variable considered for this specific analysis was gender. This allowed observation of whether or not gender can explain an adolescent's level of marijuana use. The .05 statistical level of significance was used for all comparisons. A Chi-Square analysis was conducted using diagnostic levels of drug use as the dependent variable and gender as the independent variable. The diagnostic categories included three categories of drug use; misuse, abuse, and chemical dependency. These categories are based on the findings of the Adolescent Substance Battery.

RESULTS

Urinalysis results for the sample are presented in Table 1. A total of 106 adolescents, or 36 percent of the sample tested positive for drug use. Of these, a total of eighty-nine adolescents or 84 percent tested positive for marijuana use as indicated in Table 2.

Table 3 provides a breakout of the numbers and percent of adolescents testing positive for marijuana use. The majority were living with both parents and the second largest group were living with mother. Nearly three quarters of the adolescents were males and the overall group was generally equally distributed under age sixteen and over sixteen years of age. Three out of four adolescents testing positive for marijuana use were European Americans with the rest fairly distributed among ethnic minority populations. Two-thirds of the adolescents were in grades eight through ten.

The levels of marijuana use at the time of the urinalysis testing are provided in Table 4 and the majority are at the lower end below 100 ng/ml, followed by moderate and high levels.

Table 1. Urinalysis Results

Urinalysis Results	Number	Percent
Negative	190	64
Positive	106	36
Total	296	100

Table 2. Drugs Used by Adolescents Who Tested Positive

Drugs Used	Number	Percent
Amphetamines	1	1
Benzodiazepines	1	1
Marijuana (THC)	89	84
Multi-Screens (Drugs)	10	9
Opiates	5	5
Total	106	100

Table 3. The Number and Percent of Adolescents Testing
Positive for Marijuana Use

Variable	*n*	Percent
Living Situation		
Both parents	49	55
Mother	23	26
Father	4	5
Friends	2	2
Foster/group home	3	4
Other	8	8
Gender		
Male	65	73
Female	24	27
Age		
<16	48	54
>16	41	46
Ethnicity		
African American	2	2
Asian American	3	3
European American	67	75
Hispanic American	1	1
Native American	6	6
Multiethnic	4	5
Other	6	8
Grade Level		
6	3	3
7	10	11
8	22	25
9	14	16
10	30	33
11	7	8
12	3	4

The diagnoses of the marijuana users are provided in Table 5 and about two-thirds are chemically dependent followed by about one-quarter of the adolescents diagnosed as substance abusers.

The THC mean levels of use for males and females are provided in Table 6. The mean level of marijuana use for females was 115.27 compared to 205.09 for males. The difference between the means was not significantly significant.

The results of the Mann-Whitney test are outlined in Table 7. Statistical significance was found in the relationship of gender and level of marijuana use, rejecting the null hypothesis. The independent variable of gender showed significance in relation to the difference between the two mean ranks, at the .05 level as shown.

Table 4. Marijuana Use by Levels of Use

Level of Use	Number	Percent
Low (below 100 ng/ml)	50	56
Moderate (100-250 ng/ml)	22	25
High (above 250 ng/ml)	17	19
Total	89	100

Table 5. Diagnoses of Marijuana Users

Diagnosis	Number	Percent
Chemically dependent	57	64
Substance abuser	20	23
Substance misuser	9	10
No significant problem	3	3
Total	89	100

Table 6. Marijuana Means of Males and Females

	Mean	Standard Deviation	Minimum Level	Maximum Level
Males	115.27	153.03	20	738
Females	205.09	221.20	24	750

Table 7. Mann-Whitney U-Wilcoxon Rank Sum W Test of THC by Gender
*Corrected for Ties

Mean Rank	Cases	U	W	Z	2-Tailed p
34.77	22 Females	512.0	765	–2.1825	.0291
47.12	67 Males				

DISCUSSION

The results show that generally males are more likely to smoke marijuana than females. There are gender role expectations that influence the attitude of adolescents' toward drug use and these attitudes can be an important influence on adolescent behavior. Downs suggested that adolescents have not relinquished the traditional gender-related double standard [40]. Gender role socialization of males and female adolescents is very likely to influence their attitudes and behaviors toward drug use. Traditional gender role socialization may lead to differences regarding the limits of acceptable behavior for females as compared to males. In general, females are socialized toward relationships and dependence while males are socialized toward isolation and independence. Males are often encouraged to experiment and take risks regarding drug use. Also, males are encouraged to "be a man" and deny fear and underestimate personal risk such a driving under the influence of drugs or getting drunk at a party. Females are often discouraged toward taking risks and using drugs. In addition, females are expected to have higher moral and behavioral standards and not be drinking and driving or consuming large quantities of drugs. For example, males are often responsible for the transportation in dating or party situations and are more likely to be driving during evening and weekend hours.

Johnston, O'Malley, and Bachman reported that the percentage of male and female adolescents who consume alcohol or marijuana does not differ significantly [41]. However, there appear to be more male daily marijuana users than female daily users among the adolescent population. Male problem marijuana users exhibit greater levels of uncontrolled impulsive behavior, sensitivity to feedback on behavior, overemphasis on masculinity, and difficulty maintaining personal relationships. Male users have more problems with denial, alienation, social nonconformity, discomfort, expression, and defensiveness [42], and have more legal problems.

CONCLUSION

More recent population surveys on the use of marijuana by adolescents provide data that underscore increased use and a strong resurgence that began in the early

1990s. According to Johnston, O'Malley, and Bachman [18], the annual prevalence (i.e., the proportion reporting any use in the 12 months prior to the survey) rate for marijuana use among eighth-graders had increased from 6 percent in 1991 to 16 percent in 1995, for tenth-graders had increased from 15 percent in 1991 to 29 percent in 1995, and among twelfth-graders had increased from 22 percent in 1992 to 35 percent in 1995. These researchers report that nearly one in twenty (4.6%) of high school seniors is a current daily marijuana user. These results are supported by the National Household Survey on Drug Abuse population survey that indicated significant increases between 1993 and 1994 in the lifetime, past year, and past-month prevalence of marijuana use among adolescents age twelve to seventeen. The Survey reports that the percentage of youth (age 12 to 17) using marijuana has been steadily increasing since 1992, with past-month use nearly doubling between 1992 and 1994. Among adolescents age twelve to seventeen in 1994, about 16 percent reported ever using marijuana, 14 percent reported using marijuana in the past year, and 7 percent reported using marijuana in the past month [19]. The increase in marijuana use by adolescents in the past seven years has fostered the utilization of urine drug screening for intervention and treatment programs. Schools and communities are now more knowledgeable concerning the implementation of urine testing as a means of confirming abstinence or continued drug use and making clinical decisions about intervention and gender-specific needs of adolescents who are using marijuana. Thus, a variety of programs are now using or contemplating urine screening for adolescent populations [20].

REFERENCES

1. W. James and D. Moore, The Adolescent Substance Battery: Clinical Diagnoses and Student Assistance Program-Case Management for Adolescents Using Drugs, *Journal of Child and Adolescent Substance Abuse, 3*:2, pp. 45-57, 1994.
2. Comprehensive Toxicology Services, *Drug Detection Guide,* Tacoma, Washington, personal communication, June 18, 1996.
3. H. Amaro, B. Zuckerman, and H. Cabral, Drug Use Among Adolescent Mothers: Profile of Risk, *Pediatrics, 84*:1, pp. 144-151, 1989.
4. R. Dembo, L. Williams, J. Schmeidler, and C. Christensen, Recidivism in a Cohort of Juvenile Detainees: A $3^1/_2$-Year Follow-Up, *International Journal of the Addictions, 28*:7, pp. 631-658, 1993.
5. T. Feucht, R. Stephens, and M. Walker, Drug Use Among Juvenile Arrestees: A Comparison of Self-Report, Urinalysis and Hair Assay, *Journal of Drug Issues, 24,* pp. 99-116, 1994.
6. J. Hall, S. Henggeler, M. Felice, T. Reynoso, N. Williams, and R. Sheets, Adolescent Substance Abuse during Pregnancy, *Journal of Pediatric Psychology, 18*:2, pp. 265-271, 1993.

7. L. Hancock, D. Hennrikus, D. Henry, and R. Sanson-Fisher, Agreement between Two Measures of Drug Use in a Low-Prevalence Population, *Addictive Behaviors, 16,* pp. 507-516, 1991.

8. D. Huttenbach, Adolescent Urine Drug Screening, A Cobb County Medical Society Program, *Journal of the Medical Association of Georgia, 76*:12, pp. 833-837, 1987.

9. B. Jenks, Re: Adolescent Urine Drug Screening (letter), *Journal of the Medical Association of Georgia, 77*:5, p. 285, 1988.

10. P. Kokotailo, H. Adger, A. Duggan, J. Repke, and A. Joffe, Cigarette, Alcohol, and Other Drug Use by School-Age Pregnant Adolescents: Prevalence, Detection, and Associated Risk Factors, *Pediatrics, 90*:3, pp. 328-334, 1992.

11. P. Kokotailo, R. Langhough, N. Cox, S. Davidson, and M. Fleming, Cigarette, Alcohol and Other Drug Use among Small City Pregnant Adolescents, *Journal of Adolescent Health, 15*:5, pp. 366-373, 1994.

12. D. McBride and J. Inciardi, The Focused Offender Disposition Program: Philosophy, Procedures, and Preliminary Findings, *Journal of Drug Issues, 23,* pp. 143-160, 1993.

13. F. Tennant and J. Shannon, Quantitative Urine Testing: A New Tool in Diagnosis and Beating Cocaine Abuse, *Postgraduate Medicine, 86,* pp. 107-114, 1989.

14. F. Tennant, Quantitative Urine Levels of Abusable Drugs for Clinical Purposes, *Clinics in Laboratory Medicine, 10,* pp. 301-308, 1990.

15. F. Tennant, Urine Drug Screening on Adolescents on Request of Parents, *Journal of Child and Adolescent Substance Abuse, 3*:3, pp. 75-81, 1994.

16. F. Thomas, Q. Quinn, B. Kuehl, and A. Neal, The Strategic Use of Urinalysis in the Treatment of Adolescents in Family Therapy, *Journal of Strategic and Systemic Therapies, 6,* pp. 1-11, 1987.

17. J. Valentine and E. Komorski, Use of a Visual Panel Detection Method for Drugs of Abuse: Clinical and Laboratory Experience with Children and Adolescents, *Journal of Pediatrics, 126*:1, pp. 135-140, 1995.

18. L. Johnston, P. O'Malley, and J. Bachman, *National Survey Results on Drug Use from The Monitoring The Future Study, 1975-1995. Volume I, Secondary School Students,* The University of Michigan, Institute for Social Research. National Institute on Drug Abuse. U.S. Department of Health and Human Services. Public Health Service. National Institutes of Health, 1996.

19. National Institute on Drug Abuse, *National Household Survey on Drug Abuse,* U.S. Department of Health and Human Services, U.S. Government Printing Office, Washington, D.C., 1985.

20. T. Brock, Urine Drug Screens in Adolescent Programs, in *Adolescent Substance Abuse: Etiology, Treatment, and Prevention,* Aspen Publishers, Inc., Gaithersburg, Maryland, pp. 207-218, 1992.

21. B. Finkle, Drug Analysis Technology: Overview and State of the Art, *Clinical Chemistry, 33,* pp. 13-18, 1987.

22. A. Saxon, D. Caslyn, V. Haver, and C. Delaney, Clinical Evaluation and Use of Urine Screening for Drug Abuse, *Western Journal of Medicine, 149,* pp. 296-303, 1988.

23. R. Schwartz, P. Cohen, and G. Bail, Identifying and Coping with a Drug-Using Adolescent: Some Guidelines for Pediatricians and Parents, *Pediatric Review, 7,* pp. 133-139, 1985.

24. D. Smith, M. Gutgesell, R. Schwartz, M. Thorne, and S. Bogema, Federal Guidelines for Marijuana Screening Should Have Lower Cut-Off Levels. A Comparison of Results from Immunoassay and Gas Chromatography-Mass Spectrometry, *Archives of Pathology and Laboratory Medicine, 113*, pp. 1299-1300, 1989.

25. N. Cobb, *Adolescence: Continuity, Change, and Diversity,* Mayfield Publishing Company, Mountain View, California, 1995.

26. E. Erikson, *Identity, Youth, and Crisis,* Norton, New York, 1968.

27. C. Gilligan, Adolescent Development Reconsidered, in *Mapping the Moral Domain,* C. Gilligan, J. Ward, J. Taylor, and B. Bardige (eds.), Harvard University Press, Cambridge, Massachusetts, 1988.

28. D. Dawson, Gender Differences in the Probability of Alcohol Treatment, *Journal of Substance Abuse, 8*:2, pp. 211-225, 1996.

29. S. Blume, Women and Alcohol: A Review, *Journal of the American Medical Association, 256*, pp. 1467-1470, 1986.

30. E. Gomberg, Alcoholic Women in Treatment: New Research, *Substance Abuse, 12*, pp. 6-12, 1991.

31. B. Thom, Sex Differences in Help-Seeking for Alcohol Problems: Entry into Treatment, *British Journal of Addiction, 82*, pp. 989-997, 1987.

32. J. Wallen, A Comparison of Male and Female Clients in Substance Abuse Treatment, *Journal of Substance Abuse Treatment, 9*, pp. 243-248, 1992.

33. C. Weisner, The Alcohol Treatment-Seeking Process from a Problem Perspective: Responses to Events, *British Journal of Addiction, 85*, pp. 561-569, 1990.

34. R. Dembo, L. Williams, J. Schmeidler, A. Getreu, E. Berry, L. Genung, E. Wish, and C. Christensen, Recidivism among High Risk Youths: A $2^1/2$ Year Follow-Up of a Cohort of Juvenile Detainees, *International Journal of the Addictions, 26*:11, pp. 1197-1221, 1991.

35. C. Millsaps, R. Azrin, and W. Mittenberg, Neuropsychological Effects of Chronic Cannabis Use on the Memory and Intelligence of Adolescents, *Journal of Child and Adolescent Substance Abuse, 3*:1, pp. 47-55, 1994.

36. N. Azrin, B. Donohue, V. Besalel, E. Kogan et al., Youth Drug Abuse Treatment: A Controlled Outcome Study, *Journal of Child and Adolescent Substance Abuse, 3*:3, pp. 1-16, 1994.

37. K. Kelleher, V. Rickert, B. Hardin, S. Pope, and F. Farmer, Rurality and Gender: Effects of Early Adolescent Alcohol Use, *American Journal of Diseases of Children, 146*:3, pp. 317-322, 1992.

38. E. Deykin, S. Buka, and T. Zeena, Depressive Illness Among Chemically Dependent Adolescents, *American Journal of Psychiatry, 149*:10, pp. 1341-1347, 1992.

39. American Psychiatric Association, *Diagnostic and Statistical Manual (DSM-IV),* Washington, D.C., 1994.

40. W. Downs, Using Panel Data to Examine Sex Differences in Causal Relationships Among Adolescent Use, Norms, and Peer Alcohol Use, *Journal of Youth and Adolescence, 14*:6, pp. 469-486, 1985.

41. L. Johnston, P. O'Malley, and J. Bachman, *Drug Use Among American High School Seniors, College Students, and Young Adults, 1975-1990: High School Seniors,* DHHS Publication No. (ADM) 91-1813, U.S. Government Printing Office, Washington, D.C., 1991.

42. W. James and H. Lonzak, The Role of Denial and Defensiveness in Adolescent Substance Use, *Journal of Child and Adolescent Substance Abuse,* 5:2, pp. 17-41, 1996.

Direct reprint requests to:

William H. James, Ph.D.
Research Associate Professor
Box 353600
University of Washington State
Seattle, WA 98195-3600

FOCUS ON ALCOHOL

Edited by SEYMOUR EISEMAN

PRIMARY ORIENTATION: **prevention of drug misuse**
A must for the drug educator

To adequately address and deal with the detrimental effects of alcohol, attempts must be made to learn and understand the motivations and attitudes which contribute to its use and misuse.

This essential collection represents a psychosocial perspective of the effects of alcohol while providing relatively unknown—but central research needed for a comprehensive understanding of the behaviors associated with alcohol use.

Table of Contents

Format: 6' x 9", 272 pages, Paper, ISBN: 0-89503-083-7

Price: $35.95 + $4.00 postage and handling

Baywood Publishing Company, Inc.

26 Austin Avenue, Amityville, NY 11701
call (516) 691-1270 **fax** (516) 691-1770 **orderline** (800) 638-7819
e-mail: baywood@baywood.com ● **web site:** http://baywood.com

J. DRUG EDUCATION, Vol. 29(3) 251-278, 1999

SOCIAL SKILLS, COMPETENCE, AND DRUG REFUSAL EFFICACY AS PREDICTORS OF ADOLESCENT ALCOHOL USE*[†]

LAWRENCE M. SCHEIER

GILBERT J. BOTVIN

TRACY DIAZ

KENNETH W. GRIFFIN

Cornell University Medical College

ABSTRACT

Numerous alcohol and drug abuse prevention trials have included social resistance training as a strategy for reducing early-stage adolescent alcohol use. Evaluations of these trials has shown them to be moderately effective, although the precise impact of the resistance training in comparison to other programmatic features has not been clearly identified. The current study examined the extent to which assertiveness and related social skills, personal competence (perceived cognitive mastery), and refusal efficacy predict alcohol involvement. Males were at greater risk for poor refusal skills and reported higher alcohol involvement. Cross-sectionally, youth characterized by poor social skill development reported lower refusal efficacy, lower grades, poor competence, and more alcohol use. Poor refusal efficacy was associated with more risk-taking, lower grades, less competence, and more alcohol use. Longitudinally, both poor refusal skills and risk-taking were associated with higher alcohol use. High personal competence was associated with lower alcohol use in both the eighth and tenth grades, but had no long-term effects on alcohol use. Findings highlight the close interplay between perceived competence and refusal skill efficacy, both of which should be included as essential components of school-based prevention strategies.

*Funding for this project was provided by the National Institute on Drug Abuse (P50DA-7656) and (R29-DA08909-01).

†Portions of these data were presented in May 1997 at the annual meeting of the Society for Prevention Research, Baltimore, Maryland.

Many school-based drug abuse prevention programs teach drug refusal skills as an effective means of countering peer and related pressures to use alcohol and other drugs [1-4]. The conceptual basis for social resistance skills programs rests heavily on the claim that youth require the confidence to refuse offers to drink alcohol and that teaching drug refusal and related social skills will bolster adolescents' ability to refuse explicit offers and peer pressure to drink. Specific features of resistance skills programs include teaching youth effective techniques to recognize explicit offers for alcohol, practicing refusal skills techniques (i.e., role playing), and developing cognitive scripts that can be invoked in situations where resistance skills would be effective. According to Botvin, "the main objective of resistance skills training is to provide adolescents with a repertoire of verbal and nonverbal skills that they can call on when confronted by peer pressure to use drugs in a variety of situations" [3, p. 32].

Although programs that utilize a social resistance skills approach have been shown to be effective for deterring the use of tobacco [5-7], alcohol and marijuana [8], it remains unclear as to which facet of the social skills training is most efficacious. In some cases, programs rely on general social skills training and confidence building [4], whereas other programs focus specifically on drug refusal skills as the most effective means of reducing consumption [9-11]. To better understand the potential efficacy of these prevention trials as well as move forward in the explanation of alcohol etiology, it is important to understand how much variation in consumption can be attributed to deficits in social skills (e.g., assertiveness) versus how much is determined by drug-specific resistance skills.

FINDINGS FROM SCHOOL-BASED DRUG ABUSE PREVENTION TRIALS

Over the past few years, several prevention studies have attempted to discern the relative effectiveness of different intervention components. Hansen and his colleagues, for example, conducted a program evaluation to determine the relative efficacy of a social resistance curriculum and an affective education model, the latter which emphasized inadequate coping skills and poor internal resources (i.e., low self-esteem) as determinants of early-stage drug use [10]. However, in the social curriculum a total of two out of twelve teaching modules included information directly related to social skills resistance training (a third module taught students to actively role play peer resistance techniques in front of adults). The remaining curriculum components included specific instruction on normative expectations (i.e., perceived drug use by peers and adults), motivations for and consequences of drug use, friendship formation (maintaining positive relations), and an assortment of strategies indirectly related to resistance skills (e.g., recognizing and resisting media and environmental influences). The eclectic nature of the social skills intervention makes it difficult to discern the relative effectiveness of this approach.

In a separate study, Hansen and Graham identified one prevention program in a comparative evaluation as Resistance Training, albeit four lessons (of a total of 9) focused on the consequences of using substances [9]. Information about the consequences of substance use could potentially boost the effects of the resistance training by increasing motivation to refuse drugs. In particular, the acquisition of information regarding negative consequences may provide a sound rationale for refusing peer advances to engage in behavior that is considered unhealthful. Because of the close developmental interplay between many of the instructional skills, it is difficult, in these and related studies, to disentangle the precise role that resistance skills training plays in contrast to other key program components that may directly influence behavioral consumption.[1]

RELATIONS OF SOCIAL AND PERSONAL COMPETENCE TO ALCOHOL USE

In contrast to social learning models of early-stage drug use, multi-modal or "generic" prevention programs emphasize the acquisition of social and personal competence as an effective means of deterring early-stage drug use [1-3]. The primary aim of these programs is to target an array of etiologic factors that are both directly and indirectly related to drug use in an effort to reduce risk and enhance protection. A core feature of competence enhancement programs is the view that vulnerability is comprised of a wide range of intrapersonal (e.g., coping skills) and interpersonal characteristics (e.g., social skills) that influence susceptibility to peer pressure. Accordingly, improvement in one area of functioning is likely to foster increased resilience in developmentally related areas of functioning [3]. For example, one of the hypothesized benefits of social skills/social competence training is to boost self-esteem and self-confidence, which has a positive impact on other related domains of functioning (i.e., increasing drug-specific refusal efficacy). Additional features of generic intervention strategies include practicing general assertiveness skills, as well as helping youth to acquire effective strategies to initiate social encounters with peers. Armed with greater confidence in their social skills, youth are likely to refuse offers to use alcohol and other drugs.

---

[1] Interestingly, Hansen and Graham [11] and Donaldson et al. [12] showed that programs emphasizing resistance skills training may have positively influenced skill development, but did not significantly reduce drug use. Although these researchers attribute the absence of this substantial and important relationship to invalid program theory, we theorize that other intrinsic "developmental" and motivational factors may influence the linkage between resistance skills and consumption. It is also important to note, as we have demonstrated with the use of the current data, that both etiology and prevention studies rely on similar methodologies that permit examination of the specific long-term developmental relations between skills and behavior.

THEORETICAL UNDERPINNINGS TO COMPETENCE ENHANCEMENT PROGRAMS

Bandura's model of personal efficacy and behavior change provides a general theoretical background for understanding the relationship between competence (i.e., cognitive skill appraisal), refusal efficacy, and behavior [13, 14]. According to Bandura, self-efficacy is the "conviction that one can successfully execute the behavior required to produce the outcomes" [14, p. 193]. In contrast to the more global constructs of self-esteem and self-concept, self-efficacy is part of a specific symbolic organization consisting of representations (i.e., cognitive schemata) that capture previous performance episodes and link these performance evaluations to perceived beneficial outcomes. When the outcomes repeatedly occur and result from personal effort and persistence, a cognitively mediated motivational framework is established linking effort, behavior, and response outcome to the self (i.e., cognitive expectation or efficacy expectation). Bandura further suggested that "reinforcement operations affect behavior largely by creating expectations that behaving in a certain way will produce anticipated benefits or avert future difficulties" [14, p. 193]. Positive performance outcomes that are based on mastery experiences are more likely to promote high efficacy expectancies that should generalize across many behavioral tasks (i.e., stimulus generalization), whereas negative outcomes are more likely to generate avoidance coping (i.e., dysfunctional behavior).

Self-efficacy is directly tied to skills and the perception of competence to actualize these skills. In its broadest interpretation, competence is generally regarded as the ability "to generate and coordinate flexible, adaptive responses to demands and to generate and capitalize on opportunities in the environment" [15, p. 80]. Social competence includes the ability and motivation to navigate challenging interpersonal situations and is often considered a prerequisite for adequate social relations. According to Pentz, the targeted skills in social competence prevention strategies includes ". . . both the cognitions associated with confidence and perceived mastery of social skills . . ." [4, p. 118]. Although social competence is considered by many to be multi-faceted and includes a broad range of interpersonal skills [16], an essential focus of these programs includes general assertiveness (disagreeing, making requests, confrontational skills), peer-specific assertiveness (e.g., dealing with a wide range of pressures from peers), and assertiveness for resisting peer pressure to use drugs.

In general, whether adolescents are with their immediate family or with peers, successful adjustment hinges on the focal youths' ability to direct questions to people, talk in front of a group, present information to a gathering of people, and express their opinions and dissatisfactions in potentially conflictual situations. Moreover, a growing body of developmental research has shown that in the early stages of adolescence, superior school performance, peer relations, and optimal mental health adjustment essentially hinge on successful acquisition and implementation of those skills [17-21]. Shy and rejected youth tend to avoid confrontational situations, fail to assert themselves properly, and get bullied, which may lead to a sense of perceived loss of control, depression, and other negative sequelae [22, 23]. Assertive youth, on the other hand, draw upon their interpersonal mastery to navigate difficult and stressful social situations and avoid some of the difficulties faced by their non-assertive counterparts. The perception of social competence helps youth to manage conflict, reduce anxiety, and provide confidence that is applied toward future situations.

A second distinguishing feature of generic, competence-based prevention approaches is a focus on personal skills and self-management strategies that can also effectively mitigate motivations to use drugs [3, 24]. Personal competence regards the ability to make effective decisions (including goal setting), implement self-management strategies to control anxiety (i.e., self-statements), maintain a sense of control in situations that require planning and mastery, and perceive self-confidence when problem-solving. In light of a growing body of research that shows strong predictive relations between competence and later mental health adjustment [25], we hypothesize that competent youth are more masterful (i.e., better able to execute a task), less motivated to engage in risky behavior, are less susceptible to negative social influences from peers and the media, and are more likely to either flatly refuse active drug offers or utilize assertive skills to defuse a confrontational situation.

OVERVIEW OF THE CURRENT STUDY

In the current study, we examine the long-term influences on alcohol consumption of both social resistance skills and social skills, the latter of which included measures of assertiveness, (lack of) social confidence, social confrontation, and social comfort.[2] In addition, controlling for prior alcohol use, as well as risk associated both with poor social skills and poor refusal efficacy, we also tested the predictive capability of personal competence skills (i.e., academic esteem, self-reinforcement, problem-solving confidence, and personal control [cognitive mastery]), which have also been linked to the onset of early-stage alcohol use [3, 24, 27]. To better understand the developmental and structural linkages between these skills and behavior and to avoid any bias associated with known program effects, we utilized a nontreatment cohort of youth participating in a school-based, drug abuse prevention trial. The use of a control cohort enabled

---

[2] The theoretical basis for the inclusion of these measures of psychosocial functioning in the prevention curriculum includes both Bandura's self-efficacy [13, 14] and Jessor and Jessor's problem behavior theory [26]. More complete descriptions of the rationale for inclusion of these and related measures as well as information pertaining to a series of program evaluations of the Life Skills Training intervention and its ability to reduce both alcohol and general drug consumption can be found in Botvin et al. [27-29].

us to examine the basic structural relations between skills (both social and drug refusal) and alcohol use unfettered by the intervention.

Annual assessments in the school-based drug abuse prevention trial were conducted between seventh (pretest) and twelfth grade and the current sample is drawn from the first and third annual follow-up conducted in the eighth and tenth grades.[3] One important motivation for using data obtained from this age group is the heightened vulnerability associated with this age period. The transitional period between the eighth and tenth grade is a period of major reorganization of the self-system, with concomitant changes in perceived cognitive [31], social [32], and physical competence [33]. This is also a period that coincides with changes in peer group composition and peer relations [34, 35], highlighting the importance of social competence to successful adjustment. Along these lines, self-efficacy theory holds that an important vehicle for transmission and acquisition of response outcomes is vicarious or direct modeling. Either by observation or through active participation, youth acquire insight into the basic rewards and contingencies that accompany various pro- and antisocial activities. During the early stages of adolescence, a primary source of observational learning is peer friendship networks, which gain in stature and respective importance for decision-making and social comparison.

In addition to these conceptual issues, we relied on a risk factor methodology to assess deficits in social competence. Newcomb has suggested that cumulative risk indices that include multiple risk factors are more efficient predictors of consumption, particularly given the diverse array of etiological determinants of alcohol and drug use [36]. In the current study, additive risk indices of poor social competence and poor refusal skills were constructed by summing across binary indicators of risk status (these methods are more fully described below). The risk indices are then used to predict concurrent and subsequent personal competence and alcohol use.

We also included a measure of risk-taking in an effort to model the influence of ineffective social reward systems and personality differences that may alternatively cause both alcohol use and poor competence. Evidence is accruing of moderate to strong relations of sensation-seeking (impulsivity, risk-taking, and unconventionality) as a correlate or causal determinant of alcohol consumption among younger aged populations [37-39]. In particular, youth characterized as risk-taking may take greater social risks and, as a result, increase their exposure

---

[3] The eighth grade assessment was included as our baseline for primarily two reasons. First, base rates for alcohol consumption in the seventh grade are extremely low (only 58% reported some use of alcohol) and the corresponding distributional properties (skewness and kurtosis) for the behavioral measures may strain the robustness of the estimation procedures. By the eighth grade, there was a higher mean level of consumption (2.62 vs. 2.05 for the frequency measures), more behavioral variability existed, and evidence of nonnormality was considerably reduced (skewness and kurtosis were reduced threefold). In addition, the use of the eighth grade cohort also permitted meaningful comparisons with epidemiological data obtained from a nationally representative sample of youth [30].

to antisocial behavior. The self-derogation model proposed by Kaplan and his colleagues [40] suggests that poor social controls and lack of ties to conventional institutions foster deviant subgroup bonding. Associations with a more deviant peer group introduces new behavioral standards (i.e., high risk-taking and drug use) that reflect the interests of disenfranchised youth. The effect of the deviant peer group is to subvert opportunities to acquire skills that are obtained either vicariously (observational learning) or directly via modeling in classroom situations. The effect of diminished learning opportunities is to reduce personal and social competence.

In addition to modeling these important covariates, a dummy-coded measure of gender (males = 1 and females = 0) was included at baseline to control for socialization influences. Rates of consumption differ even at this early age with males reporting higher rates of alcohol consumption as well as more intense drinking. It is important to specify socialization processes in a developmental model to account for possible gender-based differences. Finally, we included a measure of self-reported grades in the model to account for differential survey completion rates (grades are a proxy for reading comprehension). Consistent with the transition into middle school, grades and related academic concerns become more prominent foci, underscoring the importance of controlling for academic concerns [41], which may influence perceived competence.

METHOD

Sample Description

Data for the current study were obtained as part of a five-year investigation conducted between 1985 and 1991, which was designed to study the etiology and prevention of tobacco, alcohol, and other illicit drug abuse. Details of this study, implementation protocols, and findings related to the preventive intervention have been reported extensively elsewhere [27, 29, 42] and only a few key features are noted here. The parent study included fifty-six public schools and was conducted at three suburban sites including central and eastern upstate New York and Long Island. These areas present a mixture of rural, suburban, and urban locations, are predominantly (91%) White, and middle-class. Beginning with the seventh grade (Time 1) and annually thereafter students responded to one of three randomly administered, closed-ended, group-administered, self-report paper and pencil questionnaires. Students were assured of the confidentiality of their responses in writing (both on the parental consent form and the questionnaire itself), verbally at the time of administration, and through a Certificate of Confidentiality from the Department of Health and Human Services. Passive consent procedures were used and less than 1 percent of the total sample included in the investigation refused participation. Tracking of students at the different assessment points was accomplished using unique identification codes lithocoded onto questionnaires. Items included in the survey assessed a variety of psychosocial attitudinal, behavioral, and interpersonal domains related to alcohol, tobacco, and marijuana use.

Measures for the present study were obtained in the first annual posttest administered in the eighth grade (Time 3), and a subsequent follow-up data collection conducted in the tenth grade (Time 5). Two cohorts of data were available for this study, one collected annually in the fall and one collected shortly thereafter in the spring. Given the identical nature of the questionnaires, we combined these samples for the analyses.

ALCOHOL, COMPETENCE, AND SOCIAL SKILL MEASURES

The modeling procedures were conducted using the EQS structural equations modeling program [43]. Observed indicators were constrained to load on one latent construct and for the measurement portion of the analyses, factor variances were fixed at unity. Multiple-indicator, latent constructs of alcohol and competence were hypothesized at both the eighth and tenth grades, whereas the remaining measures were constructed as observed variables. Indicators of alcohol involvement included frequency of alcohol use (i.e., "how often, if ever, do you drink alcoholic beverages?"), quantity (e.g., "how much, if at all, do you usually drink each time you drink?"), and drunkenness ("how often, if ever, do you get drunk?"). Responses for the alcohol frequency item ranged from "never tried them" (1) to "more than once a day" (9); for the drinking quantity item ranged from "I don't drink" (1) to "more than 6 drinks" (6); and for the drunkenness item ranged from "I don't drink" (1) to "more than once a day" (9).

PERSONAL COMPETENCE

A latent construct of Personal Competence was reflected by four observed indicators tapping personal control in learning environments (i.e., cognitive mastery), self-reinforcement, academic esteem, and problem-solving confidence. Five items to tap personal control were taken from the thirty-item Paulhus Spheres of Control (SOC) battery [44]. Based on prior exploratory factor analyses, Paulhus obtained a ten-item subscale tapping personal efficacy and provided support for the empirical validity of this scale using confirmatory procedures. In the current study, an abridged set of five items (highest factor loadings) had reliabilities of .77 and .81, respectively, for the eighth and tenth grades. Sample items included "The things I achieve are due to my hard work and ability" and "I can learn almost anything if I set my mind to it." Responses ranged from "strongly agree" (1) through "strongly disagree" (5).

Six items to tap academic esteem were taken from the Janis and Field Feelings of Inadequacy Scale (FIS) [45]. Fleming and Watts [46] reported that a rotated factor solution for the full set of FIS items included dimensions tapping both academic (i.e., school abilities: $\alpha = .77$) and non-academic components of self-esteem (i.e., self-regard). Based on the analyses of those authors, we created a six-item scale to assess (lack of) confidence about scholastic abilities, including self-evaluations regarding understanding school assignments ("I have trouble understanding things that are given for reading assignments") and academic concern ("When I have to write a paper or do a reading assignment, I get kind of worried about it" and "I find it difficult to express my ideas in writing"). Three additional items tapped perceived academic confidence including "I find it hard to take tests in school," "I sometimes feel that teachers are picking on me," and "I have gotten pretty good grades during the past year" [reversed in scoring]. Responses for these items were rated on a 5-point scale ranging from "strongly disagree" (1) through "strongly agree" (5), resulting in higher scores indicative of lower academic esteem. Coefficient alphas were .65 and .66, respectively, in the eighth and tenth grades.

Six items to tap problem-solving confidence were taken from the Heppner and Petersen thirty-five-item Problem Solving Inventory [PSI: 47]. The PSI was originally factor analyzed by Heppner and Petersen using exploratory methods (principal components with varimax rotation) and an eleven-item scale ($\alpha = .85$) obtained tapping confidence in handling applied problems. Seven of the items with the highest loadings are used in the current study. Sample items included "I have the ability to solve most problems even though at first it looks as if there's no solution," and "With enough time, I think I can solve most problems that come up." Responses for these seven items ranged from "strongly disagree" (1) through "strongly agree" (5). Coefficient alphas were .79 and .83, respectively, for the eighth and tenth grades.

Nine items from the Heiby [48] thirty-item Frequency of Self-Reinforcement Attitudes Questionnaires were used to assess a general response set of self-reward strategies. According to Heiby, self-reinforcement is "the process of establishing and controlling overt and covert positive consequences of one's own behavior" [48, p. 1304]. Individuals with low frequency of self-reinforcement (FSR) will be characteristically low in self-confidence and self-esteem as part of their response set due primarily to the unpredictable nature of external sources of reinforcement. Heiby presents extensive criterion, face validity (interrater reliability), and reliability data (both split-half and test-retest) supporting the utility of a measure of self-reinforcement. From the original pool of thirty items, nine items were chosen with face validity for adolescent populations and used in the current study. Sample items included "When I succeed at small things, I become encouraged to go on," and "The way I achieve my goals is by rewarding myself every step along the way." Responses for those items ranged from "strongly disagree" (1) through "strongly agree" (5). Coefficient alphas were .84 and .86, respectively, for the eighth and tenth grades.

ASSESSMENT OF SOCIAL COMPETENCE

Sixteen items assessing frequency of interpersonal assertiveness were taken from the forty-item Gambrill and Richey Assertion Inventory [49]. Wills, Botvin, and Baker demonstrated the factorial validity and scale integrity of a reduced set of items and provided evidence of moderate relations to alcohol and drug use in an adolescent sample [50]. Sample items assessed the frequency (probability) of social assertiveness (e.g., "How often do you . . . start a conversation with someone you don't know" and "ask someone out for a date") and general assertion related to the defense of rights (e.g., "How often do you . . . express an opinion even though others may disagree with you" and "tell people when you think they have done something that is unfair"). Responses ranged from "never" (1) through "almost always" (5). In the current sample, internal consistency (coefficient alpha) was, respectively, .79 for the eighth and tenth grades.

Nine items assessing degree of nervousness in social situations (i.e., social comfort) were taken from the Richardson and Tasto [51] 166-item Social Reaction Inventory (SRI). Items in the SRI assess the verbal-cognitive component of anxiety in the domain of social relationships. Richardson and Tasto used principal axes factoring methods to derive seven domains including a set of items tapping social assertiveness (interactions) and visibility (expressing opinions and defense of rights). A common stem ("How nervous would you feel . . .") preceded each item and sample items included ". . . giving a speech before a group of strangers," and ". . . feeling like you are the center of attention in a group." Coefficient alphas were .88 and .89, respectively, for the eighth and tenth grade samples. Responses ranged from "not at all nervous" (1) through "very nervous" (5).

Four additional items assessing social confrontation and anger expression were also taken from the Social Reaction Inventory. These items are typically considered part of the general domain of social assertiveness but because of their specificity to anger feelings, may reflect a conceptually distinct facet of social assertiveness. Using the same stem as the nine-item social assertiveness scale, sample items included, "How nervous would you feel . . . telling someone you know that you are angry with him [her]," and ". . . if you tell someone who is embarrassing you to stop." A response format identical to the social assertiveness items was used with the social confrontation items. Based on the current data, coefficient alphas were .81 and .85, respectively, for the eighth and tenth grades.

Social (interpersonal) concern was assessed by an eight-item scale taken from the Janis and Field FIS. Based on a subset of the original FIS scale items, Fleming and Watts provided factor analytic evidence (direct oblimin rotation of principal components analysis) of a dimension of "social confidence" including items assessing self-consciousness (e.g., "I often worry about what other people think of me"), social shyness (e.g., "I find it hard to start a conversation when I meet new people"), and interpersonal concern (e.g., "I worry about whether other people like to be with me"). Responses for these items ranged from "strongly disagree" (1) through "strongly agree" (5) [46]. In the current study, coefficient alphas were .81 and .82, respectively, for the eight and tenth grades.

A thirteen-item scale was used to assess degree of confidence in social situations. A common stem ("How confident you are that you could do well in the following situations . . .") preceded each question (i.e., ". . . asking questions to avoid a misunderstanding," ". . . ending a conversation with friends without offending them," and ". . . making requests or asking favors"). Responses ranged from "not at all confident" (1) through "very confident" (5). Adequate psychometric properties and statistical relations with drug consumption measures have been demonstrated empirically and are reported elsewhere [42]. For the current study, internal consistency was .87 and .89, respectively, for the eighth and tenth grades.

The five scales assessing social competence were used to form an additive risk index. Each individual measure was dichotomized using an upper (or lower) quartile cut-point to determine risk status. Youth reporting infrequent assertiveness, high social concern, low social comfort, poor confrontational skills, and lacking confidence in their social skills were assigned a "1," whereas the remaining students in the distribution were given a "0." The resultant binary scales were then summed into a single additive index of social competence risk, with scores ranging from 0 to 5. Higher scores on this index are indicative of greater risk for poor social competence.

Refusal skills were assessed using a three-item scale. The three items (i.e., "refusing a cigarette offered by a friend" ["not at all confident" (1) to "very confident" (5)]; "say no when someone tries to get you to drink," and "say no when someone tries to get you to smoke" ["never" (1) to "almost always" (5)]) were averaged and the resultant composite dichotomized according to a risk-factor methodology. Students in the lower quartile of the composite were assigned a "1" to designate poor refusal skills (low confidence and infrequent skill implementation) and the remaining students not regarded as high-risk were assigned a "0." Coefficient alpha for the three-item refusal skills scale was .74 both for the eighth and tenth grades.

Several analyses were conducted to establish if there was behavior specificity for the alcohol and cigarette refusal items. First chi-square proportion tests were used to examine if there was a statistical overlap in the students reporting any alcohol experience who also reported some use of cigarettes (both behavioral measures were dichotomized to create measures of "use/nonuse"). Among youth reporting some use of alcohol, 41.4 percent reported experience with cigarettes and 64.8 percent reported they currently smoke (from at least a few times/year through a pack or more each day). This suggests that adolescents who use alcohol do so in combination with other drugs. The observed overlap in substances comports with epidemiological evidence from adolescent populations that underscores patterns of multisubstance use particularly involving cigarettes and alcohol [52]. In the current study, the generality of the drug-specific refusal skill items also was observed in the pattern of bivariate associations between the cigarette refusal items and alcohol consumption (average $r = -.37$), the alcohol refusal item and alcohol use ($r = -.64$), the smoking refusal items and smoking behavior ($r = -.41$). and the alcohol refusal item and smoking behavior ($r = -.37$). These relations reveal a pattern of shared variance between cigarette-specific skills and alcohol use and likewise between alcohol-specific skills and cigarette use. Based on this evidence, all three refusal items were included as an indicator of refusal skills efficacy (given the risk methodology used, high scores on the refusal skills measure indicate greater risk for poor refusal skills).

Finally, seven items taken from the Eysenck Personality Inventory were used to assess risk-taking [53]. This brief measure of risk-taking assesses a proclivity toward dangerous behaviors, excitement, and impulsivity. Sample items included "I get bored more easily than most people" and "I would do almost anything for a dare." Responses ranged from "strongly disagree" (1) through "strongly agree" (5) and in the current study coefficient alpha was .75 for both the eighth and tenth grades.

RESULTS

A total of 974 students were available for the longitudinal path analyses (8th grade: 51.4% male, mean age = 13, $SD = .51$). Not all of the students were able to finish the questionnaire in the allotted time period and we augmented missing data using the Expectation-Maximization (EM) algorithm. Based on statistical theorems proposed by Little and Rubin [54] and Rubin [55], multiple imputation methods can be used to augment missing data utilizing a maximum-likelihood estimation procedure that iteratively "fills in" missing data with predicted scores based on complete data [56, 57]. In contrast to both listwise deletion, an extremely restrictive procedure that would eliminate a large portion of usable data, and mean substitution which artificially inflates the kurtose (and produces biased estimates), EM procedures utilize full regression methods to produce unbiased estimates of model parameters [56]. Analyses showed that 61 percent of the cases had complete data, of the remaining cases 5 percent had at most one missing variable, and 6 percent had two missing; average number of missing values was five out of nineteen variables included in the analyses. Inspection of the sixty-six missing data patterns revealed these data were missing completely at random and satisfied the conditions for multiple imputation [55, 56]. Additional analyses indicated that missingness was significantly related to grades (a proxy for reading comprehension), therefore a measure of self-reported grades [ranging from "D's or lower" (1) through "mostly A's" (7)] was included both in the EM procedure and in the final model parameterization. A total of five augmented data sets were produced and corresponding statistics are point estimates averaging across the five imputed datasets.

GENDER DIFFERENCES IN ALCOHOL USE, SOCIAL SKILLS, AND COMPETENCE

Although a number of gender differences were nonsignificant, it is still worth noting that in the eighth grade male students reported more frequent alcohol use, greater consumption of alcohol, and more instances of being drunk. Male students also reported less social skills competence, more risk-taking, lower refusal skills competence, and less academic esteem. Female students, on the other hand, reported more self-mastery, more problem-solving confidence, and higher grades. The average absolute correlation between gender and the full set of eighth grade behavioral measures was $r = .06$, between gender and the eighth grade psychosocial measures was $r = .04$, between gender and tenth grade consumption was $r = .06$, and between gender and tenth grade psychosocial functioning was $r = .05$. Despite the limited predictive power of gender with respect to the model variables, gender was included in the final path model to account for socialization differences that may developmentally influence both consumption and competence.

Summary descriptive statistics (means and standard deviations) and bivariate relations (point estimates) for all of the measures used in the path model are contained in Table 1. Although not presented, none of the measures were characteristically skewed (exceeding 2.00) and the largest deviation from normality was observed in the drunkenness variable (kurtosis = 5.21 in the 8th grade). As expected, the additive measures of risk for poor social competence and poor refusal skills were inversely related to all five measures of personal competence (e.g., mastery) and positively associated with all three measures of alcohol. This same pattern of relations applied to risk-taking, which was positively associated with poor social competence and poor refusal skills and also positively associated with alcohol use. Consistent with our hypotheses, the four measures of competence were all negatively associated with alcohol use and the three measures of consumption were positively and highly interrelated.

The pattern of associations between competence and alcohol use remained consistent across time, however, there was also evidence of some temporal erosion as the magnitude of these associations diminished. The three measures of alcohol use remained moderately associated in the tenth grade, reinforcing that alcohol involvement was based on frequent and intense use (high volume per occasion) that also included frequent drunkenness.

Table 1. Summary of Descriptive Statistics and Correlations Among
All Observed Measures Used in the Model

	1	2	3	4	5	6	7	8
8th Grade[a]								
1. Gender	1.0							
2. Poor social skills	.02	1.0						
3. Risk-taking	.06	−.07	1.0					
4. Poor refusal skills	.08	.16	.17	1.0				
5. Academic esteem[b]	.03	.16	.15	.23	1.0			
6. Self-reinforcement	.01	−.24	−.04	−.22	−.17	1.0		
7. Cognitive mastery	−.06	−.28	−.04	−.29	−.31	.54	1.0	
8. Problem-solving	−.04	−.23	−.06	−.17	−.19	.37	.42	1.0
9. Grades	−.05	−.20	−.11	−.24	−.41	.24	.32	.20
10. Frequency	.06	.05	.29	.41	.16	−.20	−.25	−.18
11. Intensity	.08	.06	.25	.42	.16	−.19	−.23	−.15
12. Drunkenness	.05	.12	.23	.44	.19	−.17	−.23	−.14
10th Grade								
13. Academic esteem	.02	.13	.11	.14	.44	−.10	−.18	−.16
14. Self-reinforcement	−.02	−.14	−.10	−.13	−.20	.40	.23	.15
15. Cognitive mastery	−.09	−.15	−.13	−.18	−.20	.24	.32	.22
16. Problem solving	−.07	−.16	−.04	−.16	−.20	.23	.25	.30
17. Frequency	.10	.03	.23	.31	.12	−.11	−.17	−.05
18. Intensity	.11	.03	.22	.35	.14	−.15	−.22	−.07
19. Drunkenness	.06	.03	.23	.36	.09	.09	−.18	−.04
Mean	.50	1.25	3.23	0.26	5.01	3.37	3.35	3.36
Standard Deviation	.49	1.10	.72	.43	1.59	.65	.61	.66

[a]Statistics based on $N = 974$. Statistics are point estimates averaged over five imputed data sets.
[b]Scaled toward lower academic esteem.
Note: Significance level of $p \leq .05$ is obtained for correlations of .19 or greater (two-tailed) and $p \leq .01$ for $r \geq .25$.

PREVALENCE OF ALCOHOL USE AND TRANSITIONAL ALCOHOL USE

In the eighth grade, 36 percent of the students reported some use of alcohol, whereas in the tenth grade 64.3 percent of the sample reported experience with alcohol. There was a significant increase in the proportion of users [$\chi^2(1) = 110.0$, $p < .001$]. As an indication of the intensity of drinking, among the eighth grade nonabstaining youth, two-thirds of these youth reported having at least two or more drinks per occasion and one in five students reported having recently been drunk (ranging from 2 to 3 times per month to every day). In the tenth grade, the relative proportions for intense drinking and drunkenness increased to 83 percent and 30 percent, respectively.

9	10	11	12	13	14	15	16	17	18	19
1.0										
−.26	1.0									
−.27	.77	1.0								
−.31	.82	.82	1.0							
−.26	.09	.09	.10	1.0						
.21	−.21	−.18	−.19	−.23	1.0					
.23	−.28	−.21	−.22	−.35	.48	1.0				
.21	−.21	−.16	−.20	−.35	.36	.46	1.0			
−.15	.53	.44	.42	.12	−.14	−.23	−.17	1.0		
−.23	.52	.52	.48	.13	−.16	−.24	−.20	.70	1.0	
−.18	.56	.51	.52	.12	−.16	−.26	−.18	.72	.74	1.0
3.34	2.66	2.12	1.91	3.42	3.36	3.36	3.39	3.69	3.21	2.86
.53	1.75	1.62	1.43	.67	.65	.66	.56	1.93	1.74	1.78

RESULTS OF THE
CONFIRMATORY MEASUREMENT MODEL

The next step in the model building process included conducting the confirmatory factor analysis (CFA) to empirically determine the fit of the hypothesized model structure to the sample covariances. Figure 1 contains the standardized solution for the CFA. Three important pieces of evaluative information are provided from the CFA procedure. First, the standardized parameter loadings attest to the statistical reliability of the hypothesized latent dimensions (i.e., competence and alcohol involvement). In addition, estimates of the associations among the exogenous (observed) measures and between the exogenous measures and latent constructs yield information on construct and criterion validity. A third important piece of information provided by the CFA regards how well the sample covariances reproduce the implied (hypothesized) model. Several incremental goodness-of-fit statistics are used to gauge the fit including the Bentler-Bonett Normed Fit Index (NFI [58]), the Nonnormed Fit Index (NNFI), and the Comparative Fit Index [59], which in contrast to the two previous fit statistics is a population chi-square statistic that adjusts for sample size. All of the incremental fit indices range from 0 through 1 with values of .90 or more indicating a good fit. Incremental fit indices show the improvement in fit of the hypothesized model compared to a null or independence model that specifies no hypothesized correlations among the measures. In addition to these specific fit indices, the standardized root mean square of the residual differences is the average absolute differences between the observed covariances and the reproduced (parameterized) matrix. As an indicator of fit, the RMSR should be quite small (RMSR ≤ .05), indicating that the model has been correctly specified and that there is little residual discrepancy between the implied and sample covariance matrices.

Fit indices for all five augmented datasets underscored that the models provided a reasonably adequate fit to the data [$\chi^2(121, 974) = 631.60$, NFI = .914, NNFI = .900, CFI = .929, $p < .001$, RMSR = .04, $\chi^2/df = 5.22$].[4] Standardized parameter loadings for the observed indicators were large and significant, underscoring the statistical reliability of these measures. Based on their respective loadings, eighth grade Competence was most strongly indicated by cognitive mastery and least so by (low) academic esteem. Factor loadings for Alcohol Involvement were fairly equivalent in magnitude, reinforcing the equal contribution of these measures toward defining high-risk drinking. The pattern of factor loadings remained consistent for the tenth grade constructs. Correlations among the exogenous measures are contained in Table 2 and are discussed more extensively in the context of the structural equation model.

---

[4] The goodness-of-fit indices reported are based on the first set of maximum-likelihood estimates of the variance-covariance matrix produced by the EM algorithm applied to the raw data. Subsequent imputed datasets are obtained by bootsampling (974 cases are drawn randomly with replacement) from the parent raw data. Goodness-of-fit statistics for the four remaining imputed datasets were as follows: [$\chi^2(121) = 943.37$, NFI = .881, NNFI = .850, CFI = .894, $p < .001$, RMSR = .04], [$\chi^2(121) = 754.99$, NFI = .899, NNFI = .877, CFI = .913, $p < .001$, RMSR = .05], [$\chi^2(121) = 844.54$, NFI = .887, NNFI = .860, CFI = .901, $p < .001$, RMSR = .05], and [$\chi^2(121) = 815.02$, NFI = .896, NNFI = .872, CFI = .909, $p < .001$, RMSR = .05]. In addition, although all of the model fit indices underscore some improvement could be made to the fit of the base model (i.e., reducing the discrepancy between the sample and implied covariance structures), empirically conducted simulation studies have shown reparameterization with residual covariances to be highly unstable and sample specific. In particular, MacCallum and colleagues [60] have shown that respecification (e.g., sequential model modification) based on post hoc modification indices are unstable with sample sizes less than 1,500. Given the exploratory nature of this study, we felt inclined to leave the base model intact especially because all of the incremental model fit indices approached (or in some cases exceeded) the gold standard of .90.

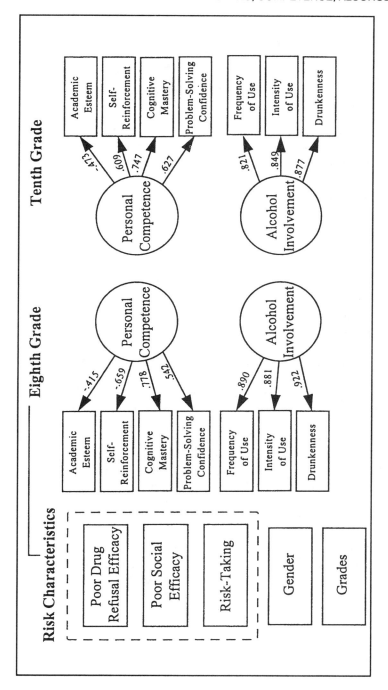

Figure 1. Confirmatory measurement model depicting associations between risk, competence, and alcohol involvement. Large circles represent latent constructs, rectangles are measured variables. Factor loadings are standardized and significance levels were determined by critical ratios on unstandardized coefficients. Factor intercorrelations corresponding to the measurement model are included in Table 2.

Table 2. Cross-Sectional (8th Grade) Associations Among Exogenous
Measures Corresponding to Final Structural Equations Model

	V1	V2	V3	V4	V5	F1[a]	F2[a]
1. Gender	1.0	−.03	.07*	.08*	−.05	−.04	.08*
2. Poor social skills		1.0	−.05	.16**	−.21***	−.42***	.08*
3. Risk taking			1.0	.20***	−.13**	−.07*	.32***
4. Poor refusal skills				1.0	−.25***	−.41***	.50***
5. Grades					1.0	.52***	−.32***
6. Personal competence[a]						1.0	−.33***
7. Alcohol use[a]							1.0

[a]Latent construct, all other measures are observed.
*$p \leq .05$
**$p \leq .01$
***$p \leq .001$

RESULTS OF THE LONGITUDINAL PATH ANALYSIS

Next, the measurement model was reconstructed and a two-wave, three-year longitudinal structural model was tested. Across-time covariances from the measurement model were reparameterized to reflect "causal" regression paths between the eighth grade predictors and tenth grade outcome constructs. Disturbance terms (residual variances that reflect variation net of prediction from the causal paths) were specified for the latent constructs in the tenth grade. Figure 2 contains the results of the longitudinal structural equation model (nonsignificant paths removed). All of the exogenous measures were allowed to freely covary, especially because specification of causal relations among contemporaneous measures are at best tenable (these correlations are contained in Table 2). The fit of this model was identical to the fit of the CFA (no post hoc parameterization was included to capture sample-specific, residual covariances).

As depicted, there were only three significant longitudinal paths: risk-taking predicted alcohol use ($\beta = .10$, $p < .05$), and poor drug refusal efficacy predicted both personal competence ($\beta = .10$, $p < .05$) and alcohol involvement ($\beta = .11$, $p < .05$). These parameter estimates are partial standardized regression coefficients and indicate the change in the outcome for a corresponding unit change in the predictor, controlling for all other measures in the model. High competence was associated with lower alcohol use at both assessments, although this relationship was smaller in magnitude in the tenth grade. Associations among the eighth grade exogenous measures (Table 2) reveal that they all were significantly associated with each other and likewise with eighth grade alcohol use.

Consistent with our research hypotheses, alcohol use was inversely associated with grades ($r = -.32$, $p < .001$) and competence ($r = -.33$, $p < .001$). As expected,

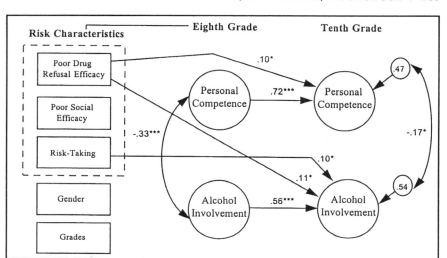

Figure 2. Longitudinal relations between social risk, competence, and alcohol use. Large circles represent latent factors and small circles with numbers reflect residual variances. Structural regression coefficients are standardized and significance levels were determined by critical ratios on unstandardized coefficients [*p < .05; **p < .01; ***p < .001].

grades were positively associated with personal competence ($r = .52$, $p < .001$). Interestingly, the correlations between competence and social skills and likewise between competence and refusal efficacy were equivalent in magnitude ($r = -.42$ and $-.41$, respectively); however, the same pattern of association was not observed between the two respective skills measures and alcohol use ($r = .08$ and .50, for social skills and refusal efficacy, respectively). These patterns, however, were consistent with the fact that higher scores on the risk indices indicated less social competence, poor refusal skills efficacy, and both of these risk conditions were related to increased alcohol use.

DISCUSSION

The primary objective of this study was to examine the relative contributions of social and personal competence and refusal skills to the prediction of adolescent alcohol use. Toward this end, we tested a two-wave, path model that included measures of social competence, drug refusal skills, personal competence, and alcohol use measured in the eighth grade and examined the long-term effects of these measures on personal competence and alcohol use in the tenth grade. The hypothesized model also included controls for risk-taking and gender, both of which may spuriously confound those relations during the early part of the adolescent development.

One of the main findings to come from this study is that only two of the early adolescent measures (high risk-taking and poor refusal skills) predicted later alcohol involvement, and both effects were relatively small. Interestingly, in their evaluation of an alcohol prevention trial, Donaldson et al. [12] reported that refusal skills did not predict alcohol use over a four-year period, although in their reported study social skills training improved refusal skills. Even though the Donaldson et al. study was a prevention study and involved a younger age group than the current study, the different findings underscore the need to identify specific and possibly age-related, causal risk processes.

One possible avenue of inquiry would include establishing whether the alcohol risk associated with the variables examined in this study is a developmentally stable process, or whether vulnerability fluctuates as conditions of risk accumulate and change over time. Younger age youth may not be exposed sufficiently to peer pressure for alcohol and drug use, but, over time, these social pressures may increase and reach a critical mass. The findings from the current study suggest that the skills associated with alcohol (and cigarette) refusal efficacy may not be static, but rather with increasing age these resistance skills gain in significance. Social skills increase in importance during adolescence as youth engage in greater social comparison and invest more in their own interpersonal competencies. Consistent with these developmental changes, refusal skills and the underlying motivations that encourage assertive behavior may become more influential processes in the development of resilience.

Somewhat unexpectedly, poor refusal efficacy was positively associated with later personal competence. In the eighth grade assessment, the zero-order relations between elements of personal competence and refusal skill were positive, indicating that higher competence was associated with higher refusal efficacy. On the basis of the zero-order relations, we speculate that, despite their initial risk status, there is some change over the three-year intervening period, and youth with poor refusal skills improve their social and personal competence (therefore individuals shift in their relative rank position). A closer inspection of the residual correlation matrix provides some support for this claim. With the exception of problem-solving confidence, all of the associations between refusal skills and the observed measures of personal competence were negative (for both the 8th and 10th grades). The tenth grade relations contained in the residual matrix reflect associations net of the effect of all predictors (with stability effects partialled). In the final structural model, the sign associated with these bivariate relations was reversed, perhaps pointing to a subsample of youth who are rapidly undergoing transitions in their skill development during the intervening period. Although SEM procedures contain many strengths for handling multivariate data with repeated measures, it is difficult to capture the full set of developmental relations with a single nomothetic model. Further analyses that dissect the sample into components reflecting stable versus changing patterns of behavior and skills should clarify these developmental mechanisms.

Our data also confirm a long-term, direct relation between risk-taking and alcohol involvement. Stacy et al. [37] has suggested that identification of high-risk youth on the basis of personality characteristics like impulsivity is an important component of designing successful interventions. Risk-taking or impulsivity may be associated with ineffective social rewards systems and poor regulation or modulation of inhibitory systems. Continued and unabated disinhibition may portend later consumption and related problems (i.e., driving under the influence, which combines risky behavior and excessive alcohol intake). The early adolescent association between risk-taking and competence provides evidence of an early developmental linkage between inhibition/reward systems and mastery evaluation. Unfortunately, the absence of a consequence measure of risk-taking to control for contemporaneous relations at follow-up prevents establishing the true causal nature of those relations.

Part of what is captured in our measure of risk-taking is an element of unconventionality and thrill seeking (e.g., fast driving, boredom, daring activities). Social control and self-derogation theories [40] suggest that unconventionality is associated with weak ties to normative institutions. Youth who lack strong ties to school and other educational environments miss out on critical opportunities to acquire competencies that are needed for successful adjustment. Social reward mechanisms for these youth that can effectively compensate for their skills deficits may include risk-taking and substance use. Future studies may want to examine the stability and predictive significance of these relations over extended periods of time in an effort to determine if personality characteristics that tie into emotional regulation and reward systems (i.e., sensation-seeking) are linked with cognitive evaluation and self-regulatory systems (i.e., competence).

Both alcohol involvement and competence were moderately stable over the three-year period, reinforcing the importance of these behaviors and skills for this age period. Rates of alcohol use in the current sample are consistent with national estimates [30] obtained from secondary school students. Slightly more than one-third of the eighth graders and roughly two-thirds of the tenth graders report some experience with alcohol (corresponding to 45.3% and 63.5% for annual use among 8th and 10th graders in the MTF study). Given the large numbers of youth reporting some alcohol use in this period and the rapid increase in usage between eighth and tenth grade period, it seems prudent to invest in strategies that reduce early onset and that can abate continued use of alcohol use during this critical age period.

Despite the absence of any long-term relations between personal competence and alcohol use, high levels of competence was cross-sectionally associated with less alcohol use, albeit the magnitude of this association diminished over time. In a separate study, Scheier and Botvin [61] examined the long-term consequences of polydrug use on cognitive and personal competence. These authors reported small, albeit significant, effects of alcohol on self-reinforcement and decision skills. Because those effects were small and the contemporaneous relations at follow-up between drug use and competence were moderate to large, these authors suggested that the effects of early-stage drug use on later competence were developmentally delayed. According to this model, early deficits in competence may not extend forward in time to sufficiently increase alcohol use, however, prolonged alcohol use through the adolescent years continues to retard skill development. It is the effect of sustained drinking and nonparticipant in socially rewarding and competitive school environments that fosters deficits in competence.

A second and no less important research goal in the current study including examining the interrelationship of social skills and competence in the early stages of adolescence. The pattern of positive associations among the competence measures and negative relations between the social risk measures and competence (including grades) were consistent with our hypotheses. The magnitude of association between the two sets of social skills (risk for poor social skills and low refusal efficacy) and competence were equivalent ($r = -.42$ and $-.41$, respectively, for social skills and refusal skills), and the moderate overlap between these constructs provides further evidence of cross-domain relations [18]. Youth with poor social skills and poor refusal efficacy also reported poor personal control (cognitive mastery), low frequency of self-reinforcement, low academic esteem, and low problem-solving confidence. Greater risk for poor refusal skills and lower personal competence also were significantly associated with alcohol use. The positive and relatively large association between grades and competence reinforces the linkage between perceptions of self-efficacy and actual performance (albeit the latter is self-reported). Both grades and competence were equivalently and moderately related to alcohol use, underscoring that alcohol-using youth reported lower grades and lower perceived mastery of important and requisite developmental skills.

Interestingly, the statistical linkage between poor refusal skills and alcohol in the eighth grade was considerably larger than the relation between risk for poor social skills and alcohol use. The individual measures comprising the index of social skills risk reflect lack of confidence in general assertiveness (i.e., defense of rights), low social confrontation, and high social concern, the latter measure ostensibly tapping social anxiety. The basis for the inclusion of social competence enhancement as part of current prevention strategies rests on the assumption that acquiring confidence in the execution of interpersonal skills will offset negative peer pressure and help youth to resist drug offers. In addition, social confidence, positive social relations, and age-appropriate assertiveness are all considered necessary (but not sufficient) for the successful transition to adulthood.

A closer inspection of the respective zero-order associations between the constituent elements of the social skills risk index and alcohol use shows these relations to be small and nonsignificant. Usually, pooling the variation of a homogeneous set of items into a single index of risk will increase their predictive strength, however, in the current analyses this was not the case. It is plausible that social skills may not present a formidable barrier against alcohol use at this early stage, but developmentally these skills may acquire greater protective strength (particularly given their comparatively larger observed relationship with personal competence). Rather than diminishing their importance for prevention, it may be prudent to reinforce these skills at an early age in an effort to reduce early-stage alcohol use and prevent further transitions from use to abuse.

IMPLICATIONS FOR PREVENTION

There are also several important lessons for prevention based on the current findings. First, the findings from the current study provide evidence that refusal efficacy has long-term deterrent capabilities and that youth who lack refusal skills are more likely to engage in alcohol use during early adolescence and this condition persists into later adolescence. Alcohol use, or for that matter any drug use, during adolescence portends negative behavioral and psychosocial outcomes that can diminish the possibility of normal adult functioning. In the face of mounting evidence obtained from evaluations of several prevention trials that resistance skills training does not obtain the same optimal goals, for example, as does normative education (i.e., altering youths' perceptions of peer and adult drug use), the current findings argue that we should continue arming these youth with appropriate social resistance skills.

In addition, the cross-sectional strength of the relations between competence, social skills, and refusal efficacy augers well for multi-modal, prevention curriculum, the latter which may be effective in reducing or delaying drug use. This is especially important given the diverse set of etiological risk factors that promote alcohol and drug use [62]. Furthermore, these findings also provide evidence that competence training can result in reduced alcohol consumption. That is, youth reporting high levels of personal competence can effectively apply these skills to offset various internal and external pressures to use alcohol and other drugs. Based on the current analyses, these pressures include a wide range of feelings of insecurity revolving around social presence (anxiety), active peer pressure to smoke or drink, and for males more than females, impulsivity.

LIMITATIONS

There are several limitations to the current study worth noting. First, the sample we analyzed represents a broad mixture of experimental alcohol use patterns, including youth reporting no alcohol use mixed with students reporting frequent, excessive, and disruptive alcohol use. The processes highlighted by the longitudinal path model, however, reflect group, rather than individual level, behavioral tendencies, and future analyses may want to exact greater precision with respect to estimation of individual differences for psychosocial functioning (i.e., competencies) as well as alcohol use (nonuse vs. use). A more specific understanding of how risk evolves over time will only help to inform prevention researchers and practitioners with respect to the broad success that can be achieved with high-risk populations.

Second, in the interest of parsimony the exogenous measures in the model represent a few of the many risk factors associated with adolescent alcohol use. Clearly inclusion of a host of social influence, motivational (i.e., expectancies), family, and personality measures are required to more accurately and fully specify the developmental influences that promulgate consumption. Among the many possible indicators of model fit, the overall R^2 value for both the cross-sectional and longitudinal model underscore that alternative models with a wider array of precursors might enhance prediction. We restricted the inclusion of control measures to satisfy the statistical requirements for ML estimation procedures. Nonetheless, alternative models should be addressed, particularly ones that identify potential mediational relations between skills and competence, which may be the appropriate hypothesized medium by which deficits in social skills promote deficits in competence and subsequent consumption.

REFERENCES

1. G. J. Botvin, Drug Abuse Prevention in School Settings, in *Drug Abuse Prevention with Multiethnic Youth,* G. J. Botvin, S. Schinke, and M. A. Orlandi (eds.), Sage, Thousand Oaks, California, pp. 169-192, 1995.
2. G. J. Botvin and E. M. Botvin, School-Based and Community-Based Prevention Approaches, in *Substance Abuse: A Comprehensive Textbook* (2nd Edition), J. H. Lowinson, P. Ruiz, and R. B. Millman (eds.), Williams and Wilkins, Baltimore, Maryland, pp. 910-927, 1992.
3. G. J. Botvin, Principles of Prevention, in *Handbook on Drug Abuse Prevention: A Comprehensive Strategy to Prevent the Abuse of Alcohol and Other Drugs,* R. H. Coombs and D. M. Ziedonis (eds.), Allyn and Bacon, Boston, Massachusetts, pp. 19-44, 1995.
4. M. A. Pentz, Social Competence and Self-Efficacy as Determinants of Substance Use in Adolescence, in *Coping and Substance Use,* T. A. Wills and S. Shiffman (eds.), Academic Press, San Diego, California, pp. 117-142, 1985.
5. D. M. Murray, C. A. Johnson, R. V. Luepker, and M. B. Mittelmark, The Prevention of Cigarette Smoking in Children: A Comparison of Four Strategies, *Journal of Applied Social Psychology, 14,* pp. 274-299, 1984.
6. B. R. Flay, Psychosocial Approaches to Smoking Prevention: A Review of Findings, *Health Psychology, 4,* pp. 449-488, 1985.
7. S. P. Schinke, L. D. Gilchrist, and W. H. Snow, Skills Intervention to Prevent Cigarette Smoking among Adolescents, *American Journal of Public Health, 75,* pp. 665-667, 1985.

8. N. Tobler, Meta-Analysis of 143 Adolescent Drug Prevention Programs: Quantitative Outcome Results of Program Participants Compared to a Control or Comparison Group, *Journal of Drug Issues, 16,* pp. 537-567, 1987.

9. W. B. Hansen and J. W. Graham, Preventing Alcohol, Marijuana, and Cigarette Use among Adolescents: Peer Pressure Resistance Training versus Establishing Conservative Norms, *Preventive Medicine, 20,* pp. 414-430, 1991.

10. W. B. Hansen, C. A. Johnson, B. R. Flay, J. W. Graham, and J. Sobel, Affective and Social Influences Approaches to the Prevention of Multiple Substance Abuse among Seventh Grade Students: Results from Project SMART, *Preventive Medicine, 17,* pp. 135-154, 1988.

11. W. B. Hansen, J. W. Graham, B. H. Woklenstein, B. Z. Lundy, J. Pearson, B. R. Flay, and C. A. Johnson, Differential Impact of Three Alcohol Prevention Curricula on Hypothesized Mediating Variables, *Journal of Drug Education, 18,* pp. 143-153, 1988.

12. S. I. Donaldson, J. W. Graham, and W. B. Hansen, Testing the Generalizability of Intervening Mechanism Theories: Understanding the Effects of Adolescent Drug Use Prevention Interventions, *Journal of Behavioral Medicine, 17,* pp. 195-216, 1994.

13. A. Bandura, *Social Learning Theory,* Prentice-Hall, Englewood Cliffs, New Jersey, 1977.

14. A. Bandura, Self-Efficacy: Toward a Unifying Theory of Behavior Change, *Psychological Review, 84,* pp. 191-215, 1977.

15. E. Waters and L. A. Sroufe, Social Competence as a Developmental Construct, *Developmental Review, 3,* pp. 79-97, 1983.

16. T. A. Cavell, The Measure of Adolescent Social Performance: Development and Initial Validation, *Journal of Clinical Child Psychology, 21,* pp. 107-114, 1992.

17. S. S. Luthar, Social Competence in the School Setting: Prospective Cross-Domain Associations among Inner-City Teens, *Child Development, 66,* pp. 416-429, 1995.

18. J. Connolly, Social Self-Efficacy in Adolescence: Relations with Self-Concept, Social Adjustment, and Mental Health, *Canadian Journal of Behavioral Science, 21,* pp. 258-269, 1989.

19. C. Frentz, F. M. Gresham, and S. N. Elliott, Popular, Controversial, Neglected, and Rejected Adolescents: Contrasts of Social Competence and Achievement Differences, *Journal of School Psychology, 29,* pp. 109-120, 1991.

20. B. L. Volling, C. MacKinnon-Lewis, D. Rabiner, and L. P. Baradaran, Children's Social Competence and Sociometric Status: Further Exploration of Aggression, Social Withdrawal, and Peer Rejection, *Development and Psychopathology, 5,* pp. 459-483, 1993.

21. K. R. Wentzel, Relations between Social Competence and Academic Achievement in Early Adolescence, *Child Development, 62,* pp. 1066-1078, 1991.

22. J. T. Parkhurst and S. R. Asher, Peer Rejection in Middle School: Subgroup Differences in Behavior, Loneliness, and Interpersonal Concerns, *Developmental Psychology, 28,* pp. 231-241, 1992.

23. J. G. Parker and S. R. Asher, Peer Relations and Later Personal Adjustment: Are Low Accepted Children at Risk? *Psychological Bulletin, 102,* pp. 357-389, 1987.

24. G. J. Botvin, Prevention of Adolescent Substance Abuse through the Development of Personal and Social Competence, in *Preventing Adolescent Drug Abuse Intervention*

Strategies, T. J. Glynn, C. G. Leukfeld, and J. P. Ludford (eds.), Research Monograph No. 47, U.S. Government Printing Office, Washington, D.C., 1983.

25. S. S. Luthar and E. Zigler, Vulnerability and Competence: A Review of Research on Resilience in Childhood, *American Journal of Orthopsychiatry, 61,* pp. 6-22, 1991.

26. R. Jessor and S. L. Jessor, *Problem Behavior and Psychosocial Development: A Longitudinal Study of Youth,* Academic Press, New York, 1977.

27. G. J. Botvin, E. Baker, L. Dusenbury, S. Tortu, and E. M. Botvin, Preventing Adolescent Drug Abuse through a Multimodal Cognitive-Behavioral Approach: Results of a 3-Year Study, *Journal of Consulting and Clinical Psychology, 58,* pp. 437-446, 1990.

28. G. J. Botvin, E. Baker, E. M. Botvin, A. D. Filazzola, and R. B. Millman, Prevention of Alcohol Misuse through the Development of Personal and Social Competence: A Pilot Study, *Journal of Studies on Alcohol, 45,* pp. 550-552, 1984.

29. G. J. Botvin, E. Baker, J. Dusenbury, E. Botvin, and T. Diaz, Long-Term Follow-Up of a Randomized Drug Abuse Prevention Trial in a White Middle-Class Population, *Journal of the American Medical Association, 273,* pp. 1106-1112, 1995.

30. L. D. Johnston, P. M. O'Malley, and J. G. Bachman, *National Survey Results on Drug Use from the Monitoring the Future Study, 1975-1994. Vol. I Secondary School Students,* DHHS Publication No. ADM 95-4026, National Institute on Drug Abuse, Rockville, Maryland, 1995.

31. D. Keating, Adolescent Thinking, in *At the Threshold: The Developing Adolescent,* S. S. Feldman and G. R. Elliott (eds.), Harvard University Press, Cambridge, Massachusetts, pp. 54-89, 1990.

32. V. C. Seltzer, *The Psychosocial Worlds of the Adolescent: Public and Private,* John Wiley & Sons, Inc., New York, 1989.

33. R. M. Lerner and T. T. Foch (eds.), *Biological-Psychosocial Interactions in Early Adolescence: A Life-Span Perspective,* Lawrence Erlbaum, Hillsdale, New Jersey, 1987.

34. B. B. Brown, Peer Groups and Peer Cultures, in *At the Threshold: The Developing Adolescent,* S. S. Feldman and G. R. Elliot (eds.), Harvard University Press, Cambridge, Massachusetts, pp. 171-196, 1990.

35. R. C. Savin-Williams and T. J. Berndt, Friendship and Peer Relations, in *At the Threshold: The Developing Adolescent,* S. S. Feldman and G. R. Elliott (eds.), Harvard University Press, Cambridge, Massachusetts, pp. 277-307, 1990.

36. M. D. Newcomb, Understanding the Multidimensional Nature of Drug Use and Abuse: The Role of Consumption, Risk Factors, and Protective Factors, in *Vulnerability to Drug Abuse,* M. Glantz and R. Pickens (eds.), American Psychological Association, Washington, D.C., pp. 255-297, 1992.

37. A. W. Stacy, M. D. Newcomb, and P. M. Bentler, Cognitive Motivations and Sensation Seeking as Long-Term Predictors of Drinking Problems, *Journal of Social and Clinical Psychology, 12,* pp. 1-24, 1993.

38. T. A. Wills, D. Vaccaro, and G. McNamara, Novelty Seeking, Risk Taking, and Related Constructs as Predictors of Adolescent Substance Use: An Application of Cloninger's Theory, *Journal of Substance Abuse, 6,* pp. 1-20, 1994.

39. M. B. Newcomb and L. MeGee, Influence of Sensation Seeking on General Deviance and Specific Problem Behaviors from Adolescence to Young Adulthood, *Journal of Personality and Social Psychology, 61,* pp. 614-628, 1991.

40. H. B. Kaplan, S. S. Martin, and C. Robbins, Pathways to Adolescent Drug Use: Self-Derogation, Peer Influence, Weakening of Social Controls, and Early Substance Use, *Journal of Health and Social Behavior, 25,* pp. 270-289, 1984.

41. R. G. Simmons and D. A. Blyth, *Moving into Adolescence: The Impact of Pubertal Change and School Context,* Aldine de Gruyter, Hawthorn, New York, 1987.

42. G. J. Botvin, *Reducing Drug Abuse and AIDS Risk: Final Report,* National Institute on Drug Abuse, Washington, D.C., 1993.

43. P. M. Bentler, *EQS Structural Equations Program Manual,* BMDP Statistical Software, Los Angeles, California, 1989.

44. D. Paulhus, Sphere-Specific Measures of Perceived Control, *Journal of Personality and Social Psychology, 44,* pp. 1253-1265, 1983.

45. I. S. Janis and P. B. Field, A Behavioral Assessment of Persuasibility: Consistence of Individual Differences, in *Personality and Persuasibility,* C. I. Hovland and I. L. Janis (eds.), Yale University Press, New Haven, Connecticut, 1959.

46. J. S. Fleming and W. A. Watts, The Dimensionality of Self-Esteem: Some Results for a College Sample, *Journal of Personality and Social Psychology, 39,* pp. 921-929, 1980.

47. P. P. Heppner and C. H. Petersen, The Development and Implications of a Personal Problem-Solving Inventory, *Journal of Counseling Psychology, 29,* pp. 66-75, 1982.

48. E. M. Heiby, Assessment of Frequency of Self-Reinforcement, *Journal of Personality and Social Psychology, 44,* pp. 1304-1307, 1983.

49. E. D. Gambrill and C. A. Richey, An Assertion Inventory for Use in Assessment and Research, *Behavior Therapy, 6,* pp. 550-561, 1975.

50. T. A. Wills, E. Baker, and G. J. Botvin, Dimensions of Assertiveness: Differential Relationships to Substance Use in Early Adolescence, *Journal of Consulting and Clinical Psychology, 57,* pp. 473-478, 1989.

51. F. C. Richardson and D. L. Tasto, Development and Factor Analysis of a Social Anxiety Inventory, *Behavior Therapy, 7,* pp. 453-462, 1976.

52. S. Bailey, Adolescents' Multisubstance Use Patterns: The Role of Heavy Alcohol and Cigarette Use, *American Journal of Public Health, 82,* pp. 1220-1224, 1992.

53. H. J. Eysenck and S. B. G. Eysenck, *Manual of the Eysenck Personality Questionnaire,* Hodder & Stoughton, London, 1975.

54. R. J. Little and D. B. Rubin, *Statistical Analysis with Missing Data,* John Wiley & Sons, Inc., New York, 1987.

55. D. B. Rubin, *Multiple Imputation for Nonresponse in Surveys,* John Wiley & Sons, Inc., New York, 1987.

56. J. W. Graham, S. M. Hofer, and D. P. MacKinnon, Maximizing the Usefulness of Data Obtained with Planned Missing Value Patterns: An Application of Maximum Likelihood Procedures, *Multivariate Behavioral Research, 31,* pp. 197-218, 1996.

57. J. W. Graham, S. M. Hofer, and A. M. Piccinin, Analysis with Missing Data in Drug Prevention Research, in *Advances in Data Analysis for Prevention Intervention Research,* L. M. Collins and L. A. Seitz (eds.), Research Monograph No. 142, National Institute on Drug Abuse, Washington, D.C., pp. 13-63, 1994.

58. P. M. Bentler and D. G. Bonett, Significance Tests and Goodness of Fit in the Analysis of Covariance Structures, *Psychological Bulletin, 88,* pp. 588-606, 1980.

59. P. M. Bentler, Comparative Fit Indexes in Structural Models, *Psychological Bulletin, 107*, pp. 238-246, 1990.
60. R. C. MacCallum, M. Roznowski, and L. B. Necowitz, Model Modifications in Covariance Structure Analysis: The Problem of Capitalization on Chance, *Psychological Bulletin, 111*, pp. 490-504, 1992.
61. L. M. Scheier and G. J. Botvin, Effects of Early Adolescent Drug Use on Cognitive Efficacy in Early-Late Adolescence: A Developmental Structural Model, *Journal of Substance Abuse, 7*, pp. 379-404, 1995.
62. J. D. Hawkins, R. F. Catalano, and J. Y. Miller, Risk and Protective Factors for Alcohol and Other Drug Problems in Adolescence and Early Adulthood: Implications for Substance Abuse Prevention, *Psychological Bulletin, 112*, pp. 64-105, 1992.

Direct reprint requests to:

L. M. Scheier, Ph.D.
Assistant Professor of Psychology
Department of Public Health
Weill Medical College of Cornell University
411 East 69th Street, KB201
New York, NY 10021

J. DRUG EDUCATION, Vol. 29(3) 279-291, 1999

ALCOHOL AND DRUG USE OF INTER-CITY VERSUS RURAL SCHOOL AGE CHILDREN

LINDA FINKE, PH.D., R.N.

JUDY WILLIAMS, M.S.N., C.S., C.A.R.N., R.N.

Indiana University School of Nursing

ABSTRACT

The purpose of this study of seventy-nine children was to determine: 1) the prevalence and type of substance use in inter-city and rural eight to twelve-year-old children; and 2) the relationships between child substance use, self-esteem, peer substance use, and family climate. The conceptual framework for the study was a modification of Kumpfer and Turner's Social Ecology Model (1991). Nineteen percent of the children had used alcohol or drugs. Thirty-three percent of the children acknowledged having friends who used substances. Inter-city children reported more alcohol and marijuana use, while the rural children reported more use of inhalants. The responses of both inter-city and rural children also indicated that there were problems with substance use and family violence in the home. Self-esteem and affiliation with drug using peers were significantly correlated with substance use of the child.

The alcohol and drug use of young school age children continues to escalate while the problem is all but ignored by parents, health care providers, school personnel, communities, legislators, and society at large. Alarms are set off concerning the record number of young school age children using alcohol and drugs, yet attention continues to be focused on the alcohol and drug use of adolescents and young adults [1-7]. Many treatment programs are aimed at junior high and high school groups, but comprehensive, effective interventions are needed to treat and prevent alcohol and drug use at much earlier age groups to bring about change and prevent future alcohol and drug use.

PREVIOUS INVESTIGATION

There is mounting evidence that children as young as eight use alcohol and other drugs [3, 4, 6, 8]. Alcohol is the drug of choice for most school age children, but Finke et al. findings indicated that rural children preferred inhalants [6]. Therefore, availability of certain substances may be a factor in drug choice. MacDonald and Blume explored decision making concerning the use of alcohol and drugs and reported that decisions to use alcohol and drugs were made as early as fifth grade [9]. Researchers have found that boys are more likely to be involved in alcohol and drug use than girls [2, 3, 10].

Research has demonstrated that the use of alcohol or drugs by family members has a significant link to the use by children. This is true for both sibling's use [11, 12] and use of parents [3, 6, 13-19]. Several researchers have found that peer use has a strong influence on the alcohol and drug use of children [1, 6, 10, 20]. Low self-esteem has also been identified with alcohol and drug use [4, 6, 10, 21, 22].

Although most study has been conducted with adolescents, there has been some investigation into prevention factors for younger children as well. Knowledge about the use and effects of alcohol and drugs has been found to be effective in preventing use by school age children [1, 10]. There is also evidence, however, that education alone is not the answer to preventing alcohol and drug use by children.

Many schools now have drug prevention education as part of the required curriculum, but few of the educational programs have been evaluated for effectiveness. For example, the "Just Say No Program" promoted by Pat Nixon during her husband's Presidency and still taught in many schools across the country has not been evaluated to determine the program's effectiveness in preventing drug or alcohol use. In fact, there are some findings that drug abuse education alone is not effective. Ennett, Tobler, Ringwalt, and Flewelling studied the Project DARE (Drug Abuse Resistance Education) [22]. DARE was created by the Los Angeles Police Department in 1983 and is still taught across the United States in elementary, junior, and senior highs. The meta-analysis conducted by Ennett et al., discovered that the effect of the DARE core curriculum on the drug resistance of children, and adolescents for that matter, was not significant. The knowledge base of the children was raised, but the increased knowledge did not predict drug resistance.

On the other hand, Donaldson, Graham, Piccinin, and Hansen evaluated a resistance skills training program involving almost 12,000 students in fifth, sixth, seventh, and eighth grades in California [23]. The theoretical basis for the program they studied was the Social Inoculation Theory which proposes that a child's decision to drink or use other drugs depends on her or his ability to resist the overwhelming situational social pressures that she or he faces [24]. The training program includes teaching refusal skills to combat the social pressures. The program was found to be effective in preventing the onset of alcohol use.

Parental monitoring or supervision of a child's behavior was found by Chilcoat and Anthony to be effective in preventing alcohol and drug use. In a large study they conducted, close supervision of children by their parents was associated with no alcohol or drug use [25]. A decrease in monitoring by parents resulted in an increased risk of starting to use drugs.

In summary, previous investigation suggests several factors that need to be explored when investigating the factors associated with the alcohol and drug use of children. These factors are sociodemographic characteristics, family members' use of alcohol and drugs, peers' use, self-esteem, and previous education about alcohol and drugs.

THEORETICAL FRAMEWORK

Ecological models suggest that behavior is the result of factors in the environment and their impact on the individual. Kumpfer and Turner developed a social ecological model to explain the use of drugs by children [26]. The Kumpfer and Turner model states that a child's family environment, school environment, and peer influences predict the self-esteem of the child which in turn predicts the child's use of drugs. Modifying the model to include a systems framework reframes the model into an interactive model. The interactive model demonstrates an interaction between the factors that explain the drug use of the child. Figure 1 depicts the researchers' model designed to predict substance use of children

CURRENT STUDY

The following reports the results of a study designed to assess and compare the alcohol and drug use of school age children in a rural and an inter-city setting, compare the use based on setting, and explore factors related to the child's use such as self-esteem, peer influences, and family member substance abuse. The purpose of the current study was twofold: 1) to examine the alcohol and drug use of school age children and 2) to compare the substance use of inter-city and rural children. The study sought to answer the following questions: 1) What is the prevalence of substance use of school age children and what substances do they use? 2) How does the substance use of inter-city school age children compare with the substance use of rural school age children? and 3) What are the relationships between child substance use, self-esteem, peer substance use, and family climate?

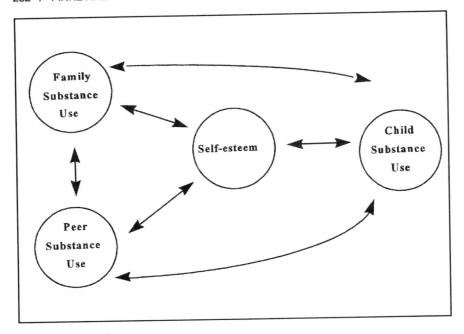

Figure 1. Child substance use model.

METHOD

The Sample

Data was collected at a rural school in Kentucky and at an inter-city summer day camp program in Indiana from seventy-nine children in all, ranging in age from eight to twelve years. The majority of children (72%) were nine or ten years old. Sixty-three percent (65%) of the children were female. The rural group was predominantly Caucasian while the inter-city group was predominantly African American. In other words, 53 percent of the total sample were Caucasian and 46 percent were minorities, predominantly African American (see Table 1).

Instruments

The children who participated in the study completed a five-part self-answer questionnaire in a multiple choice format. The children completed the questionnaire in approximately fifteen to twenty minutes. The first section of the questionnaire was designed to collect demographic data. The second section of the questionnaire contained a subscale from the Effective School Battery to examine the child's use and peer influence. National norms have been established for the

Table 1. Sample Demographics (Percent)

	Rural (n = 45)	Inter-City (n = 34)	Overall (n = 79)
Ethnicity			
Caucasian	93	0	53
African American	0	82	35
Other	7	18	11
Gender			
Female	73	53	65
Male	27	47	35
Age			
8 years or less	9	21	14
9 years	38	29	34
10 years	47	27	38
11 years	7	15	10
12 years	0	9	4
Living Arrangements			
2 natural parents	76	32	57
1 natural parent	20	53	34

subscale [27]. The third section contained questions to assess type of substance use. The fourth section was the short form of the Coopersmith Self-Esteem Inventory (SEI) to measure self-esteem [28]. The Coopersmith Self-Esteem Inventory was developed to use with school age children and has been found to have high reliability and validity [28, 29]. The last section of the questionnaire contained the first ten items of the Children of Alcoholics Screening Test (CAST) to assess family climate. The CAST is frequently used to collect information from children of alcoholics to collect information about the substance use of parents [30].

RESULTS

Sociodemographics

Of the seventy-nine school age children in the study, forty-five (57%) were from the rural community. Comparisons of rural children with inter-city children revealed significant group differences for two sociodemographic measures. Specifically, the rural and inter-city groups of children differed in race and living arrangements. The inter-city children were more likely than the rural children to identify themselves as minorities (predominantly African American), and to live with only one natural parent (53%). No significant group differences were found for sociodemographic measures of age, gender, parent education, and parent type of paid work.

Substance Use

The responses of the children indicated that a significant percent (19%) had used alcohol or drugs (see Figure 2). Fifteen percent of the inter-city children reported that they had used alcohol. Sixteen percent of the rural children and 6 percent of the inter-city children acknowledged that they had sniffed substances such as glue, gasoline, or butane. Two of the inter-city children (6%) reported that they had tried marijuana (see Table 2).

Chi-square analyses at a 95 percent confidence level were used to determine differences in substance use between the inter-city and rural groups of children. Results indicated that inter-city children were more likely than rural children to use alcohol. There was a trend for rural children to use inhalants. No significant group differences were found for other types of substance use.

Self-Esteem

The children's mean score on the Coopersmith Self-Esteem Inventory was 60.86 (see Table 2). A *t*-test for independent samples (95% confidence level for difference) indicated no significant difference between the inter-city children and the rural children in mean self-esteem scores. A significant proportion of the school age children (38% of the inter-city children and 32% of the rural children),

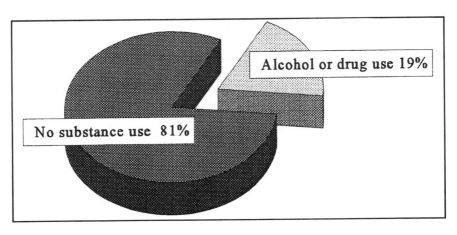

Figure 2. Substance use of school age chidlren.

Table 2. School Age Children's Responses Concerning Substance Use

	Rural (n = 45)		Inter-City (n = 34)		Overall (n = 79)	
	Mean	Std. Dev.	Mean	Std. Dev.	Mean	Std. Dev.
Self-Esteem	63.89	23.96	56.93	18.20	60.86	21.79
	Freq.	(%)	Freq.	(%)	Freq.	(%)
Family Climate						
Problem	18	40	17	53	35	45
No problem	27	60	15	47	42	55
Peer Substance Use						
Yes	11	24	15	44	26	33
No	34	76	19	56	53	67
Type of Peer Use						
Alcohol	11	24	12	35	23	29
Marijuana	3	7	10	29	13	17
Inhalants	9	20	9	27	18	23
Cocaine	2	4	6	18	8	10
Other drugs	3	7	6	18	9	11
Child Substance Use						
Yes	7	16	8	24	15	19
No	38	84	25	76	63	81
Type of Child Use						
Alcohol		0	5	15	5	6
Marijuana		0	2	6	2	3
Inhalants	7	16	2	6	9	11

however, scored below 50 on the Coopersmith Self-Esteem Inventory indicating some depression

Peer Substance Use

The children's responses indicated indeed that many of their friends used substances (see Table 2 and Figures 3 and 4). More than one-third of the inter-city children (35%) and nearly one-quarter of the rural children (24%) reported having friends who had tried alcohol. In addition, nearly one-third of the school

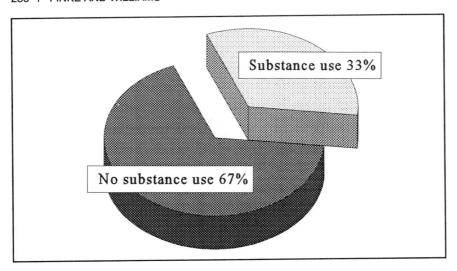

Figure 3. Peer substance use.

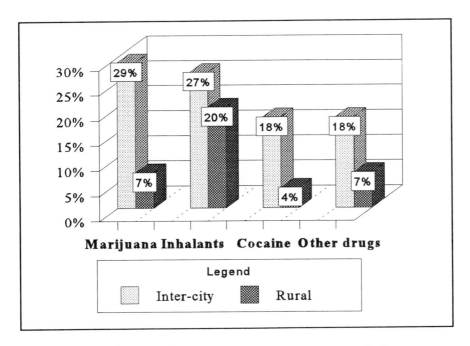

Figure 4. Type of peer substance use (excluding alcohol).

age children (32%) reported having friends who had used substances other than alcohol. Twenty-seven percent of the inter-city children and 20 percent of the rural children acknowledged having friends who had sniffed substances, such as glue, gasoline, or butane. Nearly one-third of the inter-city children (29%) and 7 percent of the rural children reported having friends who had used marijuana. Eighteen percent of the inter-city and 4 percent of the rural children reported having friends who had user cocaine or "crack." Additionally, 18 percent of the inter-city children and 7 percent of the rural children reported having friends who had used other drugs, like acid, downers, speed, or heroin.

Chi-square analyses at a 95 percent confidence interval indicated that inter-city children were more likely than rural children to have friends who had tried marijuana and cocaine. There were no significant group differences for other types of peer substance use.

Family Substance Use

The responses of both rural and inter-city children indicated that there were problems with substance use and violence in the home (see Figure 5). The CAST scores of more than half of the inter-city children (53%) and 40 percent of the rural children indicated a possible problem with parent substance use. Twenty percent of the rural children and 18 percent of the inter-city children acknowledged that they had felt alone, scared, nervous, angry, or frustrated because a parent was not able to stop drinking or taking drugs. Nine inter-city children (27%) and three rural children (7%) reported having protected another family member from a parent who was drinking or using drugs.

Chi-square analyses at a 95 percent confidence level indicated no significant difference in parental substance use between inter-city and rural children. A chi-square analysis indicated, however, that inter-city children were more likely than rural children to have protected another family member from a parent who was drinking or on drugs.

Correlations between Variables

For the seventy-nine children in this study, correlation test indicated that self-esteem had a significant relationship with child substance use ($r_{pbs} = -.25$, $p \leq .05$). The highest correlation with child substance use among the factors examined, however, was peer substance use (Phi $= .43$, $p \leq .05$). For the total sample, both family substance use ($r_{pbs} = -.33$, $p \leq .05$) and peer substance use ($r_{pbs} = -.31$, $p \leq .05$) had significant relationships with self-esteem. The relationships between self-esteem, peer substance use, family climate, and child substance use are depicted in Figure 6.

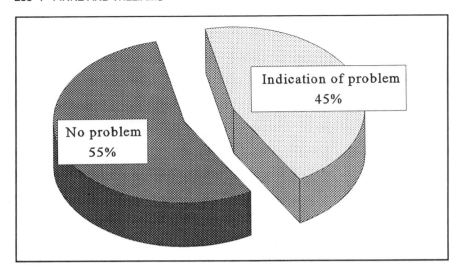

Figure 5. Children who indicated a possible problem with parent substance use.

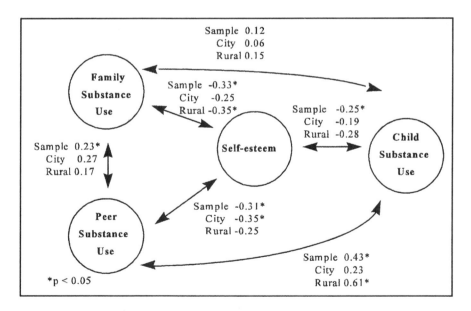

Figure 6. Relationships between self-esteem, peer substance use, family climate, and child substance use.

IMPLICATIONS AND RECOMMENDATIONS

The findings from this study are similar to the findings of other investigators. Alarmingly, 19 percent of the school age children in this study did use alcohol or drugs. They reported that 33 percent of their friends had used substances. The inter-city children tended to use alcohol and the rural children were more likely to use inhalants. The factors studied did correlate with the use of the children. Peer use and self-esteem were found to be correlated with a child's alcohol or drug use. It should also be noted that a number of the children lived in homes with one or both parents who were abusing alcohol or drugs.

Strategies are needed to prevent the alcohol and drug use of children. The prevention programs should be comprehensive and multifaceted. Furthermore, the strategies need to be early in a child's education. Hahn suggests that drug prevention educational programs are effective even in preschool [30]. The educational programs need to target not only children, but also their parents. Parents have a difficult time accepting that school age children use alcohol and drugs and even more difficulty accepting that their own children may be at risk. Parents need to be made aware of their own use and the correlation with the child's risk for use. Parents need to understand that children who are closely supervised are at less risk for alcohol and drug use. Parents have a very important role to play in preventing the alcohol and drug use of their children.

The educational programs for children need to include resistance skill training, self-esteem enhancing exercises as well as knowledge about drugs and their effect on the body and mind. The educational program would need to begin in the first year of school and continue throughout the child's education.

It is also apparent from the study and previous investigation that educational programs for children also must include survival skills for living in a home where parents or siblings abuse alcohol and drugs. Children in high risk homes need to have the coping skills to live and grow in such environments. The program would need to include knowledge about addictions, coping skills, self-esteem enhancing exercises, and physical safety skills.

Growing up in the current world can be difficult. There are many threats as well as opportunities. The biggest threat may be the effects of alcohol and drug use and abuse. It is the responsibility of all of us to give them the education and skills they need to resist the abuse of drugs and to reach their potential.

REFERENCES

1. L. Ried, O. Martinson, and L. Weaver, Factors Associated with the Drug Use of Fifth through Eighth Grade Students, *Journal of Drug Education, 17*:2, pp. 149-161, 1986.
2. J. Teets, Alcohol Usage Among Preadolescents and Adolescents, *Journal of School Nursing, 7*:3, pp. 12-17, 1991.

3. P. Bush and R. Iannotti, Alcohol, Cigarette, and Marijuana Use among Fourth Grade School Children in 1988/89 and 1990/91, *American Journal of Public Health, 83*:1, pp. 111-114, 1993.

4. K. Long and R. Boik, Predicting Alcohol Use in Rural Children: A Longitudinal Study, *Nursing Research, 42*:2, pp. 79-86, 1993.

5. L. Finke, Nursing Interventions with Children and Adolescents Who Have Substance Abuse Problems, in *Psychiatric/Mental Health Nursing Care of Children and Adolescents,* C. Evans and P. West (eds.), Aspen Publishing, Rockville, Maryland, 1992.

6. L. Finke, J. Chorpenning, B. French, C. Leese, and M. Siegel, Drug and Alcohol Use of School Age Children in a Rural Community, *The Journal of School Nursing, 12*:2, pp. 22-25, 1996.

7. L. Finke and A. Bowman, Factors in Childhood Drugs and Alcohol Use: A Review of the Literature, *Journal of Child and Adolescent Psychiatric Nursing, 10*:3, pp. 29-34, 1997.

8. M. Stevens, F. Whaley, F. Youells, and S. Linsey, Drug Use Prevalence in a Rural School-Age Population: The New Hampshire Survey, *American Journal of Preventive Medicine, 11*:2, pp. 105-113, 1995.

9. D. I. MacDonald and S. B. Blume, Children of Alcoholics, *American Journal of Drug Counseling, 140,* pp. 750-754, 1986.

10. H. Becker, M. Agopian, and S. Yeh, Impact Evaluation of Drug Abuse Resistance Education (DARE), *Journal of Drug Education, 22*:4, pp. 283-291, 1992.

11. R. Needle, H. McCubbin, M. Wilson, R. Reineck, A. Lazar, and H. Mederer, Interpersonal Influences in Adolescent Drug Use: The Role of the Older Siblings, Parents, and Peers, *The International Journal of the Addictions, 21*:7, pp. 739-766, 1986.

12. W. Gritching and J. Barber, The Impact of Quality of Family Life on Drug Consumption, *The International Journal of the Addictions, 24*:10, pp. 963-971, 1989.

13. D. Claire and M. Genest, Variables Associated with the Adjustment of Offspring of Alcoholic Fathers, *Journal of Studies on Alcohol, 48*:4, pp. 345-355, 1986.

14. L. Bennett, S. Wolin, and D. Reiss, Deliberate Family Process: A Strategy for Protecting Children of Alcoholics, *British Journal of Addiction, 83,* pp. 821-829, 1988.

15. F. Earls, W. Reich, K. Jung, and R. Cloninger, Psychopathology in Children of Alcoholic and Antisocial Parents, *Alcoholism: Clinical and Experimental Research, 12*:4, pp. 481-487, 1988.

16. J. Johnson and J. Rolf, Cognitive Functioning in Children from Alcoholic and Non-alcoholic Families, *British Journal of Addiction, 83,* pp. 849-857, 1988.

17. W. Reich, E. Felton, and J. Powell, A Comparison of the Home and Social Environments of Children of Alcoholic and Non-Alcoholic Parents, *British Journal of Addiction, 83,* pp. 831-839, 1988.

18. M. Roosa, I. Sandler, J. Beals, and J. Short, Risk Status of Adolescent Children of Problem-Drinking Parents, *American Journal of Community Psychology, 16*:2, pp. 225-239, 1988.

19. E. Werner, Resilient Offspring of Alcoholics: A Longitudinal Study from Birth to Age 18, *Journal of Studies on Alcohol, 47*:1, pp. 34-40, 1985.

20. P. D. Sarvella and E. J. McClendon, Indicators or Rural Youth Drug Use, *Journal of Youth and Adolescence, 17*:4, pp. 335-347, 1988.

21. T. Dielman, S. Leech, A. Lorenger, and W. Horvath, Health Laws of Control and Self-Esteem as Related to Adolescent Health Behavior and Intentions, *Adolescence, 19*:16, pp. 935-950, 1994.

22. S. Ennett, N. Tobler, C. Ringwalt, and R. Flewelling, How Effective is Drug Abuse Resistance Education: A Meta-Analysis of Project DARE Outcome Evaluation, *American Journal of Public Health, 84*:9, pp. 1394-1401, 1994.

23. S. Donaldson, J. Graham, A. Piccinin, and W. Hansen, Resistance—Skill Training and Onset of Alcohol Use: Evidence for Beneficial and Potentially Harmful Effects in Public Schools and in Private Catholic Schools, *Health Psychology, 14*:4, pp. 291-300, 1995.

24. _. Evans, A Social Inoculation Strategy to Deter Smoking in Adolescents, in *Behavioral Health: A Handbook of Health Enhancement and Disease Prevention,* J. D. Matarazzo, S. M. Weiss, J. A. Herd, N. E. Miller, and S. M. Weiss (eds.), Wiley Publishers, New York, pp. 765-774, 1984.

25. H. Chilcoat and J. Anthony, Impact of Parent Monitoring and Initiation of Drug Use through Late Childhood, *Journal of American Academy of Child Adolescent Psychology, 35*:1, pp. 91-100, 1996.

26. K. Kumpfer and C. Turner, The Social Ecology Model of Adolescent Substance Abuse: Implications for Prevention, *The International Journal of the Addictions, 25*:4, pp. 435-463, 1990-91.

27. G. D. Gottfredson, *The Effective School Battery, Student Survey,* Psychological Assessment Resources Incorporated, Odessa, Florida, 1985.

28. S. Coopersmith, *Self-Esteem Inventories,* Consulting Psychologists Press, Palo Alto, California, 1981.

29. J. W. Jones, *The Children of Alcoholics Screening Test: Test Manual,* Camelot Unlimited, Chicago, 1987.

30. E. Hahn, Predicting Head Start Parent Involvement in an Alcohol and Other Drug Prevention Program, *Nursing Research, 44*:1, pp. 45-51, 1995.

Direct reprint requests to:

Linda Finke, Ph.D., R.N.
Indiana University School of Nursing
1111 Middle Drive
Indianapolis, IN 46202

SUBSTANCE ABUSE PREVENTION:
A Multicultural Perspective
Edited by Snehendu B. Kar

Alcohol, tobacco, and other drugs (ATOD) abuse is a major threat to our health and quality of life. In this volume, nationally recognized substance abuse specialists, public health researchers, and community-based practitioners undertake an in-depth state-of-the-art review of substance abuse prevention intervention from a multicultural perspective.

Special emphasis is on the application of the lessons learned from fields of substance abuse and the new public health paradigm as a modus operandi for ATOD prevention in multicultural communities. The book further makes specific recommendations for prevention policy, research, professional preparation, and effective intervention strategies.

In thirteen chapters, twenty-four authors share their analyses, concerns, and conclusions in several domains including the: meaning and dynamics of multiculturalism affecting prevention intervention, relative risks and knowledge gaps across ethnic groups, social trends affecting health risks and substance abuse, lessons learned from substance abuse research and prevention, role of the media, promises and limits of the new public health paradigm for assessment, policy development, assurance of preventive services, and social action and empowerment for prevention in partnership with the public.

This pioneering volume will serve as a valuable resource to researchers, policy makers, educators, professionals and organizations interested in the health and quality of life of our communities as we approach the 21st century.

Format Information: 6" x 9", 336 pages, ISBN: 0-89503-194-9, $42.00 plus $4.00 postage and handling

Baywood Publishing Company, Inc. 26 Austin Avenue, Amityville, NY 11701
Call (516) 691-1270 Fax (516) 691-1770 **Orderline** (800) 638-7819
e-mail: baywood@baywood.com • **web site:** http://baywood.com

Critical Approaches
in the Health Social Sciences Series

The Policital Economy of AIDS

Edited by Merrill Singer

The AIDS epidemic is one that continues to sweep the globe as people worldwide, including large numbers of various medical and social groups, scramble to find explanations, medications, coping mechanisms, prevention strategies, money, and most of all, a cure. As with all epidemics, the social ways in which people respond to them, provides an often painfully revealing window on human societies. One of the most important lessons of a historical examination of epidemics is their disproportional burden on the poor or other stigmatized groups in society.

This volume, an integrated collection of seven research-based articles on AIDS by leading researchers in the field, seeks to cut through popular misunderstanding and conventional ideas about the spread and impact of AIDS by employing a political economic perspective in the analysis of the epidemic in diverse settings.

The AIDS epidemic, with its jarring mix of painful and inspiring personal stories of human suffering and resistive will, combined with a deadening and persistent cascade of faceless statistics, provides a significant challenge to the public health system, to community health workers, and to health social sciences.

It is the contention of this volume that we will fail this challenge badly if our attention remains focused on individual motivations and behaviors and ignores the wider political economy of AIDS.

248 pages, Cloth, ISBN: 0-89503-177-9
$41.00 + $4.00 p/h

Baywood Publishing Company, Inc.
26 Austin Avenue, Amityville, NY 11701
Call (631) 691-1270 • **Fax** (631) 691-1770 • **toll-free Orderline (800) 638-7819**
e-mail: baywood @baywood.com • **web site:** http://baywood.com

The newest edition in Baywood's
Policy, Politics, Health and Medicine Series

NEW

Stress at Work
A Sociological Perspective
by Chris L. Peterson

This book provides a theoretical background to occupational stress, and traces the development of models for understanding stress and the stress response. It also reports on a study of stress and ill-health in a large manufacturing organization in Australia. It examines the effects of stress, low self-esteem and poor mastery on psychological outcomes and ill-health symptoms.

This book examines a number of theoretical models in the development of the stress concept and its application. It traces the pioneering work of Hans Selye and early bio-physiological models are examined as well as the development of psychological models of stress. These are critically evaluated and sociological models are examined as providing a more effective understanding of the causes of stress, that is within a social, political and cultural context.

Table of Contents

Format Information: 6" x 9", 284 pages, Cloth, ISBN: 0-89503-190-6
$45.00 + $4.00 p/h

Baywood Publishing Company, Inc., 26 Austin Avenue, Amityville, NY 11701
call (631) 691-1270 • **fax** (631) 691-1770 • **toll-free orderline (800) 638-7819**
e-mail: baywood @baywood.com • **web site:** http://baywood.com

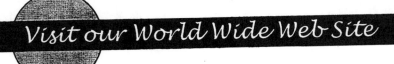

Journal of DRUG EDUCATION

INSTRUCTIONS TO AUTHORS

Submit manuscript to:

Dr. Seymour Eiseman, Editor
Department of Health Science
California State University, Northridge
Northridge, CA 91330

Manuscripts are to be submitted in triplicate. Retain one copy, as manuscript will not be returned. Manuscript must be typewritten on 8-1/2" × 11" white paper, one side only, double-spaced, with wide margins. Paginate consecutively starting with the title page. The organization of the paper should be indicated by appropriate headings and subheadings.

Originality Authors should note that only original articles are accepted for publication. Submission of a manuscript represents certification on the part of the author(s) that neither the article submitted, nor a version of it has been published, or is being considered for publication elsewhere.

Abstracts of 100 to 150 words are required to introduce each article.

References should relate only to material cited within text and be listed in numerical order according to their appearance within text. State author's name, title of referenced work, editor's name, title of book or periodical, volume, issue, pages cited, and year of publication. Do not abbreviate titles. Please do not use ibid., op. cit., loc. cit., etc. In case of multiple citations, simply repeat the original numeral. Detailed specifications available from the editor upon request.

Footnotes are placed at the bottom of page where referenced. They should be numbered with superior arabic numbers without parentheses or brackets. Footnotes should be brief with an average length of three lines.

Figures should be referenced in text and appear in numerical sequence starting with Figure 1. Line art must be original drawings in black ink proportionate to our page size, and suitable for photographing. Indicate top and bottom of figure where confusion may exist. Labeling should be 8 point type. Clearly identify all figures. Figures should be drawn on separate pages and their placement within the text indicated by inserting: —Insert Figure 1 here—.

Tables must be cited in text in numerical sequence starting with Table 1. Each table must have a descriptive title. Any footnotes to tables are indicated by superior lower case letters. Tables should be typed on separate pages and their approximate placement indicated within text by inserting: —Insert Table 1 here—.

Authors will receive twenty complimentary reprints of their published article. Additional reprints may be ordered.

Volume 29, Number 4 — 1999

JOURNAL OF

DRUG
EDUCATION

CONTENTS

Executive Editor:

SEYMOUR EISEMAN, DR.P.H.

Baywood Publishing Company, Inc.

ISSN 0047-2379

Journal of DRUG EDUCATION

EXECUTIVE EDITOR
SEYMOUR EISEMAN, DR. P.H.
Department of Health Sciences
California State University, Northridge

The *Journal of Drug Education* is a peer-refereed journal.

Journal of Drug Education is noted in: *Abstracts on Criminology and Penology; Academic Abstracts; Adolescent Mental Health Abstracts AGRICOLA; ALCONARC: ASSIA: All-Russian Institute of Scientific and Technical Information; Applied Social Sciences Index & Abstracts; Cambridge Scientific Abstracts; Cancer Prevention and Control Database; Counseling and Personnel Services Information Center; Criminal Justice Abstracts; Criminology, Penology and Police Service Abstracts; Cumulative Index to Nursing & Allied Health Literature (CINAHL);Current Contents; Current Index to Journals in Education; Dokumentation Gefahrdung durch Alkohol, Rauchen, Drogen, Arzneimittel; Drug Abuse and Alcoholism Review; EMBASE/Excerpta Medica; Health Promotion and Education Database; H.W.Wilson; International Bibliography of Periodical Literature; International Bibliography of Book Reviews; International Pharmaceutical Abstracts; Kindex Medicus; MEDLINE; National Information Services Corporation (NISC); NCJRS Catalog; National Institute on Alcohol Abuse and Alcoholism's Alcohol and Alcohol Problems Science Database, ETOH; Psychological Abstracts; Smoking and Health Database; Safety and Health at Work ILO-CIS Bulletin;* and *Sociological Abstracts*

The *Journal of Drug Education* is published by the Baywood Publishing Company, Inc., 26 Austin Ave., P.O. Box 337, Amityville, NY 11701. Subscription rate per Volume (four issues): Institutional—$175.00 Individual—$48.00 (prepaid by personal check or credit card). Add $7.00 per volume for postage inside the U.S. and Canada and $12.50 elsewhere. Back list volumes are available at $192.50. Subscription is on a volume basis only and must be prepaid. Copies of single issues are not available. No part of this journal may be reproduced in any form without written permission from the publisher.

J. DRUG EDUCATION, Vol. 29(4) 293-294, 1999

EDITORIAL: CONSENSUS STATEMENT, 14th JULY 1997 OF THE FARMINGTON CONFERENCES

The purpose of *this* statement is to define the basis for shared identity, commitment, and purpose among journals publishing in the field of psychoactive substance use and associated problems. Our aim has enhanced the quality of our endeavors in this multidisciplinary field. We share common concerns and believe that we do well to join together in their solution. To that end we accede to this document as a statement of our consensus and as basis for future collaboration.

1. Commitment to the peer review process

1.1 We are committed to peer review and would expect research reports and scientific reviews to go through this process. As regards the extent to which other material will be so reviewed, we see that as a matter for editorial discretion, but policies should be declared.

1.2 Referees *should be told* that their access to the article on which they have been requested to commit is in strict confidence. Confidentiality should not be broken by pre-publication statements on the content of the submission. Manuscripts sent to reviewers should be returned to the editor or destroyed.

1.3 Referees *should be asked* to declare to the editor if they have a conflict of interest in relation to the material which they are invited to review, and if in doubt they should consult the editor. We define "conflict of interest" as a situation in which professional, personal, or financial considerations could be seen by a fair-minded person as potentially in conflict with independence of judgement. Conflict of interest is not in itself wrong-doing.

2. Expectations of authors

2.1 **Authorship:** All listed authors on an article should have been personally and substantially involved in the work leading to the article.

2.2 **Avoidance of double publication:** Authors are *expected to ensure* that no significant part of the submitted material has been published previously and that it is not concurrently being considered by another journal. An exception

293

to this general position may be made when previous publication has been limited to another language, to local publication in report, or publication of a conference abstract. All such instances, we would expect authors should consult the editor. Editors are encouraged to develop policies concerning electronic publication. Authors are asked to provide the editor at the time of submission with copies of published or submitted reports that *are related to that submission.*

2.3 **Sources of funding for the submitted paper must be declared** *and will be published.*

2.4 **Conflicts of interest experienced by authors:** *Authors should* declare to the editor if their relationship with any type of funding source might fairly be construed as exposing them to potential conflict of interest.

2.5 **Protection of human and animal rights:** *Where applicable* authors *should* give an assurance that ethical safeguards have been met.

2.6 **Technical preparation of articles:** We will publish guidance for authors on the technical preparation of articles with the form of instruction at the discretion of individual journals.

3. **Formal response to breach of expectations by an author**

3.1 Working in collaboration with our authors, we have a responsibility to support the expectations of good scientific publishing practice. To that end each journal will have defined policies for response to attempted or actual instances of *duplicate* publicatplagiarismarism, or scientific fraud.

4. **Maintaining editorial independence**

4.1 *We are committed to independence in the editorial process. To the extent the owner or another body may influence the editorial process, this should be declared, and in that case any sources of support from the alcohol, tobacco, pharmaceutical, or other relevant interests should be published in the journal.*

4.2 *We will publish declarations on any sources of support received by a journal, and will maintain openness in regard to connections which a journal or its editorial staff may have established which could reasonably be construed as conflict of interest.*

4.3 **Funding for journal supplements:** when we publish journal supplements, an indication will be given of any sources of support for their production.

4.4 **Refereeing journal supplements:** An editorial note will be published to indicate whether it has or has not been peer reviewed.

4.5 **Advertising:** Acceptance of advertising will be determined by, or in consultation with, the editor of each journal.

Seymour Eiseman

J. DRUG EDUCATION, Vol. 29(4) 295–308, 1999

PEER-LED AND ADULT-LED PROGRAMS—STUDENT PERCEPTIONS

RACHEL ERHARD
Tel Aviv University

ABSTRACT

This research examines whether peer-led prevention programs are prefer-able to adult-led programs. Participants were 2,447 students in 94 classes, from 31 schools running drug prevention programs. The schools were divided into two groups according to the model they used in their program: fifteen schools used peer-led model, while sixteen used the adult-led model. A 46-item questionnaire was constructed in order to examine the students' perception of the programs. The results show that all the input measures (content, atmosphere, openness, discipline, facilitators' competence) and the outcome measures (satisfaction, knowledge, avoidance, curiosity, personal relationship) were perceived as more positive in the peer-led model. The differences were small, but significant. While the findings suggest that the peer-led model has a somewhat greater potential for primary prevention, the differences found do not enable us to state with certainty that this model is preferable for primary prevention purposes.

Since they were first introduced into schools, primary prevention programs on smoking, alcohol, and drugs have been constantly changing and undergoing revision (see Meyer's comprehensive survey [1]). In the past, beyond the different approaches and models they employed, these programs shared a common characteristic: they were led by adults—specialists, educational counselors, or teachers who had received appropriate training. A recent popular innovation is the replacement of adults by peers reflecting the new "therapeutic" paradigm of using people as resources [2, 3], and is regarded as particularly effective for adolescents. Young people prefer to be in the company of others of their own age group [4-7]. Writers have advanced a number of theories about why adolescents turn to peers, and at some point begin naming friends as more significant to them than parents. Blos argues that self identity emerges from psychological changes associated with narcissism and phallic conflicts [8, 9]. Erikson, from his life-crisis perspective, points out that friends offer constructive feedback and information on self-definitions and perceived commitments [10]. Social-cognition theories view peers as important because of their capacity to reinforce others [11]. The intergenerational-conflict perspective [12] or the discontinuity perspective [13] offer another view of young people's preference for their peers.

Peer groups have characteristics particularly suited to pleasant interaction: feedback tends to be more positive, goals are more likely to be shared, and a sense of freedom and openness prevails in them [14]. It is clear that adolescents influence one another, and social cognition theory provides a useful framework for understanding the mechanism underlying this influence [15]. As Kandel has indicated [16], interpersonal influence can emerge from imitation or social reinforcement, and her data suggests that both processes occur in the peer group.

Based on these theoretical considerations, the use of peer programs for primary prevention purposes has greatly expanded. This expansion sharpens the question: To what extent do adolescents prefer peer-led programs to adult-led programs?

The findings of studies that examined this question are equivocal, since many of them worked with nonintervention controls. However, some specifically stated that they had compared peer-led groups and groups receiving a different kind of intervention. For example, Luepker, Johnson, and Murray compared reduction in smoking in three schools [17]: in one the program was peer-led; in the second, teacher-led; and the third had no special program. In the school where peers were involved in the teaching, lower smoking rates prevailed over the entire three-year study. Botvin et al. report that rates of cigarette, alcohol, and marijuana use decreased following the intervention in the peer-led group, as compared to both the teacher-led and the no-treatment group [18]. Other studies did not find that peer leadership had any advantage over other types. For example, Rickert et al. [19] compared a peer-led to an adult-led AIDS education program, and found no difference in knowledge and attitudes between the two groups of participants. Prince [20], in a study of a smoking prevention program, also found no difference between peer-led and adult-led programs upon completion and after one month. The research hypothesis, that peer-leadership would be significantly more effective than adult leadership, was not substantiated. Greange [21] also reports that peer group helping, individual professional counseling, and routine counseling sessions with disruptive students all improved the behavior of these students to the same extent.

The question whether peer-led programs are preferable to adult-led programs has much practical significance in the Israeli educational system, which is now in the process of intensively introducing such programs. If the peer-led model were to be adopted, this would mean a significant change after prevention programs have been led by adults—teachers or counselors—for twenty years. This change is by no means a simple one, since peer-led programs call for an overall mobilization and a huge investment by the school system. As Tindall put it, after listing the eighteen stages of a peer-led program, implementation: ". . . involves an extensive amount of time, energy and commitment" [22, p. 138].

As a matter of fact, a survey conducted in 1995 in forty-five schools running peer-led programs showed that about 50 percent of the schools discontinued use of the model after only one year [23]. This suggests a rapid rate of burn-out among counselors due to the enormous investment of energy required to successfully carry out the program.

The effort involved in running the peer-led model would, however, be worthwhile if it had a greater prevention potential than the adult-led model. The studies noted above and others do not provide a satisfactory reply to this question since they indicate contradictory conclusions. In addition, only limited generalization can be made from these studies since the samples were very small and the reports do not include a description of other components of the program (whether the peer facilitators were from the same class/age group or older, the duration of the program, its content, other activities conducted in the framework of the program, etc.). This situation raises the possibility that the differences in the dependent variable do not arise from the specific model of leadership but rather from some other characteristic of the program (an intervening variable) which was not controlled. When there has not been control over the many elements that go to make up a "program," it is impossible to attribute any differences (before and after or between a research group and a control group) to the facilitator, regardless of whether he/she is a peer or an adult.

Therefore, in this study we have chosen to begin by describing the set of characteristics which make up a "program." In the second stage, we compare the students' perceptions, in both types of faciliation, of the inputs and outputs of the prevention program in which they participated.

The Israeli Ministry of Education is in the process of introducing substance abuse prevention programs throughout the educational system from elementary school to the end of secondary school. The Ministry has not issued a nationwide mandatory program, but has only provided guidelines for such a program. The decision as to the nature and scope of the program is an internal decision to be taken by the school. Consequently, the variety of programs is so wide that one could say that every school has one of its own. In this situation, there is a dichotomous distinction between programs led by adults and those led by peers. The former are usually led by homeroom teachers who have participated in a training program run by the school counselor. The peers also are trained, usually in concentrated seminar form, with ongoing supervisory sessions during the implementation of the program. The training consists of actual elements of the program itself: attitudes, knowledge, law, life skills, but also practices interpersonal helping skills and leading small discussion groups. This is done through lectures, films, dynamic discussions, and experimental learning led by a trained school counselor.

The question that interested us was: is there any relationship between the model used—peer-led versus adult-led—and the way the students perceive the prevention program?

METHOD

Sample

Two thousand-four-hundred forty-seven students in 94 classes, grades eight through eleven, from 31 schools running drug prevention programs, participated in the study. The schools were divided into two groups based on the model they used in their program: fifteen schools used the peer-led, while sixteen used the adult-led model. Those schools that completed running the program according to plan were included in the sample. In each school, the researchers randomly sampled three classes from the age group participating in the program. The numbers of boys and girls participating were almost identical and the differences in research results between genders and age groups were minute. Therefore, no distinction between the groups was made in presenting the findings.

Tools

1. Student Questionnaire

A 46-item questionnaire was constructed, consisting of: thirty-one closed questions on a 5-point Likert scale from 1—"not at all" to 5—"to a very great extent"; twelve questions on a nominal-dichotomous scale to check the content topics to which the student is exposed; three personal background questions (name of school; grade level; gender).

The following measures; divided into two categories, were constructed from the forty-six closed questions.

Input measures —
1. The students' perception of the program contents; whether they are interesting, varied and relevant;
2. The students' evaluation of the program facilitators (teachers or peers); whether they "did a good job," whether it would be better to invite outside specialists to lead the program or to have it led by peers/teachers;
3. Evaluation of the atmosphere during the lessons; whether it was pleasant, whether the participating students were serious about the lessons, cooperated with the facilitators and listened to them and other students;
4. Evaluation of the degree of interpersonal openness exhibited by the participating students; whether the atmosphere was conducive to an

open discussion and whether the students, even those who were rarely heard in class, were prepared to talk about themselves;

5. Evaluation of discipline; whether there was more disruption than in other lessons and whether the students regarded them as free lessons.

Outcome measures —

1. **Direct outcomes:** a) Cognitive outcomes—the students' perception that thanks to the program they had learned about drugs, understood the subject better and knew more about the damage and danger involved in their use; b) Avoidance of drug use—the degree to which the students feel that owing to the lesson they would avoid drug use in the future; c) Increased curiosity—since it is often claimed that prevention programs arouse the students' curiosity and hence their desire to experience drugs rather than to avoid them, the students' perception of this aspect was examined.

2. **Indirect outcomes:** a) Facilitators as an address—to what extent are the facilitators perceived by the students as an address to turn to for personal advice on drugs and alcohol or personal issues. It is particularly interesting to examine this outcome, since the initiators of the peer-led programs assume that faciliators will become "special friends" and will play a role in secondary prevention, namely by intervention in time of crisis; b) Improvement of interpersonal relations in class and in school. This was based on the assumption that non-academic activities conducted in the school have an added value, and the belief that peer facilitation improves relations among the students in the class, contributes to the relationships between students and teachers, and also causes students to feel they can influence what happens in the school.

3. **Satisfaction with the program**—as a generalized measure—to what extent the students enjoyed participating in the program and want more lessons of this kind.

The number of questions in each measure ranges from one to five. The alpha reliability of the measures is satisfactory, and no lower than .75.

This questionnaire, adapted to the program model, was used for two school groups. In schools where the program was peer-led we used the term "peers" in the wording, and in those where the program was teacher-led we used the term "teachers." This remark is relevant to nine questions.

2. Interview by School Counselor

A personal structured interview was conducted with each counselor in the grade levels for which she/he is responsible. The interview provided general information about the characteristics of the prevention program that had been conducted in the school.

FINDINGS

The findings are presented in three stages: first, a description of the prevention programs as they were conducted in the thirty-one schools that make up the sample, along with a comparison of the peer-led and adult-led models; next, a comparison of the students' perceptions of the input variables in the two models; and finally, a comparison of the outcome variables in both models.

Description of the Prevention Programs

This description is based on the information obtained from the structured interview with the school counselors. Drug prevention programs have many overt and hidden features, both quantitative and qualitative. Of all these, we chose to compare only the major, observable ones.

The Contents

Three types of content are generally included in drug prevention programs: *cognitive* (information on drugs and the damage they cause, legal aspects, etc.); *personal-affective* (like resistance to social pressure, assertiveness, coping with stressful situations, etc.); and *attitudinal-social* (who is a good friend, informing, publicity, etc.). Table 1 shows a list of topics generally included in prevention programs. The participants were asked whether they had covered each of the topics, and the table shows the percentage in both groups who replied in the affirmative.

Table 1. Breakdown of Topics in the Prevention Program by Model

Topics	Peer-led replying "yes" %	Teacher-led replying "yes" %
1. Information about drugs, alcohol, smoking	93	95
2. Informing	57	55
3. Decision-making	68	66
4. Social pressure	92	87
5. Advertisement	37	34
6. Legal aspects	47	65
7. Why yes/why no	80	76
8. Coping with stressful situations	76	64
9. How to say no (assertiveness)	69	53
10. Who is a good friend	53	54
11. Clarifying attitudes about drugs	64	74
12. Alcohol and driving	65	73

Comparison of the models shows that both expose the students to the same topics with minute differences. For example, in the peer-led program, a little more time is spent on personal coping skills, while the teacher-led program emphasized the legal aspects more.

The Scope of the Program

This characteristic relates to the total number of hours each student spent in the program: in class, listening to guest lectures, watching plays or films, meeting with a rehabilitated addict, etc. The disparity is very wide, ranging from the shortest program of seven hours to one of about forty hours. Although there was much variance within each group, and the schools are spread over the entire range of hours, it turns out that the average number of hours of peer-led programs was slightly less than that of the teacher-led.

Structure of Activity

The programs include classroom activity, i.e., conversations and discussions centering on a topic raised by the facilitator—peer or teacher. They may also include activities conducted outside the classroom, such as attending a play, film, lecture, meeting with an ex-addict, visit to a rehabilitation center, and the like. After investigating whether the recommended combination of these two types of activity was carried out in both groups, we found that classroom discussion constituted on the average 60 percent of the program's scope in the teacher-led model, and 65 percent in the peer-led model. We later examined the structure of the classroom discussions and found that in both groups, at least some of them were conducted in smaller formats; e.g., with half of the class. In three schools using the peer-led model and five with the teacher-led model, all of these discussions were carried out with the entire class.

Guest Lecturers

It is common practice to invite outside experts—physicians, judges, police officers, an expert on rehabilitation, etc.—to speak before participants in prevention programs. Indeed, twenty-seven out of the thirty-one schools in the sample invited outside experts. The four schools that did not invite such experts followed the teacher-led model.

Play/Films

Experiential activity such as watching a film or attending a play is recommended in the guidelines for prevention programs. In fact, all of the schools with teacher-led programs, and most (with the exception of four) of those with peer-led programs varied their programs by including a film or play.

A Meeting with a Rehabilitated Addict

Although there is much controversy about the effect of such a meeting on students' behavior, it is frequently included in drug programs. Fifty percent of the schools with adult-led programs, and 40 percent of those with peer-led programs arranged a meeting with an ex-addict.

Parental Involvement

The initiators of these programs recommended involving the students' parents in the program. This is generally done by organizing a lecture for parents only, a lecture for parents and students, inviting them to watch and discuss a play or film, or to jointly watch a play written and staged by the students themselves. Ten of the fifteen schools in the peer-led model held joint activities with the parents, but only six of the sixteen schools with teacher-led programs did so. Although the schools apparently understand how important parental involvement is, none of them offered such an activity more than once.

In summary, the above description provides a picture of currently run prevention programs. It turns out that while the scope of the programs varies greatly, they are similar in all other aspects. They have common "core contents"; hold classroom discussions along with grade level activities; the classroom discussions are held partly in smaller groups and partly with the whole class; most of the schools invite guest lecturers; most provide students with other types of experiences, such as plays or films; about half of them arrange a meeting with a rehabilitated addict, and the same rate invite the students' parents for a meeting on drugs. Among the wide range of program characteristics that we examined, we did not find a single one that was unique to one of the models compared in this study. The only exception was the mode of facilitation itself—whether the program was led by peers or by teachers. Since the programs are so similar, differences in the students' perceptions can be attributed to the model of facilitation.

Input Measures

Five input measures, described in the section on Method, were examined. Table 2 shows the means and standard deviations of the measures in the two groups and the results of t tests to examine the significance of differences between the groups.

In four of the five compared measures, students who participated in the peer-led program perceive it as more positive. The measure in which no difference was found examined classroom discipline, and its purpose was to find whether students take advantage of a situation in which a teacher facilitator is replaced by a peer. It turns out that this fear was groundless—the level of discipline in the peer-led program was no worse than in the teacher-led. It is important to note, however, that while most of the differences found between the two groups were statistically significant, they were very small. Still, since the direction of the differences is uniform, in favor of the peer-led program, we may conclude that participants in peer-led programs have a more positive perception

Table 2. Perceptions of the Input Variables—Peer-led vs Teacher-led Models
(means, standard deviations and t-test)

Measures	Peer-led		Teacher-led		t-test
	Mean	SD	Mean	SD	
Evaluation of content	3.30	0.82	3.09	0.77	−6.49*
Evaluation of atmosphere	3.32	0.78	3.16	0.73	−5.01*
Evaluation of openness	2.78	0.92	2.38	0.94	−10.42*
Evaluation of discipline	2.61	1.07	2.57	0.94	ns
Evaluation of facilitators	3.59	0.81	2.68	0.79	−28.12*

*$p < .05$.

of the input variables. The most significant difference was found in the measure "evaluation of facilitators." The students clearly have a higher estimation of peer- than of adult-facilitation. This preference is explicitly expressed in responses to the item: "All in all I think the peers/teachers did a good job"—while 60 percent of the students in peer-led programs replied "to a great extent/to a very great extent," only about half as many (30%) responded in this vein in regard to teacher facilitators. The same was true of the statement "Activities of this kind are better led by outside lecturers rather than by peers/teachers"—64 percent of those in teacher-led programs agreed with this statement in contrast to 27 percent of those in peer-led programs.

The class atmosphere and the degree of the students' readiness to be open about their personal lives were also perceived more positively in the peer-led model, although, as stated previously, the differences were relatively small. One might have expected to find more closeness and intimacy as a result of peer facilitation, particularly in the small discussion groups, than was borne out by the findings. However, a tendency towards greater openness is clearly shown. While 30 percent in the peer-led model agree that "the atmosphere in the lessons was open and many students talked about themselves," only half that number (about 15%) in the teacher-led group responded in the same way.

It is interesting that although both groups covered largely the same topics, these were perceived more positively in the peer-led group. This may be because of the slightly different emphases given to the topics in that group, i.e., somewhat more attention to interpersonal subjects (like assertiveness and coping with stress) may have enhanced the program's relevance and interest. Perhaps it was not the "what"—the topics themselves—but rather the "how"—the way they were put across, that made the difference. It is also possible that the peers used more dynamic and creative methods of facilitation.

All of the above indicates that all the basic conditions—the program inputs: facilitators, contents, and atmosphere—were perceived more positively by students in the peer-led model. The question now is whether these positive "opening conditions" were translated into more positive outcomes in the peer-led model.

Outcome Measures

Six measures, described in the section of Method, were used to examine the program outcomes. Table 3 presents the means and standard deviations of these six measures in the two groups and t-tests to examine the significance of the differences between them.

Significant differences, albeit small ones, between the two models were found in each of the six measures. While in five of them, the outcomes of the peer-led model are more positive, in the measure "facilitators as an address" the opposite is true. In general, the students in programs led by their peers were more satisfied. A higher percentage of these students replied that they enjoyed participating in the lessons and were interested in participating in similar programs.

The three outcomes, defined by us as direct, are higher in the peer-led model: the students perceive that they learned more and that they would avoid drugs in the future. An interesting finding related to the concern that the student's curiosity to experiment with drugs would be enhanced. Most of the students, from both groups, reported that the program had not caused them to think about trying drugs. It should be noted in this context that the mean correlation between this measure and the measure of acquired information about drugs is 0.1, which means there is no connection between drug-related knowledge and increased curiosity. This finding may provide an answer to those fearful of the damage that may be caused by a program on drug use. However, the surprising finding is that only 40 percent of the students in the teacher-led program,

Table 3. Perceptions of the Outcome Variables—Peer-led vs Teacher-led Models (means, standard deviations and t-test)

Measures	Peer-led		Teacher-led		
	Mean	SD	Mean	SD	t-test
Evaluation of knowledge	3.21	1.04	3.08	1.00	−3.16*
Evaluation of motivation	2.70	1.16	2.50	1.09	−4.36*
Increased curiosity	1.69	1.05	2.12	1.18	9.45*
Facilitators as an address	1.74	0.95	2.07	1.04	8.17*
Improved relations	2.62	0.94	2.36	0.89	−7.17*
Satisfaction	3.47	1.08	3.16	1.09	−7.23*

*$p < .05$.

compared to 61 percent in the peer-led, replied that their curiosity about trying drugs had not been whetted. On the other hand, 13.3 percent in the adult-led program, compared to 8.2 percent in the peer-led, replied that the program to a great extent/to a very great extent made them curious to try out drugs. This would indicate that the adult-led programs arouse greater curiosity and that in this sense the peer-led programs have an advantage.

Of those outcomes we defined as indirect, the measure "facilitators as an address" turned up an interesting finding in both groups. As a rule, most of the students do not regard facilitators—peers or adults—as an address to turn to for personal advice. This finding refutes the basic assumption of the peer-led model, namely that thanks to the peers' role in the program, they would be perceived by their classmates as a "special friend." The findings clearly show that this anticipated role change did not materialize. The peers most likely retain their original role as classmates. On the other hand, the programs actually helps the teachers to make a more significant change in their role, and a higher rate of students replied that following the program they would turn to them for personal help. Once they see the teacher as someone who deals not only with academic topics, but is also involved with the "here and now," students may feel closer to him/her.

Similarly, the second indirect outcome—improved interpersonal relations in the school—was attained to a limited extent. It seems neither of the two models has a significant effect on this sphere of school life. Nonetheless, the peer-led model was perceived as making a somewhat greater contribution to this aspect as well.

To sum up, students in a peer-led drug program express somewhat more satisfaction than those in a teacher-led program. The perceived direct outcomes in the peer-led model—the program imparts knowledge, does not arouse curiosity and prevents future drug use—are somewhat higher than those in the adult-led model. The indirect outcomes of the program are perceived as relatively low: the contribution to improved relations is relatively scant, and the facilitators, be they adults or peers, do not become an address to turn to for personal advice.

DISCUSSION

The research findings to some degree validate the basic assumptions underlying the peer-led model. The students explicitly state that they prefer their classmates as facilitators of a prevention program to adults. They are more satisfied with the program, and a higher percentage of those in a peer-led program would like more lessons of this kind.

The interesting question is, then, to what extent these positive attitudes towards peers and satisfaction with the program are reflected in the outcomes envisioned for the activity. In other words, are the outcomes of the program, as reported on by the students, significantly higher in the peer-led model than in the teacher-led program? Does the students' satisfaction with their peers' facilitation contribute to the effectiveness of the program? Is the peer-led model really more effective in primary prevention of drug use?

In an attempt to come up with a cautious reply to these questions, we refer to the measure "avoidance of drug use" ("More students will avoid drug use after having listened to the lessons"). In other words, the way the students perceive the program's prevention potential will serve as an indirect measure of the perceived effectiveness of the program. Although the two models differ significantly in this measure, the raw size of the difference is small and, in itself, is an insufficient basis for the claim that the peer-led model is more effective in preventing adolescents' drug use. In my view, the peer-led program is nevertheless somewhat preferable since it is less likely to cause damage by stimulating curiosity. While the teacher-led program clearly aroused curiosity about drugs among 13.3 percent of the students, the peer-led program had a similar effect on only 8.2 percent. One should also bear in mind that participants in the peer-led model replied that they had learned more about the damage and dangers of drug use than those in the teacher-led model. For all of the above reasons, one can state, with great caution, that the peer-led model possesses a somewhat greater potential for primary prevention than the teacher-led model.

The potential for secondary prevention—turning to the program facilitator for help in time of crisis—was low in both models. Neither the peers nor the teachers were perceived by the adolescents as an address to turn to for personal help. The assumption that after the program the peers would become "special friends" was refuted. The overwhelming majority of students continue to perceive the peer facilitators in their old role as classmates, not as an address for personal help. Instead, as a result of the program, the teachers were perceived by some as persons they would ask for personal advice or help. This may suggest that teachers may be perceived as more accessible to students when they deal with non-academic topics such as drug use.

I should like to comment on the main limitation of this study. The comparison made here, between two models, was a rigorous one. The "facilitator factor," which was used to differentiate between the two programs is only one characteristic among many. Controls on the program characteristics were only general. Future studies should have, if possible, more stringent control over many other characteristics of the program, to enable researchers to state with greater confidence that any differences found originate in the model of facilitation.

In summary, while the findings suggest that the peer-led model has a somewhat greater potential for primary prevention, the differences found do not enable us to state with certainly that this model is preferable for primary prevention purposes. Nonetheless, the adolescents' clear preference for peers as facilitators should be taken into account in order to enhance the effectiveness of prevention programs.

REFERENCES

1. A. Mayer, Primary Prevention Approaches to Reducing Substance Misuse, *Adolescent Substance Misuse,* T. P. Gullotta, G. R. Adams, and R. Montemayor (eds.), Sage, Newbury Park, California, pp. 140–172, 1995.
2. C. Painter, *Friends Helping Friends,* Educational Media, Minneapolis, Minnesota, 1989.
3. F. Reissman, Restructuring Help: A Human Services Paradigm for the 1990s, *American Journal of Community Psychology, 18:*2, pp. 221–230, 1990.
4. B. B. Brown, S. A. Eicher, and S. Petrie, The Importance of Peer Affiliation in Adolescence, *Journal of Adolescence, 9,* pp. 73–96, 1986.
5. R. Montermayor and E. Hanson, A Naturalistic View of Conflict between Adolescents and Their Parents and Siblings, *Journal of Early Adolescence, 5:*1, pp. 23–30, 1985.
6. R. Montermayor and R. Van Komen, The Development of Sex Differences in Friendships and Peer Group Structure among Adolescence, *Journal of Early Adolescence, 5:*3, pp. 285–294, 1985.
7. J. M. Reisman, Friendship and Its Implications for Mental Health or Social Competence, *Journal of Early Adolescence, 5:*3, pp. 383–391, 1985.
8. P. Blos, The Second Individuation of Adolescence, *The Psychoanalytic Study of the Child, 22,* pp. 162–186, 1967.
9. P. Blos, *The Adolescence Passage: Development Issues,* International Press, New York, 1979.
10. E. H. Erikson, *Identity, Youth and Crisis,* W. W. Norton, New York, 1968.
11. B. R. McCandless, *Adolescents: Behaviors and Development,* Dryden Press, Hinsdale, Illinois, 1970.
12. K. Davis, The Sociology of Parent-Youth Conflict, *American Sociological Review, 5,* pp. 523–545, 1940.
13. R. Benedict, Continuities and Discontinuities in Cultural Conditioning, *Psychiatry, 1,* pp. 161–167, 1938.
14. R. Larson, Adolescents' Daily Experience with Family and Friends: Contrasting Opportunity Systems, *Journal of Marriage and the Family, 45:*4, pp. 739–750, 1983.
15. A. Bandura, *Social Learning Theory,* Prentice-Hall, Engelwood Cliffs, New Jersey, 1977.
16. D. B. Kandel, *Peer Influences in Adolescence,* Paper presented at the meeting of the Society for Research of Child Development, Boston, 1981.
17. R. V. Luepker, C. A. Johnson, and D. M. Murray, Prevention of Cigarette Smoking: Three-Year Follow Up of an Educational Program for Youth, *Journal of Behavioral Medicine, 6:*1, pp. 53–62, 1983.
18. G. J. Botvin, E. Baker, N. L. Renick, A. D. Filazzola, and E. M. Botvin, A Cognitive Behavioral Approach to Substance Abuse Prevention, *Addictive Behavior, 9,* pp. 137–147, 1984.
19. V. I. Rickert, J. M. Susan, and A. Gottlieb, Effect of Peer Counselor AIDS Educational Program on Knowledge, Attitudes and Satisfaction of Adolescents, *Journal of Adolescent-Health, 12:*1, pp. 38–43, 1991.

20. F. Prince, The Relative Effectiveness of a Peer-Led and Adult-Led Smoking Intervention Program, *Adolescence, 30*:117, pp. 187–194, 1995.
21. N. Greange, *The Effects of Individual and Peer Group Counseling on a Sample of Disruptive High School Students,* Unpublished doctoral dissertation, University of the Pacific, Stockton, California, 1982.
22. J. A. Tindall, *Peer Programs: Planning Implementation and Administration*, Accelerated Development, Bristol, Pennsylvania, 1995.
23. R. Erhard, *Peer-Led Programs—Primary Prevention of Substance Misuse*, Ministry of Education, Psychological and Counseling Services, Jerusalem, 1995.

Direct reprint requests to:

Rachel Erhard
Tel Aviv University
School of Education
Ramat Aviv, 69978 Tel Aviv
Israel

J. DRUG EDUCATION, Vol. 29(4) 309–322, 1999

"I'VE HAD TOO MUCH DONE TO MY HEART": THE DILEMMA OF ADDICTION AND RECOVERY AS SEEN THROUGH SEVEN YOUNGSTERS' LIVES

WELSEY LONG

COURTNEY VAUGHN

University of Oklahoma

ABSTRACT

Aware of the dearth of in-depth studies on recovering adolescent addict/ alcoholics, we conducted a year-long qualitative study of seven formerly-addicted youth committed to recovery. The research question was: how do addicted youth become and remain sober? Bending to social stress, including racism and ethnic prejudice, three participants relapsed. However, personal commitment augmented by familial, community, spiritual, and educational support encouraged four to remain sober. Learning from both those who failed and succeeded, the theoretical concepts of surrender, social stress, and resiliency helped to interpret the participants' patterns of response and better understand adolescent recovery.

Investigating the topic of drug and alcohol addiction among adolescents in the United States can be a depressing business. As one young woman so prophetically told us, "I've had too much done to my heart." Most of these youngsters either drop out or are expelled from school and end up in prisons, mental hospitals, or treatment centers. But few recover while they are still young, if ever at all. Perhaps in search of hope and aware of the few in-depth studies of recovering adolescent addict/alcoholics, we conducted a longitudinal qualitative study of seven formerly-addicted youth committed to recovery [1-4].

DESIGN

After spending many hours with the residents, teachers, counselors, and administrators of a nationally acclaimed residential school and long-term treatment center for addicted youth, we selected seven teenage participants

309

who seemed highly committed to changing their lives: two Euro-American males; one African- and one Jordanian-American male; two Euro-American females; and one American-Indian female. Patients are released, usually after several months, when the center's staff believes they have a relatively decent environment in which to live and a chance to live sober and productive lives. The program stresses the Twelve Steps of Alcoholics Anonymous (AA) which emphasize cultivation of a spiritual life and rigorous self assessment, resulting in changing past destructive behavior and living a "golden rule" existence. (For the Twelve Steps of AA, see Appendix A.)

We conducted an ethnographic-phenomenological investigation into the experiences of these youngsters, in particular their prior existence in a drug- and alcohol-infested world, demises, and subsequent struggles to change. First, we conducted extensive phenomenological interviews with each one, generating a life history and extensive responses to questions relating to their efforts to become and remain sober [5-7]. Throughout a twelve-month period we conducted several more interviews with each youngster, occurring both before and after being released from treatment. Creating an ethnographic element to the study we spent hours socializing with and observing the participants at the treatment center and conducting interviews with various counselors, teachers, and family members to determine the trustworthiness of the participants' stories [8].

After having transcribed, coded, and patterned the data, we found that the life of each participant was similar and yet unique [8]. Two distinct groups existed: three relapsed while four remained clean and sober. The experience of the participants making up each of these categories produced thematic responses to the research question: how do addicted youth become and remain sober? They emerge by implication in the following individual portraits and are identified and interpreted in the next section.

THREE RELAPSE

Melinda

Melinda was fifteen years old when we first met her. Her mother was a full-blood Navajo who never knew her own parents. The older woman spent much of her childhood in foster homes and orphanages, and during this time experienced sexual abuse. Eventually, she was adopted by a white family. Melinda's mother was never married to her estranged father, an alcoholic of mixed racial ancestry: Cherokee, German, Filipino, and Guatemalan. Currently, he is living in Guam with a wife and children.

When Melinda was ten, her mother married a man who became Melinda's adoptive father. The couple had one other child, a boy several years younger than Melinda; but they divorced a few years after his birth. Her adoptive father is a recovering alcoholic and attends numerous AA meetings. Her mother drinks only occasionally but is addicted to over-the-counter mini-thins. During our study Melinda's mother was very depressed; she had not held down a full-time job since her divorce. Melinda's mother was emotionally homebound, remaining in her room as much as possible and relying on Melinda's grandmother for financial support. When at home Melinda provided all the nurturing needs for her younger brother, as it was not uncommon for her mother to go for days without speaking. "She said she couldn't handle us kids," Melinda told us, "and her solution was just to go to her room and not to look at it." Melinda desperately "wanted them [Melinda's mother and stepfather] back together because it really hurt and everything because I missed my dad, and it wasn't the same."

Melinda was a good student until her mother and stepfathers' divorce. At thirteen, she started using drugs and alcohol to be accepted by her peers and to make her problems "go away." As a user, Melinda experienced blackouts, ran away from home, and was involved in delinquent behavior. Eventually, her mother banished her from the house, and her adoptive father forced her into treatment.

There, Melinda seemed to accept the discipline and demands of schoolwork and recovery. Yet, her mother rarely came to see her, and Melinda suspected that "she [only] wants me back home for cleaning." Melinda begged her adoptive father to take her after she completed the program. He refused.

Feeling that she had no hope for a loving home, after many months of treatment, Melinda ran away and was never found. Melinda's father said she called her brother several times and then was never heard from again. The authorities believe she may be dead.

Ali

When we first met Ali he was seventeen years old. Born in Jordan, when Ali was four, he, his four siblings, and his parents had moved to the United States where they became financially successful. Although his parents were Christian, they were also traditionally Middle Eastern, stressing the importance of the extended family and deference to familial male authority figures.

In school Ali excelled until his encounter with drugs in the ninth grade. He started using marijuana and nicotine, as do so many youth, but it was not long before he experimented with acid, cocaine, crank, crystal methane, and crack cocaine. He began stealing money and salable goods to buy drugs. He even robbed his uncle's and parents' homes. He was caught, tried, and sentenced to drug treatment.

When attempting to explain why he began using, he recalled that certain students routinely called him ethnic names such as "camel jockey."

No one noticed me. I was a good wrestler and didn't get any attention from that. Our school was big on wrestling, and I thought this would make me more popular. When a guy who was kicked off the wrestling team invited me to his house I thought this was the beginning for me. All they did was get high, and before long I was getting high with them.

Ali was quite productive and successful in treatment. Yet his family was filled with shame and visited him only sporadically. After leaving treatment it appeared as though Ali was in recovery. He continued to attend AA meetings and work toward a GED. However, he was refused entrance back into public school. Perhaps to ease the blow, his parents bought him an expensive new car, and he was soon a noticeable target for the opportunistic people who have been known to attend Twelve Step meetings. He was approached by two white females who asked for a ride home. Ali consented, only to discover the women were drug dealers. Ali smoked crack two weeks after becoming involved with them and was selling drugs the next week. He was caught and sentenced to serve time in a penitentiary. Now released, he is again using and selling drugs.

Anthony

When we first met Anthony, an African-American, he was eighteen years old. His father and mother were no longer together, and he was not certain if they were ever married. Apparently, however, his father and mother had provided for themselves and five children, but that had all ended when his parents severed their relationship. Then ten years old, Anthony, his mother, and the children moved into a low income housing project, and Anthony's life changed dramatically.

Anthony's mother became addicted to drugs and he was surrounded by numerous other youngsters who engaged in delinquent behavior. He began drinking and using marijuana and other drugs, as did the other children living in his mother's home. Perhaps in search of another family, Anthony also joined a gang.

Amazingly, Anthony did attend public school until he reached the tenth grade, but, as he put it. "I wasn't getting anything from school but high." At seventeen he was court ordered to treatment as a result of drug- and alcohol-related felony convictions.

While in treatment Anthony worked toward completing his high school diploma, and his counselors believed that he showed signs of authentic recovery. After leaving the center, the pressure to provide money for his family, ironically, the lack of family support, and his own needs to appear successful drove him back to dealing drugs. He was arrested and fled prosecution after being released on bail. Today, he has been recaptured, tried and convicted and, at the time of this writing, is in prison.

FOUR REMAIN SOBER

Jessica

Jessica was sixteen when our study began. A Euro-American female, she was one of two children born to her mother and father. Her mother worked in a bank and her biological father, who is now deceased, was an oil field worker. An alcoholic, he had spent time in the penitentiary for numerous drunk driving convictions and eventually died of a heart attack, most probably brought on by excessive drinking. Jessica was only eleven at the time. Probably, financial destitution led Jessica's mother to remarry. That relationship was not successful, and the couple separated when Jessica was eleven.

The death of Jessica's father and the introduction of her mother's new husband and his three children into their household had a disastrous affect on her already fragile state. She fought regularly with her stepbrother who tried to kill her on one occasion. One night he reached for a gun which he thought was loaded and pointed it to "my head and pulled the trigger, and there weren't any bullets in it."

Incidences such as these characterized Jessica's fall into oblivion. Jessica had already begun to drink when she was ten. She added marijuana, crank, cocaine, crack cocaine, acid, ecstasy, PCP, and crystal methane to the list. More dramatic than her drug and alcohol use was that she "never paid for it. The only thing I've ever bought was a six-pack of beer." One night Jessica overdosed and was taken to a hospital. She had been found in a hotel room with eight adult men who were arrested for drinking and having sex with a minor.

Jessica was sent to treatment for the third time, where she did well. After graduation from the facility Jessica moved in with her mother who insisted to local school officials that Jessica be re-admitted to high school. Moreover, Jessica's mother drove her fifty miles to attend support group meetings. Grateful, Jessica told us:

> I don't know what I would do without my mother. We used to have so many fights and problems. She told me she loved me, and she wanted me to stop using drugs. . . . My mother works at the bank and every one in town knows her. She told my teacher that I would be glad to talk about drugs and how they almost ruined my life. It's kind of funny that I speak to students every two weeks about staying away from drugs.

Jessica was proud that she was asked to provide drug education for her school. "I was scared at first but so many of those people didn't know the first thing about drugs. In rural towns people mostly drink. It was amazing to hear myself trying to talk people out of trying drugs. These group meetings were kind of like A.A. for me."

As the months wore on, Jessica's popularity increased not only with her peers but with parents in the town. Jessica was singled out at a school assembly by the principal and her homeroom teacher for her work with drug education. Jessica was surprised by the recognition and was even more gratified when the principal announced that the school almost refused to re-enroll her. "I think my assisting in the drug groups helped me. Even if I wanted to get high . . . I don't. I would disappoint so many people. People look up to me, and I couldn't do that to them."

John

Characterized as nobody's child, John, a Euro-American, was eighteen years old when we first interviewed him. His mother, who had two children, died when John was six, and he was sent to live with a grandfather. His grandfather died shortly thereafter, and an aunt took him in. After a short stay, John was shuffled off to his grandmother' house. She became ill and a neighbor, Jake, took John in and became his legal guardian.

The instability of John's life and the availability of drugs led him into early delinquent activities. As a preteen John began using marijuana, and at thirteen John was participating in gang-related felonious acts. Eventually, he was arrested for destruction of property, assault and battery, theft, and petty larceny and sentenced to a drug treatment program. John's guardian supported him through these and other arrests and two treatment center stints. "I was involved with gangs, guns, and drugs all while I'm staying in his home, and he was patient with me, never pressuring me. He asked me if I wanted help with my drug use. If needed he would get me into treatment or counseling." John believed that God sent this father figure to him.

John admitted that he turned his life around while in drug treatment. But he believed that *any* positive focus, such as religious convictions or pursuance of a college degree, could insure sobriety and a productive life; for example, he did not think that regularly attending Twelve Step meetings, as stressed in treatment, was the only means of remaining sober. According to John, young people such as he "involve themselves in gangs [and drugs] because of the sense of security that is involved in it and the sense of love that they feel from other people. They probably haven't gotten it in any of their life." For John, replacing the emptiness with devout religious convictions has keep him focused and sober.

John was proud that he graduated from the treatment program in six months, faster than anyone before him. But he was also quick to give most of the credit to God. John had taken high school courses while in treatment and, after leaving, returned to public school. After graduating John enrolled in a nearby community college. His career interests included physical therapy and the ministry. In college, John met a fellow student to whom he later proposed. The wedding was canceled when John's fiancee became pregnant by another man. John dropped out of school, stopped attending church (but was still a devout Christian), and quit his full-time job. He became a door-to-door vacuum cleaner salesman for a while and, at the time of this writing, is seeking other employment.

Mick

Mick was eighteen years old when we began our study. A Euro-American male, he was the younger of two boys born to working class parents. Mick grew up in a violent home. He father regularly beat the boys and their mother. Mick sadly remembered, "we didn't know what he was going to be like when he came in, . . . if he was going to flip out about what happened at work today, or if he was going to bring some candy to us." The couple divorced when Mick was twelve.

Mick's family also has a history of alcohol and drug abuse. His maternal aunt and grandfather were alcoholics; while his father was a heavy drinker and smoked marijuana. With his older brother, Mick started experimenting with drugs at the age of twelve, smoking pot which they obtained from their father's "stash." By the time Mick was sixteen he was addicted to crack cocaine and involved with gangs. From the seventh to tenth grades Mick was a terrible student. Yet, a part of him always wanted to do well. He repeated the tenth grade three times before deciding to quit. Soon after, he was arrested for grand larceny and sentenced to drug treatment.

Also following a somewhat non-traditional path, after a short stint Mick was discharged from the treatment center for not following facility rules. But instead of being placed back into the streets, the facility allowed him to enroll in the adult inpatient program. Mick was grateful because he was still on probation for robbery, breaking and entering, and drug possession, and total suspension from the facility would have forced him back into court where he could have been sentenced as an adult to time in a penitentiary. Encouraged by a few older men serious about recovery, while in the adult center Mick diligently worked the Twelve Steps and attempted to find employment.

After leaving treatment Mick attributed his success to the fear of going to prison (which was imminent if he continued using) and his dedication to the A.A. program. Also, following a suggestion from his parole officer, Mick enrolled in a local junior college. Proud of himself, he told us, "I get pumped about going to school. I love that, man. I love being able to say, 'hey, I'm going to college. . . . I go to work' . . . makes me feel good to be productive and have an organized lifestyle."

For the first time in his life Mick believed he had a future. "I pray every day that I won't ever use again. I no longer crave drugs or alcohol. There was a time if I smelled drugs it took all I had to stop from trying to get some. Prayer has taken that away from me. I think I've beat my addiction but I got to keep going to meetings." Accompanying Mick from time to time is a newfound woman friend. Time will tell whether, as in John's case, the relationship will threaten or strengthen Mick's new sober life.

Lisa

When we first interviewed Lisa, a Euro-American female, she was sixteen years old. She was the oldest of three girls. Her two younger sisters had also been involved with drugs. Their mother and father were no longer together. They divorced when Lisa was eleven. Both of her parents used heroine intravenously throughout her childhood. Her father was a violent man, physically abusing her mother. She and the two girls would move to a battered woman's shelter when the beatings became too regular or severe. Lisa's father and mother finally quit using after being arrested, convicted, and sent to prison for selling drugs.

During her short life, Lisa had been raped and involved with gangs; also, she has had three abortions. She was first raped by her father's best friend while her supposed protector lay comatose in the next room from a near heroine overdose. Eventually, the state took Lisa and her sister into protective custody and placed them in foster homes. Lisa remembered growing up in poor neighborhoods and attending public schools most of her academic years. She attended a private, religious school for a time, but even this restrictive environment could not protect her from herself. At eleven, Lisa had started using when she sniffed gasoline while walking home from school. Five years later she was committed to treatment after a near heroine overdose.

After Lisa completed the treatment center program she choose to live in a half-way house. Lisa was afraid to move in with her mother or father, both of whom had been released from prison. Lisa worked hard to develop a positive self image and eventually told us, "For the first time in my life I actually love myself, . . . and no one is ever going to use me again. I won't let them." Then out of prison, her father attended a half-way house family group session, and Lisa told him, "'Your drug addiction almost killed you and Momma. You never considered me and Jill [her sister]. We went from foster home to foster home, and you never tried to change and come get us. I forgive you but I would never do my kids like you done us.'" Lisa and her father seemed to come to an understanding. Eventually, Lisa and her entire family began attending A.A. and N.A. meetings.

In addition, Lisa returned to school, although while in treatment she had taken and passed the GED exam. She went out for and made the girls' softball and volleyball teams. "I never attended school, and I wanted to prove to myself that I could be successful and graduate from high school." Also a pep club member, Lisa enjoyed being a student and making friends. For once she felt like a "normal" girl. "If these people knew of my past they would die. I'm doing so well no one knows I go to A.A. and N.A. meetings, or that I am in recovery. . . . For the first time I feel so normal. I was so crazy to use drugs. I almost ruined my life."

During the last few weeks of the study Lisa experienced the urge to use. She quit attending public school, got a job, and moved back into a half-way house, where her father was also living. Although Lisa had enjoyed school immensely, the pressure of appearing but not feeling normal and the easy access to drugs wore her down. "Passing" may have helped her stay sober, but it seemed to have accentuated, not ameliorated, Lisa's divided self [9].

PATTERNS OF RESPONSE

Race and Ethnicity:
Acceptance versus Nonacceptance

The three participants who relapsed shared similar situations and characteristics that made sobriety difficult. All three were non-white, which hindered their being socially accepted whether they used or not. Ali had frequently been called "sand nigger" at school; and his subsequent need to be validated by whites led him to "start buying drugs and giving them away so that students would like me." Similarly his need to be associated with beautiful white girls led him back to using. After being arrested the last time Ali lamented, "I feel so stupid. I should have known that a woman in her thirties wouldn't want a man not even twenty. She needed someone with a car. Access to money, and crazy enough to supply her needs."

Like Ali, Melinda wanted the approval and acceptance of her peers. She had attended a suburban school with few non-white students. A small number of American Indians were enrolled in Melinda's school, but they wore long hair, occasionally dressed in a manner that indicated their culture and heritage, and were involved with their tribes' ceremonies and other activities. Melinda did not identify with them because she was reared "like a Caucasian." Culturally, Melinda had difficulty deciding where she belonged. Her adopted father was white, her mother was a fair-skinned American Indian, and her biological father had a mixed non-white ancestry. "It was hard making and keeping friends, and I thought and still do that a lot of it had to do with my race." When one of Melinda's few close friends began socializing with other students, Melinda became afraid that she would lose her friendship. The new friend was a year older than Melinda and was already using drugs and alcohol, mainly beer and marijuana. Melinda remembered, "At first I was afraid to use, but they started teasing me and calling me names, and I felt I had to . . . I thought they would stop being my friends."

Also focusing on race, Anthony attributed being African American and poor to his entry into drug use. He spoke about how difficult it was for blacks to find decent employment and how the school district so easily gave up on him. "I went to school one day and the principal told me in his office that he felt I was causing problems for student and staff." The principal then informed him he would be going to school half a day three days a week, and he would not return until his office contracted his mother. One month later the call had never come. "If I was white there is no way this would have happened. Because I'm black they treat me any kind of way." Anthony never went back to school until he was forced into the drug treatment school. There, he seemed eager to continue his education. Nevertheless, after his release, he was bitter and frustrated. "When you're not high white people think you are; when you're not stealing, white people think you are; when you're looking for work, white people think you ain't." When reflecting on Anthony's words, he may have been saying, "I'll never make it."

The white students, on the other hand, seemed better able to blend back into their communities. Jessica flourished at her public school and was even accepted as a reformed user. Somewhat different from Jessica, Lisa feared exposure, telling us, "I thought there would be problems when I returned to school. I thought people would remember me. It had been a year and a half since I went there. Nobody noticed me. I guess it's because I looked like every other kid at school." Her ability to hide her past addiction and appear normal, white, and middle class, for a time enabled her to work on her recovery without setbacks.

Mick and John had no problems resuming their school lives when they returned to their communities. Mick's probation officer even helped him enroll. "It was easier than I thought. I don't think no one remembered me. . . . Everyone I used to get high with got kicked out, dropped out, or graduated. I picked up where I left off when I used to go there. Hanging in the halls, meeting with babes, and hanging out on weekends." Public education also welcomed John back.

> They didn't ask any questions. I went with my transcript from the [treatment] facility school, and, in about five minutes, I was in a counselor's office enrolling. I don't think no one at the school [students] knew of my past. There are so many kids at the school, no one probably noticed me because I wasn't causing any problems.

The larger communities also seemed willing to accept Jessica, Lisa, Mick, and John. John's legal guardian gave him a party after he was released from treatment. Neighbors and family were invited to show they had missed John, and that they supported his efforts to get help. "I was kinda glad for the party. I was wondering how my next door neighbors were going to act when I got out. The party made it easier for me to fit back in. I was able to hang out with people my age without people thinking I'm trying to corrupt their son or daughter." Mick and Lisa had the same good fortune with their neighbors. People who knew of their past never mentioned it. Lisa commented, "I just didn't want a whole lot of people in my business. . . . No one asked questions, even though they knew where I had been. It was not long before I was a normal teenager. I didn't have to go through any problems with friends and neighbors as the facility staff said I might." Mick had the same experience. "I knew everyone knew of my drug treatment but no one mentioned it. Friends and neighbors acted as if I didn't have a problem. They accepted me back as if I wasn't the boy who used to steal from them and be high and drunk all the time."

Family Stress/Family Support

As already suggested, Melinda, Anthony, and Ali had limited family support, succor that may have shielded them emotionally from a racist world. Melinda commented. "I wanted her [Mom] to come and visit so bad. I wanted her to know how I was doing, and how I was working on trying to get home. . . . She came once during my stay and only stayed thirty minutes. Me and my father pleaded with her to stay, and she wouldn't." Melinda's hope was that her mother would see how well she was progressing and look forward to her daughter's return home. Melinda's step-father was only partially supportive.

Ali's family appeared to be emotionally supportive when he first arrived in treatment. They attended some group meetings. But during one group therapy session Ali's father stated, "it is uncommon for persons from Jordan to involve themselves with drugs, and Ali has shamed the family." Ali's face lowered, and after his family left, he prayed they would never return. Ali's prayer was at least partially answered because his father, two brothers, and sister did not return for some time, claiming their heavy work schedules precluded it. After Ali's release it seemed to him that his father was unable to forgive Ali for committing criminal acts and being a drug addict. And yet the older man lavished his son with expensive gifts such as a new car.

After leaving treatment, Anthony experienced a general lack of family support. When Anthony graduated from the drug treatment facility family and friends had a party celebrating his return home. Thoughtlessly, they served alcohol and drugs. His brother stated that it took some doing to get Anthony to take a drink, but his mother convinced him that he could because of the party; but she cautioned him to stop the next day.

Conversely, the families of the four recovering youngsters were involved in the participants' treatment and continued to be so after their children's graduations. Jessica's mother explained, "I come because I want to continue to learn about addiction and how I can continue to help Jessica. When I think I have all the answers, I might quit coming." And John's guardian still attends family meetings, even though John no longer participates.

With the exception of John, those still sober are attending A.A. and N.A. meetings with their parents. Mick said, "my family [members] challenge each other. Me, my brother and both my parents are recovering. We ride to the meetings together. I'm only able to go twice a week, but the others attend a least three a week." The support and encouragement of his family being involved with A.A. makes it easier for him. "I used to get high with my brother, steal drugs from my father's 'stash,' and get drunk with my mother. Now that we're all sober I don't have anybody to get high with, plus we would all know if somebody slipped [relapsed]." As Lisa put it, "If we all stick together and support each other, one day at a time we'll beat this drug stuff."

Spirituality

The four who remained sober had hit a personal "bottom" and as a result they surrendered to a "higher power," something that seemed to encourage their sobriety [10-11]. Mick prayed "everyday for strength not to use again. People who don't use don't know how tough it is to stay clean. People, places, smells, and stuff remaind you of the times when you were using, and your mind makes you start thinking of using. Whenever this happens I just start praying." Lisa reiterated that "everyday you have to fight for your sobriety. Your mind makes you think you can do it one more time and quit again. You have to have something just as powerful as drugs to fight for you, and that is God. If I didn't pray everyday and believe God helps me, I know I would be using." Jessica rejoined, "no matter what situation I was in I knew I could pray, and God would help me. When I finally decided to stop I asked God to help me with my drug problem, and He did. I pray because without Him I know I would be using again and back to my old ways." John concluded, "I knew if I was to change my life permanently, I had to have a real relationship with God."

CONCLUSION

Social stress literature suggests that if the stress level of a recovering person's daily life reaches a perceived intolerable level, s/he will return to using. And this is exactly what happened to three of the participants. Conversely, positive environmental conditions (stress modifiers) enabled four of the participants to enjoy recovery. These participants became resilient, developing the capacity to survive and even thrive despite great personal tragedy. They accomplished this by being provided with and seeking out protective factors such as educational, familial, community, and spiritual support [12-16].

Interestingly John and Lisa even suffered considerable losses of their protective factors as time went on. Yet they made adjustments and survived without using. This suggests that resiliency can be internalized over time even when key external or environmental support wanes. The participants' spiritual convictions were particularly helpful during this regrouping process. They "came to believe" that some magnificent universal force loved and cared for them [9]. Hopefully, that damage done to their hearts is on the mend.

APPENDIX A

Twelve Steps of Alcoholics Anonymous

1. We admitted we were powerless over alcohol—that our lives had become unmanageable.

2. Came to believe that a Power greater than ourselves could restore us to sanity.

3. Made a decision to turn our will and our lives over to the care of God as we understood Him.

4. Made a searching and fearless moral inventory of ourselves.

5. Admitted to God, to ourselves, and to another human being the exact nature of our wrongs.

6. Were entirely ready to have God remove all these defects of character.

7. Humbly asked Him to remove our shortcomings.

8. Made a list of all persons we had harmed and became willing to make amends to them all.

9. Made direct amends to such people wherever possible, except when to do so would injure them or others.

10. Continued to take personal inventory and when we were wrong promptly admitted it.

11. Sought through prayer and meditation to improve our conscious contact with God as we understood Him, praying only for knowledge of His will for us and the power to carry that out.

12. Having had a spiritual awakening as the result of these steps, we tried to carry this message to alcoholics who still suffer, and to practice these principles in all our affairs.

REFERENCES

1. W. DeJong, Relapse Prevention: An Emerging Technology for Promoting Long-Term Drug Abstinence, *The International Journal of the Addictions, 29,* pp. 681–705, 1994.

2. A. S. Friedman, N. W. Glickman, and M. R. Morrissey, Prediction to Successful Treatment Outcome by Client Characteristics and Retention in Treatment in Adolescent Drug Treatment Programs: A Large Scale Cross Validation Study, *Journal of Drug Education, 6,* pp. 149–16, 1986.

3. V. Johnson and R. J. Pandina, Effects of the Family Environment on Adolescent Substance Use, Delinquency, and Coping Styles, *American Journal of Drug and Alcohol Abuse, 17,* pp. 71–88, 1991.

4. R. A. Siegel and A. Ehrilich, Comparison of Personality Characteristics, Family Relationships, and Drug-Taking behavior in Low and High Socioeconomic Status Adolescents Who Are Drug Abusers, *Adolescence, 24,* pp. 925–936, 1995.

5. R. Tesch, The Contribution of a Qualitative Method: Phenomenological Research, Paper presented at the meeting of the American Research Association, New Orleans, Louisiana, 1988.

6. L. Barritt, A. Belkman, and K. Mulderij, *Researching Education Practice,* University of North Dakota, Center for Teaching and Learning, Grand Forks, North Dakota, 1985.

7. C. Moustakas, *Phenomenological Research Methods,* Sage, Thousand Oaks, California, 1994.

8. R. Bogden and S. Biklen, *Qualitative Research for Education,* Allyn and Bacon, Boston, 1982.

9. N. K. Denzin, *The Alcoholic Society: Addiction and Recovery of the Self,* Transaction Publishers, New Brunswick, 1993.

10. H. M. Tiebout, The Ego Factors in Surrender in Alcoholism, *Quarterly Journal of Studies on Alcohol, 15,* pp. 610–621, 1954.

11. J. Nowinski, *Substance Abuse in Adolescents and Young Adults: A Guide to Treatment.* Norton and Company, New York, 1990.

12. C. S. Lindenberg, S. C. Gendrop, and H. K. Reiskin, Empirical Evidence for the Social Stress Model of Substance Abuse, *Research in Nursing and Health, 16,* pp. 351–362, 1993.

13. A. D. Kanner, J. C. Coyne, C. Schaefer, and R. S. Lazarus, Comparison of Two Modes of Stress Measurement: Daily Hassles and Uplifts versus Major Life Events, *Journal of Behavioral Medicine, 4,* pp. 1–39, 1981.

14. N. Garmezy, Stressors of Childhood, in *Stress, Coping and Development in Children,* N. Garmezy and M. Rutter (eds.), McGraw-Hill, New York, 1983.

15. E. E. Werner and R. S. Smith, Protective Factors and Individual Resilience, in *Handbook of Early Childhood Intervention,* Meisels and Shonkott (eds.), Cambridge University Press, Cambridge, 1990.

Direct Reprint requests to:

Welsey Long
Department of Educational Leadership
University of Oklahoma
Norman, OK 73019

J. DRUG EDUCATION, Vol. 29(4) 323-335, 1999

PREVENTING ALCOHOL ABUSE:
AN EXAMINATION OF THE "DOWNWARD SPIRAL"
GAME AND EDUCATIONAL VIDEOS*

MICHAEL CZUCHRY
Fayetteville State University, North Carolina

TIFFINY L. SIA
Institute of Behavioral Research

DONALD F. DANSEREAU
Texas Christian University

ABSTRACT

Downward Spiral is a board game developed by the authors to illustrate the dangers of continued substance abuse. Previous work has found that college students and probationers find the game interesting, enjoyable, useful, and realistic [1]. In the current study, college students either played Downward Spiral, watched educational videos on substance abuse, or completed a set of questionnaires unrelated to alcohol and drug abuse. Those students who either played the game or watched the videos rated both as beneficial. However, students who watched videos had somewhat higher levels of consumer satisfaction. Students who played the game rated it as smoother, and they felt more positive following the session than students who watched videos. Both videos and the game increased students' intentions to limit alcohol consumption compared to students who served as controls. Individuals in the game group also indicated significantly greater intentions to change their alcohol behavior than those in the other groups.

Although there is evidence that both drug treatment and drug abuse prevention programs can be successful [2-6], the National Institute on Drug Abuse and the National Institute on Alcohol Abuse and Alcoholism have repeatedly called for

*This work was supported by the Texas Christian University Research and Creative Activities Fund and the National Institute on Drug Abuse (DA08608). The interpretations and conclusions, however, do not necessarily represent the position of Texas Christian University, NIDA, or the Department of Health and Human Services.

323

the development of approaches that will bolster the effectiveness of both types of programs. One critical determiner of how impactful a program will be is the motivation and engagement level of the participant [7-10]. To date, the most well known technique for enhancing engagement is motivational interviewing [11]. In using this technique, a counselor works one-on-one with a client to identify core issues and prepare him or her for change. Although this approach appears to be successful, new approaches are needed, especially for group settings.

In this regard, we have developed a set of activities directed at facilitating an openness to treatment and willingness to change for probationers who have been remanded to drug abuse treatment [12]. These group activities are part of a 5-year NIDA sponsored project called Cognitive Enhancements for Treatment of Probationers (CETOP). The activities are oriented toward enhancing self-esteem, facilitating the recognition of a need for change, as well as providing new strategies that residents may use to make treatment more positive and worthwhile. Initial investigation of one of the activities designed to facilitate motivation to change—a board game called the Downward Spiral [13]—has found that college students and probationers find the game interesting, enjoyable, useful, and realistic [1]. The game, which is a sole-survivor type of game for five to six people, uses drug-related consequences, facts, and quotes to illustrate the continuing dangers of abuse. Players assume the role of someone who is committed to continuing drug and alcohol abuse. In the course of playing the game they experience vicariously how substance abuse can affect their characters' health, social support network, self-esteem, and financial legal situation (for a more detailed description of the game, see [1]).

The use of games as instructional and therapeutic tools is certainly not a new idea. Educators have long theorized that games may provide engaging, motivating formats for promoting learning outcomes. Research on the effectiveness of games (often computer games) for instructional purposes generally support their motivational benefits (for a review, see [14]). Games appear to be as beneficial as traditional forms of instruction, and in some cases (games that focus on math, physics, or language learning) appear to facilitate learning to a greater extent than other methods. Although games are widely accepted as having therapeutic effects and are implemented regularly [15], little research has been conducted to examine their effectiveness in treatment and prevention settings.

We suggest that the rich experiential base provided by games can be especially impactful when combined with factual and/or motivational information. Researchers have stressed the importance of integrating both episodic (experience based) and semantic (factual) types of information for meaningful personal change to occur [16]. Programs that attempt to influence attitudes and behavior through informational or emotional appeals often lack experience-based knowledge and are consequently relatively ineffective [8, 17]. In addition to providing a mechanism for integrating multiple types of information, games may provide a more palatable, indirect vehicle for communicating with participants by delivering messages through the "side door." This peripheral approach may thus avoid problems that arise from direct attacks on a person's alcohol and drug-related attitudes that sometimes actually increase intentions to abuse [18].

We also suggest that, as a consequence of becoming naturally engaged in aspects of the game (e.g., developing a winning strategy, anticipating what will happen next), individuals may be less resistant to the serious content of the game. The engaging, indirect characteristics of games may provide a powerful means for influencing attitudes and behavior. Although it has been suggested that individuals need to be receptive and interested in a message for it to have an impact [19], research has shown that it is sometimes possible to change attitudes in an indirect, peripheral fashion, and this may be especially true for certain individuals such as those with low need for cognition [20]. Advertisers, for example, will sometimes use sex appeal to capture the attention of their audience, resulting in increases in sales even if viewers are paying little attention to information about the product itself.

Our previous work on Downward Spiral has been primarily exploratory in nature, the main question being whether students and probationers would be open to the board game format. In the current study, students either played the game, watched two videos on the dangers associated with alcohol and other substance abuse, or completed a set of questionnaires unrelated to substance abuse issues. The videos selected for inclusion are currently shown by the Alcohol and Drug Education and Awareness Program at Texas Christian University (TCU) for students who have received alcohol violations. In addition to examining the perceived effectiveness of the activities, we also examined the impact that these activities have on behavioral intentions toward alcohol-related issues.

METHOD

Participants

One hundred eighty-seven Texas Christian University students, recruited from undergraduate psychology classes, received experimental credit for completing the experiment. Of these, two (1.1%) were not included because they did not complete the materials appropriately, and two (1.1%) were not included because their ages (ages 42 and 56) were outside of the target population (i.e., college students aged 18–24). The final sample ($N = 183$) had an average age of 19.40 and 68 percent were female.

Stimulus Materials

Downward Spiral

The game was designed as a sole-survivor game in which the goal is to outlast other players or recover. The game focuses primarily on alcohol-related consequences (though we do include some consequences that involve marijuana, cocaine, or heroin use). Players roll three dice and move the number of spaces indicated. The colored square they land on determines the type of consequences they receive (e.g., health, social support, self-esteem, or financial legal). Players take a card and read the consequence, points lost, and fact or quote to other players (see Figure 1 for examples of consequence cards), and then record on their score sheet the points or possessions lost (see Figure 2). Players can earn back points when they land on educational squares by remembering facts, quotes, or consequences received by other players.

Educational Videos

The educational videos selected are currently used by the Alcohol & Drug Awareness Program at Texas Christian University. The first video, *Cruel Spirits: Alcohol & Violence,* is used in each session and depicts alcohol-related consequences that occur in a variety of situations, such as at Mardi Gras in New Orleans. The focus of the first video was on alcohol, although it also targets the relationship between alcohol and violence. The second video, *America Hurts:*

Self-concept	Health
After a drinking episode, I tell myself that I've got to change. But after awhile, I forget about my promises, and it's not until I do something stupid again that I remember my broken promises.	I got drunk and decided not to use a condom and had unprotected sex. I caught a curable venereal disease and have to get treatment. It was pretty embarrassing and not very pleasant.
Lose 3 Personal Accomplishment points	Lose 4 Physical points
Quote	
Change is not made without inconvenience, even from worse to better.	
Richard Hooker (1554-1600) English theologian	**Fact**
	One out of five students abandon safe sex practices when drunk.

Figure 1. Examples of game cards used in Downward Spiral.

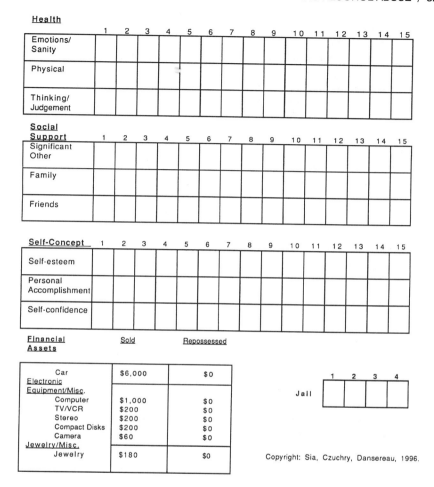

Figure 2. Examples of the score sheet used in Downward Spiral.

The Drug Epidemic, provides several case studies of individuals who abuse drugs and how their drug use becomes the driving force in their lives.

Dependent Measures

Consumer Satisfaction Questionnaire

The consumer satisfaction questionnaire was developed to assess the extent to which the activities were interesting, enjoyable, and useful. Students rated the following items on 8-point Likert scales:

1. How interesting was participating in this activity?
2. How much did you enjoy participating in this activity?
3. How much did you learn about the possible consequences of drug and alcohol use?
4. Do you think this activity is an effective way to learn about alcohol and drug related consequences?
5. To what extent do you feel this activity might help students consider the consequences of irresponsible drinking?
6. To what extent do you think that this activity could help students who do have alcohol problems?
7. To what extent would you like to do more of the activity you just participated in?
8. To what extent would you recommend this activity to people you know?
9. To what extent would you recommend this activity to be used in colleges?

A principal component analysis computed on the nine items revealed one factor that included all items (coefficient alpha = .95).

Session Evaluation Questionnaire

The *Session Evaluation Questionnaire* (SEQ) [21] is an established clinical assessment that uses semantic differential scales (e.g., shallow vs. deep) to evaluate both the effectiveness of the session and the feelings of participants. Prior research has established four factors: session depth (valuable, deep, full, powerful, and special), session smoothness (good, safe, easy, relaxed, pleasant, smooth, and comfortable), post-session positivity (happy, pleased, definite, confident, friendly, and involved), and post-session arousal (excited, moving, wakeful, fast, aroused, and energetic). The coefficient alphas (based on ratings from all sessions) for these factors in the current study were as follows: session depth = .82, session smoothness = .76, positivity = .79, and arousal = .74.

Behavioral Intentions Measure

The behavioral intentions measure was developed to examine students' intentions to engage in responsible alcohol related behaviors. Participants read the following instructions prior to completing the questionnaire:

> Alcohol continues to be a major concern on college campuses across the nation. Whether students drink or not, they are likely to be confronted with negative consequences associated with alcohol at some point during their college years. We would like to find out about the sort of activities that TCU students would be willing to do to help with alcohol-related problems. For the following activities, please *indicate how likely you would be to engage in each activity.* Answer the questions as if we were to actually call upon you to carry them out.

Students rated the likelihood that they would engage in each of the following activities on 8-point Likert scales (anchored at 0 with "very unlikely I would do this" and at 7 with "very likely I would do this"):

1. Talk to an incoming first year student about the negative consequences associated with alcohol use?
2. Talk to your friends about alcohol related issues?
3. Participate in a group discussion about alcohol related issues?
4. Lead a seminar to address alcohol related problems on campus?
5. Tell a friend they are drinking too much?
6. Become a peer counselor at the drug and alcohol education center?
7. Encourage a friend to go to the counseling center to deal with an alcohol-related problem?
8. Listen to a prominent speaker talking about the dangers of alcohol use?
9. Intervene when you see someone drinking too much?
10. Set limits on how many alcoholic drinks you will have at a party?
11. Make changes in your alcohol consumption?

A principal components analysis with varimax rotation was conducted on these eleven items and three factors emerged with eigenvalues greater than 1.0. The first factor (scale), social prevention, had a coefficient alpha of .78 and included the items lead a seminar, talk to an incoming first year student, become a peer counselor, talk to friends, and participate in group discussions. The second factor (scale), intervene, had a coefficient alpha of .79 and included the items tell a friend they are drinking too much, encourage a friend to go to the counseling center, intervene when you see someone drinking too much, and listen to a prominent speaker. The final factor (scale), control, had a coefficient alpha of .46 and included the items set limits on how many alcoholic drinks you will have at a party and make changes in alcohol consumption. Because of the low coefficient alpha for the control factor, these two items were examined separately.

Procedure

Students were randomly assigned to three activities (game, video, and questionnaire) as they arrived to the experiment. Participants were taken to the experimental rooms where they received five minutes of general instructions and then either played Downward Spiral, watched two videos depicting the dangers associated with alcohol and other drug use, or completed a set of unrelated questionnaires for sixty-five minutes. Students then completed the consumer satisfaction, SEQ, and behavioral intentions measures.

RESULTS

Consumer Satisfaction

An ANOVA with Activity (video vs. game) as the between-groups factor and the consumer satisfaction factor as the dependent variable, revealed a significant main effect for Activity, $F(1, 119) = 6.91$, $p < .05$. As can be seen in Table 1, students who watched videos had higher levels of consumer satisfaction than students who played the game. Due to a violation of homogeneity of variance for this analysis, a Mann-Whitney U Test was conducted. This analysis was also significant, $Z = -2.41$, $p < .05$.

Session Evaluation Questionnaire (SEQ)

A MANOVA with Activity (video, game, questionnaire) as the between-groups factor and Session Depth and Session Smoothness as the multiple dependent variables revealed a significant multivariate effect for Activity, $F(2, 180) = 12.13$, $p < .05$. Univariate effects were significant for Session Depth, $F(2, 180) = 12.74$, $p < .05$, and Session Smoothness, $F(2, 180) = 9.97$, $p < .05$ (see Table 2 for means and standard deviations). Tukey's HSD post-hoc tests revealed that students who watched videos ($p < .05$) or played the game ($p < .05$) rated the session as significantly *more* deep than students who filled out questionnaires. Students who watched videos rated the session as significantly *less* smooth than students who played the game ($p < .05$) or filled out questionnaires ($p < .05$).

A MANOVA with Activity (video, game, questionnaire) as the between-groups factor and Positivity and Arousal as the multiple dependent variables revealed a significant multivariate effect for Activity, $F(2, 180) = 5.92$, $p < .05$. Univariate effects were significant for Positivity, $F(2, 180) = 4.82$, $p < .05$, and Arousal, $F(2, 180) = 6.67$, $p < .05$ (see Table 2 for means and standard deviations). A Kruskal-Wallis test, conducted due to a violation of homogeneity of variance for the univariate analysis of positivity, was also significant, chi-square $(2, N = 183) = 11.25$, $p < .05$. Tukey's HSD post-hoc tests revealed that students who played the game felt more positive compared to students who watched videos ($p < .05$) or filled out questionnaires

Table 1. Means and Standard Deviations for
the Consumer Satisfaction Factor

Activity	M	SD	N
Video	4.75*	1.21	63
Game	4.07*	1.62	58

*$p < .05$

Table 2. Means and Standard Deviations for the Session Evaluation
Questionnaire (SEQ) Factors

Factor	Activity	M	SD	N
Session Depth	Video	5.33$_a$	1.09	63
	Game	5.04$_a$	1.04	58
	Questionnaire	4.44	.87	62
Session Smoothness	Video	5.01	.78	63
	Game	5.72$_a$	.88	58
	Questionnaire	5.46$_a$	.99	62
Positivity	Video	4.58$_a$	.79	63
	Game	5.08	1.12	58
	Questionnaire	4.62$_a$	1.00	62
Arousal	Video	3.74$_a$	1.05	63
	Game	3.63$_a$	1.11	58
	Questionnaire	3.10	.96	62

Note: For each factor, means that share a subscript are not significantly different from each other ($p < .05$).

($p < .05$). Students who played the game ($p < .05$) or watched videos ($p < .05$) felt more aroused compared to students who filled out questionnaires.

Behavioral Intentions Measure

A MANOVA with Activity (video, game, questionnaire) as the between-groups factor and the Social Prevention and Intervene factors as the multiple dependent variables was conducted (see Table 3 for means and standard deviations). No effects were significant.

A MANOVA with Activity (video, game, questionnaire) as the between-groups factor and the Limit and Change items as multiple dependent variables revealed a significant multivariate main effect for Activity, $F(2, 179) = 4.00$, $p < .05$. Univariate effects were significant for both Limit, $F(2, 176) = 4.86$, $p < .05$, and Change, $F(2, 176) = 5.28$, $p < .05$. Tukey's HSD post-hoc tests were conducted. Students who played the game ($p < .05$) or watched videos ($p < .05$) planned to set greater limits on alcohol consumption at parties compared to students who filled out questionnaires. Students who played the game ($p < .05$) planned to make more changes in their personal alcohol consumption compared to students who watched videos or filled out questionnaires.

Table 3. Means and Standard Deviations for the Behavioral Intentions Measure

Factor	Activity	M	SD	N
Social Prevention	Video	4.01$_a$	1.49	63
	Game	3.88$_a$	1.77	58
	Questionnaire	3.76$_a$	1.53	62
Intervene	Video	4.95$_a$	1.35	63
	Game	4.62$_a$	1.43	58
	Questionnaire	4.65$_a$	1.43	62
Limit	Video	5.44$_a$	1.49	63
	Game	5.75$_a$	1.77	58
	Questionnaire	4.73	1.53	62
Change	Video	3.57$_a$	1.35	63
	Game	4.88	1.43	58
	Questionnaire	3.63$_a$	1.43	62

Note: For each factor, means that share a subscript are not significantly different from each other ($p < .05$).

DISCUSSION

Students rated both watching videos and playing Downward Spiral as beneficial. However, students who watched videos had somewhat higher levels of consumer satisfaction. One possible explanation may be the comparison levels students may have been using in making their ratings. In the video group, ratings may have been made in comparison to other educational videos (potentially those seen during high school health classes). Since the videos used in this study had been selected for use by the alcohol and drug education and awareness program at TCU they were likely to be more interesting and impactful than the typical videos used in high school. On the other hand, students who played Downward Spiral probably have not had as much exposure to educational games, and thus may have been comparing the game to more entertainment-oriented games such as Monopoly.

In terms of session effectiveness, perhaps it is not surprising that students who watched videos or played the game rated the sessions as being deeper and more arousing compared to students who completed questionnaires. It is interesting, however, that students who played the game also rated the session as smoother and felt more positive in comparison to students who watched videos. These benefits may stem from the greater interaction game players had with their peers. We anticipate that the smoothness and positivity of the session will lead to increased openness to further discussions about substance abuse issues.

It does not appear that the game or videos altered students' behavioral intentions toward social prevention or intervention. Students who played the game or watched videos did not intend to get more involved in proactive activities, such as becoming a peer counselor, than students who served as controls. However, those who watched videos or played the game did intend to make personal changes. Students who engaged in either activity intended to set greater limits on the number of alcoholic drinks they would have at parties, and students who played the game also intended to make general changes in their alcohol consumption. These findings are especially important given the difficulty prevention programs have had in altering behavior, especially as it pertains to alcohol consumption [8]. It is important to note that, in the current study, we were measuring behavioral intentions and not actual behaviors. This was mostly due to the difficulty of observing and recording behavior which was illegal for most participants. In fact, great care was taken to protect the anonymity of all participants. Fortunately, behavioral intentions are known to correlate highly with actual behavior [22, 23], and thus the current findings are encouraging.

As mentioned in the introduction, games offer a potentially powerful means for altering an individual's attitudes and behavioral intentions because games are naturally engaging and because they may be able to deliver information through the "side-door." In contrast, direct frontal approaches appear to have problems. Bensley and Wu [18] suggested that following a direct anti-alcohol message, students often intend to drink more to re-establish their own sense of control and freedom. On the other hand, the game and, to a lesser extent, the videos examined in the current study appear to increase intentions to monitor alcoholic consumption.

The current findings are also encouraging because an important component was not included. In experiential types of learning, it is important to give participants an opportunity to synthesize and share any insights that may have occurred over the course of the activity [24]. Such discussions would be expected to benefit both students who watched videos or played the game. In the residential treatment setting, we have scripted the debriefing following the game. First, participants engage in small group discussions to determine who won and why. Such a decision is often ambiguous because the game typically ends before a clear winner emerges. The criteria used to determine who won is then shared with the entire group (several groups play simultaneously). Then, participants share any insights or discoveries with the group. This post-game process may be the most powerful aspect for eliciting change. We are currently investigating the debriefing aspect of the game with students who have received alcohol violations and must attend educational meetings at the TCU Alcohol and Drug Education Center. Students in one group read an information packet on the dangers of alcohol and other drug use, watch a video (one of the videos included in the current study), and then engage in a scripted discussion with their counselor. Students in the other group play Downward Spiral instead of watching the video. We expect that the game will facilitate the group discussion that follows as well as increase students' intentions to make personal changes in their alcohol consumption.

The current study is encouraging. It suggests that a game board format may be useful in the prevention setting. However, additional research is required to further examine the viability of the game. The videos examined in the current study also appear effective. Research is being conducted to examine the extent to which the current findings will generalize to other populations. In addition, the game is currently being implemented along with a set of other activities directed at facilitating an openness to treatment and willingness to change in a residential drug abuse treatment facility.

REFERENCES

1. M. Czuchry, T. L. Sia, D. F. Dansereau, and S. M. Dees, Downward Spiral: A Pedagogical Game Depicting the Dangers of Substance Abuse, *Journal of Drug Education, 27*:4, pp. 373-387, 1999.
2. M. D. Anglin, Treatment of Drug Abuse, in *Drugs and Crime,* M. Tonry and J. Q. Wilson (eds.), University of Chicago Press, Chicago, Illinois, pp. 393–460, 1990.
3. D. D. Simpson, Effectiveness of Drug-Abuse Treatment: A Review of Research From Field Settings, in *Treating Drug Abusers Effectively,* J. A. Egertson, D. M. Fox, and A. I. Leshner (eds.), Blackwell Publishers of North America, Cambridge, Massachusetts, pp. 41-73, 1977.
4. D. D. Simpson and S. B. Sells, Effectiveness of Treatment for Drug Abuse: An Overview of the DARP Research Program, *Advances in Alcohol and Substance Abuse, 2,* pp. 7–29, 1982.
5. W. B. Hansen, School-Based Alcohol Prevention Programs, *Alcohol Health & Research World, 17*:1, pp. 54–60, 1993.
6. W. R. Miller, The Effectiveness of Treatment for Substance Abuse: Reasons for Optimism, *Journal of Substance Abuse Treatment, 9,* pp. 93–102, 1992.
7. W. R. Miller, Increasing Motivation for Change, in *Handbook of Alcoholism Treatment Approaches: Effective Alternatives,* R. K. Hester and W. R. Miller (eds.), Pergamon Press, New York, 1989.
8. P. E. Nathan, Failures in Prevention: Why We Can't Prevent the Devastating Effect of Alcoholism and Drug Abuse, *American Psychologist, 38,* pp. 459–467, 1983.
9. D. D. Simpson and G. W. Joe, Motivation as a Predictor of Early Dropout From Drug Abuse Treatment, *Psychotherapy, 30*:2, pp. 357–368, 1993.
10. D. D. Simpson, G. W. Joe, G. Rowan-Szal, and J. Greener, Client Engagement and Change During Drug Abuse Treatment, *Journal of Substance Abuse, 7,* pp. 117–134, 1995.
11. W. R. Miller and S. Rollnick, *Motivational Interviewing: Preparing People to Change Addictive Behavior,* Guilford, New York, 1991.

12. S. M. Dees and D. F. Dansereau, *A Jumpstart for Substance Abuse Treatment: CETOP Readiness Activities, a TCU/CETOP Manual for Counselors,* Institute of Behavioral Research, Texas Christian University, Fort Worth, Texas, 1997.

13. T. L. Sia, M. Czuchry, and D. F. Dansereau, *The Downward Spiral of Substance Abuse,* Copyrighted instructional game, Department of Psychology, Institute of Behavioral Research, Texas Christian University, Fort Worth, Texas, 1996.

14. J. M. Randel, B. A. Morris, C. D. Wetzel, and B. V. Whitehill, The Effectiveness of Games for Educational Purposes: A Review of Recent Research, *Simulation & Gaming, 23*:3, pp. 261–276, 1992.

15. E. T. Nickerson and K. B. O'Laughlin, It's Fun—But Will It Work? The Use of Games as Therapeutic Medium for Children and Adolescents, *Journal of Clinical Child Psychology,* pp. 78–81, Spring 1980.

16. D. F. Dansereau, S. M. Dees, and D. D. Simpson, Cognitive Modularity: Implications for Counseling and the Representation of Personal Issues, *Journal of Counseling Psychology, 41*:4, pp. 513–523, 1994.

17. M. S. Goodstadt, Prevention Strategies for Drug Abuse, *Issues in Science and Technology, 3,* pp. 28–35, 1987.

18. L. S. Bensley and R. Wu, The Role of Psychological Reactance in Drinking Following Alcohol Prevention Messages, *Journal of Applied Social Psychology, 21*:13, pp. 1111–1124, 1991.

19. W. J. McGuire, Personality and Attitude Change: An Information-Processing Theory, in *Psychological Foundations of Attitudes,* A. G. Greenwald and T. C. Brock (eds.), Academic Press, New York, 1968.

20. R. E. Peety, J. R. Priester, and D. T. Wegener, Cognitive Processes in Attitude Change, in *Handbook of Social Cognition: Volume 2: Applications,* R. S. Wyer, Jr. and T. K. Srull (eds.), Lawrence Erlbaum Associates, Hillsdale, New Jersey, 1994.

21. W. G. Stiles and J. S. Snow, Dimensions of Psychotherapy Session Impact Across Sessions and Across Clients, *British Journal of Clinical Psychology, 23,* pp. 59–62, 1984.

22. I. Ajzen and M. Fishbein, *Understanding Attitudes and Predicting Social Behavior,* Prentice-Hall, Englewood Cliffs, New Jersey, 1980.

23. M. Kim and J. E. Hunter, Relationships among Attitudes, Behavioral Intentions, and Behavior, *Communication Research, 22*:3, pp. 331–364.

24. S. Kohn, Specific Programmatic Strategies to Increase Empowerment, *The Journal of Experiential Education, 14*:1, pp. 6–12, 1991.

Direct reprint requests to:

Donald F. Dansereau
Department of Psychology
Texas Christian University
Box 298920
Fort Worth, TX 76129

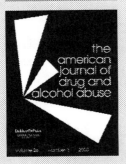

J. DRUG EDUCATION, Vol. 29(4) 337-357, 1999

FACTORS IN MARIJUANA CESSATION AMONG HIGH-RISK YOUTH*

MICHELLE D. WEINER

STEVE SUSSMAN

WILLIAM J. McCULLER

KARA LICHTMAN

University of Southern California

ABSTRACT

The rise in marijuana use among high school students has generated considerable concern. The apparent failure of current marijuana control efforts may be due in part to ignorance about why students use marijuana and what influences them to consider quitting. This article utilized both open-ended and multiple-choice surveys as well as health educator-led focus groups to assess issues related to marijuana use and cessation among a population of high-risk youth. A total of 842 students participated, assessed as two separate samples from eleven continuation high schools in southern California. Approximately 70 percent of the students are current marijuana users. Interpreting results across both samples, it is apparent that interest in quitting marijuana use among continuation high school students is high. Over half of the marijuana users surveyed have tried to quit and failed. Still, several social images associated with marijuana smokers are positive and subjects express a lack of confidence in the efficacy of marijuana cessation clinic programs. Subjects believe that either self-help or punitive methods are the most effective types of marijuana cessation activities. A reportedly high rate of failed quit attempts suggests that effective marijuana cessation programs are needed in this population. Future programs must address both reasons users resist change, including use of marijuana as a stress reliever, and the particular motivations that subjects report regarding why they desire to quit using marijuana, including legal, vocational, and health consequences.

*This article was supported by a marijuana supplement to a grant awarded by the National Institute on Drug Abuse (#DA07601).

337

Since the early part of this decade, the use of marijuana by teenagers has been on the rise [1, 2]. According to NIDA's Monitoring the Future study, the percentage of eighth graders reporting marijuana use in the past thirty days rose from 9.1 percent in 1995 to 11.3 percent in 1996. Similarly, the percentage of tenth graders using marijuana in the past thirty days rose to 20.4 percent, up from 17.2 percent the previous year. Overall, marijuana use has increased more than 250 percent among eighth graders and 150 percent among tenth graders since 1992. Additionally, data from the Drug Use Forecasting annual report indicate that the percentage of adult arrestees under the age of twenty testing positive for marijuana increased from 10 percent in 1989 to 72 percent in 1996 [3]. These disturbing trends in marijuana use suggest that current cessation strategies must be revisited and more effective programs need to be designed.

A first step in developing successful marijuana cessation programs is to understand why adolescents use marijuana [4]. The existing literature on the etiology of marijuana use indicates several correlates or predictors of initial and continued marijuana use. Among these are previous marijuana use behavior, use of other drugs, and various psychosocial variables [5]. Specific psychosocial variables that are linked to marijuana initiation and use include: peer and adult use [e.g., 6-11]; peer pressure to use [12]; weak parental attachments [13-15]; parental marijuana use, behaviors, and attitudes [e.g., 7]; drug use offers [13]; positive marijuana use outcome expectancies [13, 16]; attitudes favorable to marijuana use [17]; and subjective expected utility of the effects of marijuana use [18].

Another variable of interest that relates to the etiology of marijuana use pertains to the specific functional meanings of marijuana use to the adolescent. It is essential that researchers understand the needs that marijuana use fulfills if alternative ways to meet these needs are to be offered. One way of assessing the functional meanings of marijuana use is to ask adolescents directly why they use it [19]. An abundant literature is available on why people use cigarettes [e.g., 19, 20]. Since cigarette smoking and marijuana use are known to be associated [21, 22], one can hypothesize that reasons for cigarette use may be similar to reasons for marijuana use. A study by Perry, Murray, and Klepp [19] found that 56 percent of the variance in cigarette smoking behavior of 2,587 ninth- and tenth-graders was accounted for by six functional meanings of tobacco use: 1) a coping mechanism for dealing with boredom and frustration; 2) as a way to have fun; 3) a strategy to reduce stress; 4) a transition marker or a claim on a more mature, adult status; 5) a way of gaining admission to the peer group; and 6) a way to maintain one's own personal energy, to feel centered or renewed. It seems likely that marijuana use may serve these same functions.

In considering ways to aid people with marijuana cessation, it is also important to understand why people might decide to quit. Some research suggests that the most compelling reasons for quitting marijuana may be related to physiological and psychological effects of the drug. For example, Bailey, Flewelling, and Rachal investigated whether predictors from a social context domain (e.g., peers' use of drugs) or a drug-specific domain (e.g., perceived consequences of drug use on psychological and physiological functioning) would better distinguish between those who became regular users of marijuana versus those who experimented with its use but never became regular users [23]. Using a sample of 456 high school students, they found that those who reported never having gotten "stoned" from marijuana use, and those who believed that the physical and mental adverse effects of marijuana were important, were less likely to continue to use marijuana. In another study of adult marijuana users seeking treatment for marijuana [24], two reasons related to the negative physiological effects of marijuana, "self-control" and "health concerns," received the highest ratings on a "Reasons for Quitting" scale. Receiving lower ratings were social context variables such as "self-image," "not socially acceptable," and "legal problems." These findings suggest that the primary reasons people quit using marijuana are related to drug-specific physiological and psychological effects.

Other evidence suggests that social influence may be an important variable to examine when investigating why users quit marijuana. Kandel and Raveis found that marijuana use cessation for a group of people twenty-eight to twenty-nine years old who had been active marijuana users at age twenty-four to twenty-five was predicted by marriage after age twenty-four to twenty-five for both sexes [25]. It is possible that the satisfying social interactions associated with nonuse may eliminate reliance on marijuana for this purpose.

Given current understanding of why young people use and stop using marijuana, a variety of intervention approaches have been tried. These include participation in school and school-plus-community based prevention programs [e.g., 26-29]; Marijuana Anonymous, a 12-step cessation program modeled after Alcoholics Anonymous [5]; and clinic-based approaches [24]. Unfortunately, these approaches have achieved limited success [5]. One possible reason for this is that these action-oriented programs may be presented to adolescents who have not yet decided to quit using marijuana. Borrowing from research on the stages of self-change in cigarette smoking cessation [30, 31], it is important to identify the percentage of adolescent marijuana users who are contemplating quitting their use and need assistance in quitting behavior versus those who need help to move from precontemplation to contemplation. Reasons for quitting information is more relevant for those in the stage of precontemplation, whereas action-oriented strategies are more relevant for those in the stage of contemplation [30].

THE PRESENT STUDY

The present study involves continuation high school students as subjects. In California, continuation or alternative high schools serve students who are unable to remain in the comprehensive school system for behavioral, emotional, or other reasons such as substance abuse [32]. Among this population, rates of marijuana use are consistently higher than they are among comprehensive (regular) high school students [32, 33]. In southern California, approximately 41 percent of continuation high school students report weekly marijuana use in comparison to only 9 percent of comprehensive high school students. Given the widespread use of marijuana within this group, this is an appropriate sample in which to study reasons for use and cessation of marijuana.

Two samples of youth from continuation high schools participated in this study. The first sample participated in focus groups to generate reasons for marijuana use, reasons for quitting marijuana use, and cessation strategies. In addition, close-ended survey questions addressed students' stages of change, their willingness to participate in various marijuana cessation programs, the perceived effectiveness of different types of cessation programs, and the credibility of potential sources of information on marijuana.

The second sample responded to close-ended questions regarding why people use or do not use marijuana. Specifically, students rated a list of reasons people may use marijuana, a list of reasons people may not use marijuana, and identified social images associated with people who use marijuana. This line of inquiry was intended to reveal functional meanings of the use of marijuana.

METHODS

Sample One

Subjects

A total of 453 students from ten Los Angeles area continuation high schools completed surveys in October and November of 1996. Table 1 presents the demographic characteristics of the sample. Current drug use is also presented in Table 1. Seventy-four percent of the sample reported using marijuana at least once in the last thirty days (335 of the 453 subjects).

Data Collection and Instruments

Parents were informed of the study, and a non-participation consent form could be signed and returned to exclude those students whose parents did not wish them to volunteer. Students and parents were ensured that participation in the study was completely voluntary, and that students could withdraw from the study at any time. They were also informed that responses would be kept anonymous. This protocol received Internal Review Board approval because

Table 1. Demographic and Drug Use Characteristics of Two Samples of Adolescents at High Risk for Drug Use (Samples One and Two)

Response Category		Sample One (n = 453) Mean (SD)	Sample Two (n = 389) Mean (SD)
Age		16.8 (0.83)	16.6 (1.03)
Alcohol Use		1.79 (2.09)	1.98 (2.76)
Cigarette Use		3.50 (3.97)	3.93 (4.21)
Marijuana Use		2.85 (3.28)	3.01 (3.66)
"Hard" Drug Use		0.62 (1.37)	0.50 (1.57)
		Percent (%)	Percent (%)
Gender	Male	53.9	61.3
	Female	46.1	38.8
Ethnicity	Asian/Pacific Islander	2.6	6.8
	Black/African American	8.8	9.1
	Latino/Hispanic	50.8	47.0
	Native American	1.6	1.8
	White/Non-Latino	32.9	29.0
	Other	3.2	6.3
Lives with both parents	Yes	55.7	53.7
	No	44.3	46.3
Currently a parent	Yes	13.8	11.6
	No	86.2	88.4
Currently married	Yes	2.7	3.0
	No	97.3	97.0
Currently working	Yes	27.9	27.6
	No	72.1	72.4

Notes: Drug use scale reflects frequency of drug use in the last month where 0 = 0 times; 1 = 1 to 10 times; 2 = 11–20 times; 3 = 21–30 times. . . . 10 = 91–100+ times.

responses were anonymous and no biochemical data was collected. In addition, questions regarding marijuana use were not considered particularly sensitive among this high risk, older adolescent sample. Previous studies, particularly of cigarette smoking, indicate that biochemical validation is not necessary when collecting anonymous data [28]. Parental and student decline totaled 5 percent. An additional 12 percent of the population was recorded absent on the day of testing.

An extended focus group protocol was used to gather the data. First, a twenty to thirty minute pretest was administered to classrooms of continuation high school students (n = about 15 subjects per class). Once the pretest was complete, a focus group discussion was conducted to generate reasons these youth use marijuana, why they would quit marijuana use, and what activities might be useful for facilitating cessation of marijuana use. Focus group discussion is theorized to promote expression of new ideas, unbiased by the constraints of self-report demanded by a questionnaire format [34]. Because 74 percent of the sample reported marijuana use in the last thirty days (and such items are not particularly sensitive within this sample) and continuation school classroom size is half that of the regular school system, whole classes were involved in the focus groups to minimize disruption to the school. Although samples of six to eight youths are typically recommended when engaging in focus groups, previous work suggests that a sample size of fifteen is not too large to obtain numerous quality responses to focus group questions [4, 34].

Pretest questions were designed to collect demographic and drug use data and information relevant to marijuana use cessation (see Tables 1 through 4). Current drug use reflected frequency of use in the last thirty days. Marijuana use stages of change data were also collected. Of the response categories, two assessed "precontemplation," three assessed "contemplation," one assessed "action," and one assessed "maintenance."

Pretest items also were designed to assess various intervention strategies. Specifically, a cessation strategies rating list was used to determine the degree to which students felt the proposed cessation activity would work. Students also indicated their preference for either in-school or out-of-school programs and endorsed the health educator characteristics or background they would find most trustworthy.

Subjects then participated in a 30-minute focus group discussion. A total of thirty-one focus groups was formed (31 classes). Verbal responses were recorded verbatim (in writing) by the health educator and were later content coded. Previous work with this population included use of audiotapes or having focus group observers or the health educator (i.e., the group facilitator) write down information. This group of youth tends to be less verbal than general populations of youth. A simple recording of information by the health educator was found to provide nearly identical information as the other methods. Thus, use of the health educator was considered adequate for the present study.

Focus group responses were independently coded by two coders. The first coder, a forty-two year old white male (the second author), coded responses into mutually exclusive and exhaustive categories. For the "why use marijuana" item, thirty categories were developed. A second coder, a twenty-five year old African American male (the third author), coded responses into those same categories. A total of fourteen categories accounted for 88 percent and 90 percent of all responses coded by the first and second coders, respectively. The rank order of the categories was identical across coders, with three exceptions (79% agreement): 1) the "relieve boredom" category was coded as occurring in fourteen versus fifteen groups; 2) the "fun" category was coded as occurring in

Table 2. Ratings of the Perceived Effectiveness of Ways to Stop Marijuana Use Among a High-Risk Population (Sample One)

Asked of students: How effective are the following as ways to stop marijuana use?

Response Category	Mean	SD	Rank
Quit in private, on your own, without any policies	2.15	1.14	1
Inpatient (rehab) stay	2.40	1.10	2
Jail time	2.40	1.16	2
Fines	2.47	1.11	4
Driver's license suspension	2.54	1.15	5
12-step meetings or counseling	2.57	1.06	6
Education about the effects of marijuana	2.64	1.00	7
Public service work	2.78	1.01	8
School suspension	2.92	1.11	9
Do nothing	3.14	1.16	10

Notes: Response scale is: 1 = very effective; 2 = somewhat effective; 3 = a little effective; and 4 = not effective. The minimally significant difference for any two means within this sample is 0.05 (two-tailed, $p < 0.05$).

eleven versus twelve groups; and 3) the "parents use it" category was coded as occurring in five versus six groups by the first and second coder, respectively.

For the "why quit marijuana" item thirty categories were developed. A total of seventeen categories accounted for 90 percent and 87 percent of responses, respectively. The rank order of the categories was identical, with three exceptions (79% agreement): 1) the "don't like becoming stupid" category was coded as occurring in seven versus five groups; 2) the "something bad happened" category was coded as occurring in five versus six groups; and 3) the "for the sake of the children" category was coded as occurring in four versus two groups, respectively.

For the "what are some cessation activities" item, seventeen categories were developed. A total of nine categories accounted for 88 percent and 86 percent of the responses, respectively. The rank order of the categories was identical, with two exceptions (78% agreement): The "discussion of bad consequences" category was coded as occurring in eleven versus seven groups, and the "sports activity" category was coded as occurring in nine versus five groups, respectively. In all cases of disagreement, the rank order of a category differed by one to three ranks. Discrepancy of any coding was subsequently resolved through discussion and consensus between the two coders, and those categories comprising at least 85 percent of all responses across groups constitute the present focus group data.

Table 3. Credibility of Information Sources on Marijuana Among a High-Risk
Population (Sample One)

Response Category	%	Rank
I would be more likely to believe information about marijuana from someone if . . .		
The speaker had personal experience with drugs	47.7	1
None of the above	28.2	2
The speaker was the same age group as me	9.5	3
The speaker was the same ethnic background as me	6.3	4
The speaker was from the same neighborhood as me	4.4	5
The speaker held the same political beliefs as me	2.3	6
The speaker was the same gender as me	1.6	7
Whose opinion about marijuana would be most trustworthy to you		
An ex-user	64.3	1
A parent	16.0	2
A scientist	7.6	3
Other relative	4.3	4
A teacher	2.4	5
A religious leader	2.4	5
A police officer	1.2	7
An entertainer (singer, actor)	1.4	8
Someone in the government	0.5	9
A social activist	0.0	10

Table 4. Results of Focus Groups in Thirty-One Classrooms (Sample One)

Groups Asked: Why Use Marijuana?[a]	No. of Groups Identifying This Category as a Response
To get high/baked	21
Relieve stress/forget problems/coping	21
Feels good/makes you happy/makes you laugh	18
Relaxation	16
Relieve boredom/adventure/novelty/curiosity	14
Medical reasons (ADD, headaches, nausea, glaucoma, appetite, pain)	14
Peer pressure/friends use it/to fit in	13
Fun/recreational	11
To be cool/a rebel/an adult/get an image	8
Stimulate/expand/open your mind	6
Tastes/smells good	5
Parents use it	5
Religious/spiritual experience	4
Helps one sleep	4

[a] The most popular fourteen categories are listed, which accounted for 88 percent of all focus group responses to this item.

Table 4. Cont'd.

Groups Asked: Why Quit Using Marijuana?[b]	No. of Groups Identifying This Category as a Response
To avoid getting in trouble/jail/probation	23
Job (e.g., join the military, high-paying job)	19
Drug testing	18
Too much money	11
Bored/sick of using it	11
Don't's like becoming stupid/unmotivated/ lazy/having a lack of energy	7
Medical problem/health	7
Family pressure	6
Getting fat	6
School problems	5
General: something bad happened	5
Memory loss	4
Someone asked them to (e.g., boy/girlfriend)	4
For sake of children	4
Pregnancy	3
Lessened effect	3
Sports	3

[b] The most popular seventeen categories are listed, which accounted for 90 percent of all focus group responses to this item.

Groups Asked: What Are Some Cessation Activities?[c]	No. of Groups Identifying This Category as a Response
Discussion of bad consequences (e.g., lungs, arrests, money, lack of energy, memory problems)	11
Counseling/12-step groups/listen to recovery panels or speakers who have stopped/ discussion of getting stupid from use	9
Sports activity involvement	8
Involvement in other activities	6
Discussion of negative effects on friends or family	5
Setting goals	4
Heard about death related to use	3
Group discussions	3
Getting a job/training	2
Church	2

[c] The most popular seventeen categories are listed, which accounted for 88 percent of all focus group responses to this item.

Sample Two

Subjects

A total of 389 students from nineteen Los Angeles area continuation high schools completed surveys in October and November of 1996. Ten of the nineteen schools from which data were collected overlapped with Sample One schools but different classrooms within schools were sampled. Table 1 presents the demographic and drug use characteristics of this sample. The same demographic and behavioral items were used for Sample One, and these two samples of subjects, while from different continuation high school classrooms, are quite similar on demographic and behavioral characteristics. Sixty-four percent of the sample (250 out of 389) reported using marijuana at least once in the last thirty days.

Data Collection and Instruments

As in the first sample, an anonymous, non-participant consent form protocol was used. Decline and absentee rates were identical to the first sample and, as with the first sample, biochemical validation was not used. A 10-page self-report questionnaire was administered. Questionnaire items assessed individual reasons to use marijuana, reasons not to use marijuana, and social images associated with marijuana use (see Tables 5 through 7). Students were supplied with seventeen reasons why someone might use marijuana and were asked to rate each on a 5-point rating scale, from "not important" to "extremely important." A sixth response scale option, "I would not use marijuana for any reason," was added for non-smokers. Supplied reasons included, for example, "Marijuana use is an expression of individuality and freedom," "Marijuana use is fun," and "Marijuana use helps one to cope with stress." Item options and responses are listed in Table 5.

Subjects were also supplied with seventeen reasons why someone might not use marijuana and then rated these items using the same scale as in the previous section. Examples included, "Marijuana use can make one an outcast." "Marijuana can make you feel paranoid," "Marijuana is addictive," and "Marijuana can hurt one's motivation to do things." Item options and responses are listed in Table 7.

Social images associated with marijuana were assessed by providing a list of forty-two characteristics, including "sophisticated," "silly," "street smart," "free," "wise," and "environmentalist." Twenty-one of the items were intended to reflect positive social images and twenty-one were intended to reflect negative social images. Students were asked to circle all responses that they associated with a marijuana user.

Demographics, drug use, and quitting-related items were adapted from previous work in which they have demonstrated adequate psychometric properties [1, 8, 11, 15, 18, 32]. The other items were adapted from the findings of

Table 5. Reasons You Might Use Marijuana (Sample Two)

Response	Mean (SD)	Rank
Marijuana use helps one to relax.	3.58 (1.38)	1
Marijuana use is fun.	3.38 (1.53)	2
Marijuana can improve one's appetite.	3.23 (1.58)	3
Marijuana has some beneficial effects such as medicinal and economic.	3.22 (1.48)	4
Marijuana use helps one to cope with stress.	3.18 (1.45)	5
Marijuana is a less dangerous drug than some legal drugs such as alcohol or tobacco.	3.05 (1.59)	6
Marijuana use can improve one's ability to have good sex.	2.85 (1.61)	7
Marijuana use enhances artistic creativity.	2.82 (1.50)	8
Marijuana is not addictive.	2.51 (1.56)	9
Marijuana use is an expression of individuality and freedom.	2.36 (1.39)	10
Everyone uses marijuana.	2.30 (1.51)	11
Marijuana laws are not enforced.	2.17 (1.49)	12
Marijuana use can help bolster one's motivation to do things.	2.09 (1.35)	13
Marijuana use can make someone feel trusting of others.	2.05 (1.37)	14
Marijuana use can make one's clothes smell good.	1.82 (1.36)	15
Marijuana use helps one to fit in/belong.	1.79 (1.20)	16
Marijuana use can improve one's memory.	1.71 (1.16)	17

Notes: Response scale is: 1 = not important; 2 = a little important; 3 = somewhat important; 4 = very important; and 5 = extremely important. The minimally significant difference between any two means in this sample is 0.17 (two-tailed, $p < 0.05$).

Table 6. The Twenty-five Most Popular Social Images
Associated With Marijuana (Sample Two)

Social Image	Percentage Who Generated This Category as a Response
Funny/Humorous	61
Mellow	57
Crazy	53
Happy	52
Silly	50
Spaced Out	50
Burned Out	45
Open-minded	43

(Cont'd.)

Table 6. (Cont'd).

Social Image	Percentage Who Generated This Category as a Response
Wild	43
Cool	41
Stupid .	41
Peaceful	40
Free	38
Creative	37
Rebellious	34
Street smart	33
Moody	31
Sexy	31
Tough	29
Popular	28

Table 7. Reasons Not to Use Marijuana (Sample 2)

Response	Mean (SD)	Rank
Marijuana injures one's memory.	2.96(1.59)	1
Marijuana use can hurt one's motivation to do things.	2.84(1.57)	2
Marijuana use can make someone feel paranoid.	2.68(1.51)	3
Marijuana can make you eat too much.	2.65(1.54)	4
Marijuana use can dull one's ability to have good sex.	2.53(1.64)	5
Marijuana is addictive.	2.51(1.60)	6
Marijuana use can make one's clothes smell bad.	2.50(1.58)	7
Marijuana use is expensive.	2.49(1.47)	8
Marijuana use dulls one's senses.	2.48(1.54)	9
Marijuana laws are enforced.	2.43(1.59)	10
Marijuana is a dangerous drug.	2.38(1.59)	11
Marijuana use can add to one's stresses.	2.31(1.56)	12
Marijuana use can make one tense.	2.30(1.51)	13
Marijuana use can make one an outcast.	2.20(1.45)	14
Marijuana use is not fun.	2.18(1.54)	15
Few people really use marijuana.	2.14(1.51)	16
Marijuana use is an expression of dependence.	2.01(1.38)	17

Notes: Response scale is: 1 = not important; 2 = a little important; 3 = somewhat important; 4 = very important; and 5 = extremely important. The minimally significant difference between any two means in this sample is 0.17 (two-tailed, $p < 0.05$).

previous reasons for cigarette smoking [8, 19, 20, 31], reasons for marijuana use [2, 5, 9, 17, 18], and marijuana cessation [5, 12, 23-25] work.

RESULTS

Sample One

A majority of the subjects who used marijuana in the last thirty days have considered quitting marijuana (267 of 335 respondents or 80%), and 52 percent reported that they had previously tried to quit; those who reported never using marijuana were excluded from this analysis. Among marijuana users ($n = 335$) responding to a question designed to identify the stages of change for marijuana cessation, 36.8 percent of the respondents reported being in the precontemplation stage, 25.9 percent of respondents were in the contemplation stage, 4.7 percent were in the action stage, and 32.6 percent were in the maintenance stage. Together the last three groups represented 63.2 percent of the total sample. Thus, approximately two-thirds of the sample reported a current desire to quit or had already quit marijuana use. Finally, when responding to a multiple-choice item that asked students whether they thought they would ever quit using marijuana, only 23.7 percent of the marijuana using sample indicated that they did not think they would ever quit.

Despite an interest in marijuana cessation, subjects rejected the notion of organized marijuana cessation programs. In a close-ended question asking subjects if they would participate in a "quit marijuana" program at their school, 62.2 percent of subjects using marijuana said "no." Moreover, 68.9 percent of marijuana users also indicated that they would be unwilling to participate in a "quit marijuana" program outside of school. Instead, most marijuana users (80.6%) believe they could quit using marijuana on their own.

Ratings of the perceived effectiveness of various ways to stop marijuana use indicated subjects' desire to quit marijuana without an organized program. Results did not differ between nonusers only and the full sample, so both users and nonusers were included in this analysis. "Quit in private, on your own, without any policies" received the highest mean rating (2.15, $sd = 1.14$) for effectiveness out of a list of ten different cessation strategies, using a scale where "1 = very effective" and "4 = not effective." Other methods of achieving marijuana cessation that received relatively high ratings for effectiveness were either restrictive or punitive. "Inpatient stay" received the second highest mean effectiveness rating and "jail time" the third highest effectiveness rating (see Table 2). "Fines" and "driver's license suspension" (2.54, $sd = 1.15$) received the fourth and fifth highest effectiveness ratings, respectively. The method that received the lowest effectiveness rating was "do nothing" (see Table 2).

It is important not only to discern methods of cessation that are acceptable to the target audience, but also to determine the most credible sources to relay information about marijuana. For this reason, students were asked to identify whom they would be most likely to believe as an information source about marijuana. Computation of simple frequencies and percentages indicated that people with previous drug experience were the most credible source, a category endorsed by almost half the sample (47.7%) (see Table 3). Moreover, when asked whose opinion about marijuana would be most trustworthy from a list of ten choices, over half the sample (64.3%) selected an ex-user, again emphasizing the weight of personal testimony about drug use. The next most frequently selected source, a parent, accounted for only 16 percent of the responses (see Table 3).

In order to design effective cessation programs, the most basic information that is needed is to understand why people use marijuana and why people quit using marijuana. Results of thirty-one focus groups indicated that "getting high" and "stress coping," both mentioned by twenty-one groups, were the most common reasons people offered for using marijuana (see Table 4). The second and third most commonly offered reasons for marijuana use were related to the experience of good feelings by using marijuana: "Feels good/makes you happy/makes you laugh" was mentioned by eighteen groups and "relaxation" was mentioned by sixteen groups. Two categories, "relieve boredom/adventure/novelty/curiosity" and "medical reasons," were mentioned by fourteen groups each.

The most frequently mentioned reason for quitting marijuana use, cited by twenty-three focus groups, was "To avoid getting in trouble/jail/probation." The category of "job" was mentioned by nineteen groups and a possibly related item, "drug testing," received eighteen mentions. Two of the top five most frequently mentioned categories by the focus groups, "too much money" and "bored/sick of using it," each were mentioned by eleven of the focus groups.

Focus groups also were asked to generate cessation activities for people trying to quit marijuana. The most popular response was "discussion of bad consequences" with eleven groups identifying this as a cessation activity. A similar item, "counseling/12-step groups/listen to recovery panels or speakers who have stopped/discussion of getting stupid from use," was the second most frequently mentioned cessation activity with nine groups endorsing it. "Sports activity involvement" (8 groups), "involvement in other activities" (6 groups), and "discussion of negative effects on friends or family" (5 groups) comprised the third, fourth, and fifth of the five most frequently mentioned activities, respectively.

Sample One analyses were recalculated as a function of gender or ethnicity (white/non-white). Either chi-square or ANOVA models were calculated. No differences in self-reported frequency of marijuana use as a function of gender or ethnicity were found. Few gender differences were found. Females reported education, 12-step meetings, and inpatient stay as more effective strategies than males ($F = 5.50$, 7.09, and 6.50, respectively; all $p < 0.02$; R^2 varied from 0.01 to 0.02).

Few ethnic differences were found. Non-whites were found to provide fewer reports of being in precontemplation (29% versus 51%) and more reports of being in maintenance (21% versus 8%); fewer reports of not being able to quit marijuana in the future (19% versus 31%); and fewer reports of not wanting to participate in a "quit marijuana use" program outside of school (65% versus 77%); although non-whites also gave more reports of not knowing where to get help (22% versus 16%) (Chi-squares = 15.72 ($df = 3$), 6.12 ($df = 2$), 7.93 ($df = 2$), and 7.04 ($df = 2$), respectively; all $p < .05$). Also, non-whites reported education, public service work, school suspension, and fines as more effective strategies than whites, although they reported quitting on one's own as less effective ($F = 16.56$, 5.98, 6.33, 4.05, 7.20, respectively; all $p < .05$; R^2 varied from .01 to .04).

Sample Two

In this sample, close-ended items were used to identify reasons for marijuana use, reasons not to use marijuana, and social images associated with marijuana use. Subjects first used a scale of 1 = not important to 5 = extremely important to rate seventeen possible reasons for marijuana use. "Marijuana use helps one relax" received the highest mean importance rating (3.58, $sd = 1.38$) and was significantly more important than all other reasons rated. The second most important reason was "marijuana use is fun"; however, this reason was only marginally different from the reason rated third most important, "marijuana can improve one's appetite" or the reason rated fourth, "marijuana has some beneficial effects such as medicinal and economic," but it was rated significantly higher than the reason rated fifth, "marijuana use helps one to cope with stress." Finally, "marijuana is a less dangerous drug than some legal drugs such as alcohol or tobacco" followed stress-coping as the sixth most important reason one might use marijuana. It was the last of the reasons to receive a rating between "somewhat" and "very" important (see Table 5).

Subjects also were asked to indicate all social images that they associated with marijuana users from a list of forty-two possible social images (see Table 6). Positive images comprised three of the four most frequently cited social images. "Funny/humorous" was the most frequently identified social image associated with marijuana users, cited by 61 percent of the sample. "Mellow," "crazy," and "happy" were the second, third, and fourth most frequently mentioned social images and were endorsed by 57 percent, 53 percent, and 52 percent of the sample, respectively. Only two more social images were mentioned by at least half of the sample: "silly" and "spaced out" were both endorsed by 50 percent of the sample. Thus, three of the six most popular social images associated with marijuana were positive in nature.

Respondents next rated a list of seventeen items of their important reasons not to use marijuana. Again, a scale of 1 = not important to 5 = extremely important was used to rate items. "Marijuana injures one's memory" received the highest mean importance rating (2.96, sd = 1.59); however, it was not significantly more important than the second most important reason, which was related to reduced motivation. "Paranoia" received the third highest importantce rating and was rated marginally less important than "reduced motivation." "Marijuana can make you eat too much" and "marijuana use can dull one's ability to have good sex" were the fourth and fifth most important reasons not use marijuana (see Table 7).

Sample Two analyses were recalculated as a function of gender or ethnicity (white/non-white). Either chi-square or ANOVA models were calculated. In this sample, males were more likely than females to report marijuana use in the last thirty days (71% versus 54%; chi-square (df = 2) = 10.96, $p < .001$). Also, whites were more likely than non-whites to report marijuana use in the last thirty days (79% versus 57%; chi-square (df = 2) = 16.27, $p < .001$). Few gender differences were found regarding reasons for using marijuana. Males rated artistic creativity and as a means to make one feel trusting of others as more important reasons than females (F = 4.18 and 6.16, respectively; $p < .05$; R^2 = .02). Regarding reasons for not using marijuana, females rated marijuana as a dangerous drug, adding to one's stresses, making one tense, hurting one's motivation to do things, being addictive, and making one eat too much as more important reasons (F ranged from 3.80 to 6.22, all $p < .05$, R^2 ranged from .01 to .02).

Regarding ethnic differences in reasons for using marijuana, whites reported it being fun as a more important reason than non-whites (F = 11.66, $p < .001$, R^2 = 04). Regarding reasons for not using marijuana, non-whites rated all reasons as more important than whites except for marijuana as an expression of dependence, as expensive, and that marijuana laws are enforced (these 14 significant Fs ranged from 5.31 to 18.70, all $p < 0.02$, R^2 ranged from 0.02 to 0.06).

DISCUSSION

These data confirm that many continuation high school students are interested in marijuana use cessation. In Sample One, over half the users had tried to quit using marijuana before. Thus, it seems that adolescent marijuana users are interested in changing their behavior and many have already tried to stop using marijuana without success. The failure adolescents face when they try to quit using marijuana may be a result of their belief that they can quit using marijuana without help. For example, more than three-fourths of Sample One subjects believed that they could quit marijuana use on their own. Further, quitting on one's own was rated as the most effective way to stop using marijuana.

However, given that over half of Sample One have already failed in a marijuana cessation attempt, it seems that adolescents may need outside assistance to achieve marijuana cessation.

Unfortunately, adolescents seem resistant to joining organized marijuana cessation programs. Only a minority of subjects who were marijuana users responded that they might be willing to participate in a "quit marijuana" program either at school (38%) or outside of school (31%). If subjects are resistant to organized programs, these findings may explain, in part, the limited success that school and community marijuana cessation programs have had [5]. Lack of belief in the efficacy of cessation programs may keep individuals from participating in them and, among those that do participate, decrease the potential for behavior change by inhibiting a full commitment to the program principles.

Besides quitting on their own, results indicated that subjects believed that restrictive or punitive type programs, such as inpatient stay and jail time, are the most effective ways to achieve marijuana cessation. Thus, subjects seemed to suggest that either a person may exhibit self-control to achieve marijuana cessation or, failing that, must be restricted from opportunities to use marijuana by relatively "painful" methods. In addition to inpatient treatment and punitive measures, these data provide some other clues to the type of marijuana cessation program that might appeal to adolescents. Many smoking cessation programs have likely failed because they begin in the action stage of trying to achieve cessation. However, without helping the patient move from precontemplation where indifference to quitting is exhibited to contemplation where the person decides he or she would like to quit, change in smoking behavior will not occur. If this framework is applicable to marijuana smokers, movement from precontemplation to contemplation stages would likely involve consideration of the costs relative to benefits of use. Primary costs indicated by subjects include legal (e.g., jail time), emotional, economic (e.g., fines, too much money), being unmotivated or having less energy, being overweight, becoming silly or "spaced out," having memory problems, becoming paranoid and becoming addicted to marijuana (according to Tables 2, 4, 6, and 7). These costs should be incorporated into introductory marijuana use cessation sessions to encourage users to take action to quit.

Data from focus groups in Sample One and close-ended items in Sample Two indicated that having fun and stress relief were main reasons for marijuana use. Perhaps, providing alternative ways to cope with physical or psychological discomfort may be important to achieving marijuana cessation in adolescents. The other key reason for using marijuana was related to having fun. Thus, alternative recreational activities or ways to alleviate boredom may be essential to effective cessation programming. Subjects reported getting involved in other activities such as sports or a job as major cessation activities. This suggests that adolescents believe that marijuana use is at least partially a way to relieve boredom or spend free time.

Data provide some insight on the credibility of various sources of information about marijuana. People who have had personal experience with drug use are the most believable to high-risk adolescents. This finding should be used to inform future programming since it suggests that information about the negative effects of drug use will be most believable if it is relayed by an ex-user.

Few gender differences were found. Males did rate some reasons for using marijuana as more important than females, and females did rate some reasons for not using marijuana as more important than males. Also, non-whites rated most reasons for not using marijuana as more important than whites. These results are consistent with the findings that males and whites are more likely to have used marijuana in the last thirty days. Also, these results are consistent with other recent literature that attitudes towards marijuana use, rather than lifestyle factors, most strongly covary with use [35]. More research with larger samples is needed to better explore how gender and ethnic differences are associated with reasons for use and nonuse of marijuana.

While caution should be used in generalizing these data to non-high-risk adolescents, and the reasons for using and quitting marijuana use items need more research to address their psychometric qualities completely, the results of this study provide several avenues for future research on adolescent marijuana cessation. It is clear that marijuana use cessation is a challenge for adolescents and they need guidance in quitting marijuana use. Based on the credibility of different sources about marijuana and marijuana use, the best person to deliver this or any message about marijuana use is someone with personal experience with the drug. Programs designed to aid cessation should focus on the negative effects of marijuana and should offer alternative ways to relieve negative physical and psychological conditions such as stress.

REFERENCES

1. L. D. Johnston, P. M. O'Malley, and J. G. Bachman, National Survey Results on Drug Use from the Monitoring the Future Study, 1975-1995 (Vol 1, Secondary School Children; Vol. 2, Young Adults), National Institute on Drug Abuse, Rockville, Maryland, NIH Publication No. 94-3810, 1996.
2. R. Mathias, Marijuana and Tobacco Use Up Again among 8th and 10th Graders, *National Institute on Drug Abuse (NIDA) Notes, 12*:2, pp. 12–13, 1997.
3. CESAR Fax, *Younger Arrestees in U.S. Favor Marijuana; Older Arrestees Stay with Cocaine,* Adapted from 1996 Drug Use Forecasting Annual Report on Adult and Juvenile Arrestees, 6:26, Drug Use Forecasting program (DUF), National Institute of Justice (NIJ), 1996.
4. S. Sussman, R. Petosa, and P. Clarke, The Use of Empirical Curriculum Development to Improve Prevention Research, *American Behavioral Scientist, 39*:7, pp. 838–852, 1996.

5. S. Sussman, A. W. Stacy, C. W. Dent, T. R. Simon, and C. A. Johnson, Marijuana Use: Current Issues and New Research Directions, *Journal of Drug Issues, 26*:4, pp. 695–733, 1996.
6. J. A. Andrews, H. Hops, S. C. Duncan, and E. Tidlesley, Risk and Protective Factors of Heavy and Problem Substance Use among Adolescents, Poster presentation at the 14th Annual Scientific Sessions of the Society of Behavioral Medicine, San Francisco, California, 1993.
7. J. S. Brook and M. Whiteman, Paternal Determinants of Male Adolescent Marijuana Use, *Developmental Psychology, 17*, pp. 841–846, 1981.
8. W. B. Hansen, J. W. Graham, J. L. Sobel, D. R. Shelton, B. R. Flay, and C. A. Johnson, The Consistency of Peer and Parent Influences on Tobacco, Alcohol, and Marijuana Use among Young Adolescents, *Journal of Behavioral Medicine, 10*, pp, 559–579, 1987.
9. D. B. Kandel, Adolescent Marijuana Use: Role of Parents and Peers, *Science, 181*, pp. 1067–1069, 1973.
10. National Commission on Marijuana and Drug Abuse, *Marijuana: A signal of Misunderstanding*, First Report of the National Commission on Marijuana and Drug Abuse, U.S. Government Printing Office, Washington, D.C., 5266-0002, Core Report and Two Appendices, 1972.
11. S. Sussman, C. W. Dent, T. R. Simon, A. W. Stacy, E. R. Galaif, M. A. Moss, S. Craig, and C. A. Johnson, Immediate Impact of Social Influence-Oriented Substance Abuse Prevention Curricula in Traditional and Continuation High Schools, *Drugs and Society, 8*, pp. 65–81, 1995.
12. M. S. Goodstadt, G. C. Chan, M. A. Sheppard, and J. C. Cleve, Factors Associated with Cannabis Nonuse and Cessation of Use: Between and Within Survey Replications of Findings, *Addictive Behaviors, 11*, pp. 275–286, 1986.
13. P. L. Ellickson and R. D. Hays, On Becoming Involved with Drugs: Modeling Drug Use Over Time, *Health Psychology, 11*, pp. 377–885, 1992.
14. M. D. Newcomb and P. M. Bentler, Substance Use and Abuse among Children and Teenagers, *American Psychologist, 44*:2, pp. 242–248, 1989.
15. J. Richardson, K. Dwyer, K. McGuigan, W. B. Hansen, C. Dent, C. A. Johnson, S. Y. Sussman, B. Brannon, and B. Flay, Substance Use among Eight-Grade Students Who Take Care of Themselves After School, *Pediatrics, 84*:3, pp. 556–566, 1989.
16. A. W. Stacy, M. D. Newcomb, and P. M. Bentler, Social Psychological Influences on Sensation Seeking from Adolescence to Adulthood, *Personality and Social Psychology Bulletin, 17*:6, pp. 701–708, 1991.
17. A. W. Stacy, P. M. Bentler, and B. R. Flay, Attitudes and Health Behavior in Diverse Populations: Drunk Driving, Alcohol Use, Binge Eating, Marijuana Use and Cigarette Use, *Health Psychology, 13*:1, pp. 73–85, 1994.
18. K. E. Bauman, *Predicting Adolescent Drug Use: Utility Structure and Marijuana*, Praeger, New York, 1980.
19. C. L. Perry, D. M. Murray, and K.-I, Klepp, Predictors of Adolescent Smoking and Implications for Prevention, *Morbidity and Mortality Weekly Report, 36*:4S, pp. 41S–45S, 1987.
20. S. M. Hunter, J. B. Croft, I. A. Vizelberg, and G. S. Berenson, Psychosocial Influences on Cigarette Smoking among Youth in a Southern Community: The Bogalusa Heart Study, *Morbidity and Morality Weekly Report, 36*:4S, pp. 17S–23S, 1987.

21. R. Jessor, Adolescent Development and Behavioral Health, in *Behavioral Health: A Handbook of Health Enhancement and Disease Prevention*, J. D. Matarazzo, S. M. Weiss, J. A. Herd, N. E. Miller, and S. M. Weiss (eds), John Wiley & Sons, New York, pp. 69–90, 1984.

22. J. E. Donovan, R. Jessor, and F. M. Costa, Syndrome of Problem Behavior in Adolescence: A Replication, *Journal of Consulting and Clinical Psychology, 56*:5, pp. 762–765, 1988.

23. S. L. Bailey, R. L. Flewelling, and J. V. Rachal, Predicting Continued Use of Marijuana among Adolescents: The Relative Influence of Drug-Specific and Social Context Factors, *Journal of Health and Social Behavior, 33*, pp. 51–66, 1992.

24. R. S. Stephens, R. A. Roffman, and E. F. Simpson, Adult Marijuana Users Seeking Treatment, *Journal of Consulting and Clinical Psychology, 61*:6, pp. 1100–1104, 1993.

25. D. B. Kandel and V. H. Raveis, Cessation of Illicit Drug Use in Young Adulthood, *Archives of General Psychiatry, 46*, pp. 109–116, 1989.

26. G. L. Botvin, E. Baker, L. Dusenbury, E. M. Botvin, and T. Diaz, Long-Term Follow-Up Results of a Randomized Drug Abuse Prevention Trial in a White Middle-Class Population, *Journal of the American Medical Association, 273*, pp. 1106–1112, 1995.

27. S. T. Ennett, N. S. Tobler, C. L. Ringwalt, and R. L. Flewelling, How Effective is Drug Abuse Resistance Education? A Meta-Analysis of Project DARE Outcomes Evaluations, *American Journal of Public Health, 84*, pp. 1394–1401, 1994.

28. W. B. Hansen, School-Based Substance Abuse Prevention: A Review of the State of the Art in Curriculum, 1980-1990, *Health Education Research, 7*:3, pp. 403–430, 1992.

29. C. A. Johnson, M. A. Pentz, M. D. Weber, J. H. Dwyer, N. Baer, D. P. MacKinnon, and W. B. Hansen, Relative Effectiveness of Comprehensive Community Programming for Drug Abuse Prevention with High-Risk and Low-Risk Adolescents, *Journal of Consulting and Clinical Psychology, 58*:4, pp. 447–456, 1990.

30. J. O. Prochaska and C. C. DiClemente, Stages and Processes of Self-Change of Smoking: Toward an Integrative Model of Change, *Journal of Consulting and Clinical Psychology, 51*:3, pp. 390–395, 1983.

31. C. C. DiClemente, S. K. Fairhurst, M. M. Velasquez, J. O. Prochaska, W. F. Velicer, and J. S. Rossi, The Process of Smoking Cessation: An Analysis of Precontemplation, Contemplation, and Preparation of Stages of Change, *Journal of Consulting and Clinical Psychology, 59*:2, pp. 295–304, 1991.

32. S. Sussman, A. W. Stacy, C. W. Dent, T. R. Simon, E. R. Galaif, M. A. Moss, S. Craig, and C. A. Johnson, Continuation High Schools: Youth at Risk for Drug Abuse, *Journal of Drug Education, 25*:3, pp. 191–209, 1995.

33. U.S. Department of Health and Human Services (U.S. DHHS), Tobacco, Alcohol and Other Drug Use among High School Students-United States, 1991, *Morbidity and Mortality Weekly Report* (MMWR), Centers for Disease Control, Atlanta, Georgia, *41*, pp. 698–702, 1992.

34. S. Sussman, D. Burton, C. W. Dent, A. Stacy, and B. R Flay, Use of Focus Groups in Developing an Adolescent Tobacco Use Prevention Program: Collective Norm Effects, *Journal of Applied Social Psychology, 21*, pp. 1772–1782, 1991.

35. J. Bachman, L. Johnston, and P. O'Malley, Explaining Recent Increases in Students' Marijuana Use: Impacts of Perceived Risks and Disapproval, 1976 through 1996, *American Journal of Public Health, 88,* pp. 887–892, 1998.

Direct Reprint requests to:

Steve Sussman
Institute for Health Promotion and Disease Prevention Research
University of Southern California
1540 Alcazar Street
CHP 209
Los Angeles, CA 90033

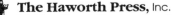

J. DRUG EDUCATION, Vol. 29(4) 359–371, 1999

EFFECTIVENESS OF REFUSAL SKILLS SOFTWARE

RAY BRYSON, PH.D.

La Quinta, California

ABSTRACT

This research explores the potential of making social skills training more accessible to schools by the use of computer-aided instruction. An easy-to-use software program called *Refusal Challenges,* which targets important social skills with effective training methods, was tested. The dependent measure was demonstration of refusal skills strategies. One-hundred-eighty-eight male and female eighth-grade students were stratified according to pre-treatment refusal skill level, gender, and teacher. They were then randomly assigned from the stratified blocks to either the computer-based refusal skills training group or a control group. Repeated measures analyses of variance indicated a significant and meaningful time by treatment interaction for refusal skills scores. The difference between treatment and control groups remained significant and meaningful at both the post-test and follow- up testing.

INTRODUCTION

Social Skill Deficits and Chemical Abuse

A number of studies have demonstrated relationships between social skill deficits and the tragic and costly abuse of chemicals such as tobacco, alcohol, marijuana, and heroin [1-3]. Being able to refuse tobacco, alcohol, and other drugs competently is particularly important during adolescence, since it is a time of declining parental influence, ascending peer influence, and increased mortality associated with risky behavior [4, 5].

Social Skills Training and Substance Abuse

Social skills training has been successful at remedying social skills deficits related to chemical abuse. Many consider it an essential component when dealing with drug abuse. Flay stated that "providing students with behavioral skills

359

with which to resist the influences of tobacco, alcohol and other drugs is a fun-damental component of almost all prevention program" [6]. Interactive refusal skills training has been shown to reduce youth drug, alcohol, and tobacco use [7-9]; improve social problem solving, interpersonal skills for managing pres-sures, assertiveness, and self-control [10]; prevent smoking relapse [11]; and improve alcohol treatment programs [12-14].

Tobler, in her meta-analysis of 143 adolescent drug prevention programs, found that peer programs which include social skills and personal coping skills training had the greatest effect size on most outcome measures (knowledge, atti-tude, drug use, and skills) for the average adolescent [15]. In her 1993 follow-up meta-analysis of 120 school-based drug-prevention programs, Tobler found that interactive instruction was the best way to teach these skills [16]. She found that good interactive programs that offered only ten hours of instruction could reduce drug use in a school by 10.6 percent.

Problems Implementing Social Skill Training in Schools

The most prevalent locations for social skills training are public school classrooms [10]. However, the drawbacks of universal classroom-based social skills training include a lack of trained staff willing to teach social skills, logistical problems in providing quality rehearsal opportunities, inability to efficiently track student progress, and difficulty dealing with individual differ-ences. Consider the difficulty in providing quality role-playing opportunities during a one hour class with thirty students. A teacher would have less than two minutes to observe and give feedback to each student, provided there were no distractions. Students would most likely be limited to practicing with an untrained peer.

Tobler stated that these problems should be addressed by assuring that all students are provided social skills training in small interactive groups by highly trained group leaders. She recommended that school districts provide aggres-sive teacher training in the use of interactive group process skills, as well as hire large numbers of extra leaders [17]. She also realized that districts often lacked the will or resources needed to bring this about.

Current Role of Computers in Behavior Change

Software can potentially reduce some of the above mentioned roadblocks to implementing classroom-based social skills training. A properly designed pro-gram can simulate quality individualized training (immediate corrective feedback, varied situations, individualization, simulated realism, privacy, and tracking) without the need for individual trainers. Computer programs can also provide geographic and temporal flexibility, provide homework, reinforcement, assignments, and substitute sessions. Sampson explained how computers could help social skills trainers use their time more efficiently [18]:

. . . a therapist generally has a finite amount of time available to spend with a client. Instead of having the therapist provide information on how to engage in assertive behavior, the computer completes this task. The counselor then has more time to discuss the nuances of assertive behavior or explore with the client the elements of his or her belief system which make it difficult to use the assertive skills they have learned.

Computer-based learning demands active participation by the learner. It can adjust for different learning rates. It can provide detailed evaluation and immediate feedback. Many people find it less threatening and more private than other methods. It also has the capacity to simulate real-life situations.

These advantages have led to a modest amount of development and research of computer programs designed to improve social skills or change other behaviors. Some of the issues computer programs have addressed include sexual behavior, aggression, conflict resolution [19], employment related social skills [20, 21], peer relations [22-24], and chemical abuse [25-27].

Despite the potential benefits, research and use of drug prevention social skills training software is rare. Weaver reviewed thirty-one computer and videodisk-based drug prevention products. He concluded that most of them suffered from a number of drawbacks, such as never having had their effectiveness researched, not being part of a comprehensive social skills training program, and not using social skills training or behavioral methods [28]. The social simulation software the author usually gave general feedback or scores at the end of an entire simulation, which was neither immediate nor detailed enough to reinforce specific choices.

School drug programs need interactive media products which are based on valid treatment methods, tested for effectiveness, and capable of being easily and universally implemented. The computer program *Refusal Challenges* was developed to meet this need.

METHOD

Participants

Refusal Challenges was tested with 188 male and female eighth-grade students in a rural Southern California middle school. They attended nine different classrooms, taught by three different teachers. Due to the demographics of the community, the overwhelming majority of the participants were Hispanic.

Instruments

The scale Gilchrist et al. developed for measuring the verbal skill components most predictive of adolescents refusing smoking was used to measure the effectiveness of *Refusal Challenges*. These factors were able to predict sixth-grade smoking behavior fifteen months after assessment with 80 percent accuracy. Interrater agreement was .84 to .93 during its development and use. The scale has been used with participants of various racial and ethnic backgrounds [29].

Gilchrist's instrument describes a risky situation then prompts the participant to list things one could say or do. The participant's written responses are coded and scored by a trained judge according to whether the responses indicate or include: a) resistance to pressure; b) direct refusals; c) I-statements; d) use of value judgments, opinions or self-disclosure; e) consequential thinking; f) factual health information to support refusal; g) recommendations of alternative behaviors; h) general compliance; i) direct compliance; or j) aggression. Positive ratings on each skill component add to the overall score, while negative responses lower the score.

Procedures

The steps of the experiment were as follows: a) pretest; b) pretest scoring; c) stratified blocking of participants; d) random assignment of participants from stratified blocks; e) computer intervention; f) posttest; g) follow-up test; and h) statistical analysis.

Pretest

Participants took the pretest measurement of refusal skills. Tests were administered by their language arts teachers, who read a written set of testing directions to the participants. Participants read the one- to two-line prompts and wrote responses independently. The instrument did not have a time limit. Students who lacked the reading and writing skills to complete the pretest did not have their papers included in the research in any way.

Stratified Blocking of Participants

Participants were assigned to stratified blocks according to gender, classroom teacher, and refusal skills scores. They were stratified by gender in light of evidence that girls benefit more from social skills training than do boys [30]. They were stratified by classroom teacher to control for effects of other classroom activities and experiences throughout the year. They were blocked according to refusal skill scores to insure pretest equality on the dependent variable.

Random Assignment of Participants

Participants from each stratified block were randomly assigned to either the computer-aided instruction group or a control group. There were ninety-four participants (49 females and 45 males) assigned to the control group and ninety-four participants (49 females and 45 males) to the treatment group. Of these participants, six did not complete the program, leaving 182 participants. Of these, ninety participants (46 females and 44 males) were from the control group and ninety-four participants (48 females and 44 males) were from the treatment group. Neither participants nor classroom teachers were aware of group membership.

Experimental Treatment

Participants progressed through all levels of the social skills computer program *Refusal Challenges.* No other social skills training was provided by the computer lab teacher. Interview with regular classroom teachers at the conclusion of the school year indicated that social skills were not taught in any of the students' classrooms during that school year.

Participants were given the directions to open *Refusal Challenges,* read the directions, follow the instructions, and notify the instructor when finished. Participants were all able to complete the program independent of teacher instruction. No special skills were needed on the part of the computer teacher. When finished, students were given unrelated computer assignments. They were given sufficient time to complete the program. Participants were able to work on the program for up to one hour a day. Most participants completed the computer program within two days. They worked in pairs.

While the treatment group was using *Refusal Challenges,* the control group used novel, unrelated computer programs in the same room. Work stations were separated by partitions so participants in the control group were not influenced by the treatment group. Since participants were already accustomed to being introduced to new computer programs in the lab, the experimental situation did not appear unusual to participants in either the control or experimental groups.

The program design of *Refusal Challenges* focused on integrating each of implementation, successful refusal skills methods, and effective computer-based training design. Factors identified as making a program implementation-friendly include: a) cost effectiveness; b) time efficiency; c) ease of use for teachers and students; d) compatibility with common school computers; e) ability to assess student progress; f) flexibility of use; and g) consistency with already adopted methods [31]. To be educationally effective the program was designed to: a) use established social skills training techniques; b) focus on common teenage problems which lead to trouble; c) include a variety of realistic peer challengers; d) teach skills components which will increase the probability of students resisting trouble; e) require progressively more complex use of the skill components; f) decrease use of ineffectual social behaviors; g) use multiple types of reinforcement, cueing, and feedback which realistically blend into the simulation; h) build self-efficacy in the ability to use these skills; and i) use effective computer-based instruction methods.

The social skills training techniques used in this program included written instruction, modeling, cueing, a diverse rehearsal, corrective and instructive feedback, and reinforcement of correct responses. The skill components targeted in this program included those determined empirically to be highly predictive of refusal of unhealthy choices [29] and used by most refusal skills trainers [32]. These refusal skill components were introduced by the computer program in the following order:

1. *Inquire.* One gets information about the situation by observing and asking questions until one decides if there is trouble.
2. *Decide.* One decides to comply, refuse, or leave the situation.
3. *Refuse.* If there is trouble, one refuses it directly.
4. *State Reasons.* One gives reasons for refusing. This may include explaining the possible consequences of the action.
5. *Suggest Option.* One proposes alternative behaviors. If the alternative is rejected, one may explain the merits of the alternative.
7. *Leave Option Open.* If the person still refuses the alternative, one invites the person to change their mind later.
8. *Assert.* If pressure persists, one may choose to assertively get the challenger's attention.
9. *Leave.* If the challenger does not listen and continues to exert pressure, one then leaves.

The program began with complete directions for playing the game given by a computerized image of a peer helper. This peer helper explained the program's goals, how to make selections, how to input responses, and how to use the help tools.

Students role-played twelve high risk situations with computer-simulated peers. The computer-simulated challengers represented a realistic balance of gender and ethnic backgrounds. In order to make the challengers realistic, all images were digitized video stills of student models. The peer challenger tried to talk students into doing something risky or unhealthy.

The risk situations involved holding stolen, goods, stealing food, stealing and drinking alcohol, drinking beer, taking pills, smoking cigarettes, chewing tobacco, smoking marijuana, ditching school, writing graffiti on a wall, and fighting. Each situation became progressively more challenging: with fewer cues given, higher levels of pressure, and more skill components required. The skills of each level built towards the next. The first levels used one skill component. The later levels required up to seven skill components.

With each challenge the students were given a list of up to five choices. With each choice the "friend" simulated on the computer realistically responded. If students make incorrect choices (making dishonest excuses, delaying, ignoring, insulting or complying), negative points were put on a scoreboard. Clues and feedback were given until a correct choice was made.

Once the correct choice was made, positive points were given on a scoreboard and the participants typed exactly what they would say. The simulation then continued to the next skill component.

After a level was completed, users were rewarded with applause and congratulations. The congratulations reminded the students of the simultation's goals. The program then played back the correct part of the interaction, complete with the student's written responses. New situations and skill components were then introduced and/or modeled.

Posttest and Follow-up

Posttest and follow-up tests were given to all students attending the nine participating classrooms. The same format and directions were given to participants as were used for the pretest by their classroom teachers. The posttest was given one and two days after treatment. Follow-up testing was done six months following treatment. Tests were scored by the same judge who had scored the pretests, who remained blind to group membership of cases.

Apparatus

A site license for the software *Refusal Challenges* was purchased from PsySoft for $299. Participants used color Power PC Macintosh 5200s. However, the software is able to run on any Macintosh computer with 4 MB of RAM or any computer running Windows 3.1, 95, or 98. Furniture was designed and built by Synergistics Inc. to allow participants to work without visual contract with others.

ANALYSIS

Following the pretest, a *t*-test of the results was conducted to check for the existence of differences prior to treatment. To test whether or not changes in refusal skills scores over time were the result of treatment, a repeated measures analysis of variance was used to measure the effect of the interaction of treatment and time. A polynomial test of order was conducted to test the treatment's effect at each point of measurement. Assumptions for repeated measures analysis of variance were conducted via a Greenhouse-Geisser Epsilon test.

RESULTS

As the table below shows, there was no significant pre-treatment difference between the control and the treatment groups on the variable.

The mean of refusal skill levels (SKIL_1, SKIL_2, SKIL_3), of the treatment group, as measured by the Gilchrist's measurement of refusal skills, climbed dramatically and maintained a meaningful increase at the six-month follow-up (μ = 24, μ = 39, μ = 35). On the other hand, the mean of refusal skills of the control group only rose slightly between pretest, posttest, and follow-up (μ = 25, μ = 26, μ = 27).

Table 1. Independent Samples T-Test On Skill_1

Group	N	Mean	SD
T	92	24.196	9.141
C	90	24.656	8.946
Separate Variances	T = −0.343	df = 180	Prob = 0.732
Pooled Variances	T = −0.343	df = 180	Prob = 0.732

Table 2. Repeated Measures ANOVA for SKIL

Source	SS	df	MS	F	P
GROUP	5871.703	1	5871.703	34.064	0.000
Error	27062.238	157	172.371		
Time	5048.260	2	2524.130	37.084	0.000
Time*GROUP	4084.662	2	2042.331	30.005	0.000
Error	21372.755	314	68.066		

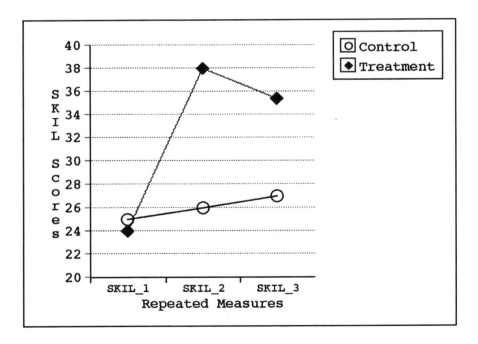

Figure 1. Mean changes for refusal skill by group.

Table 3. Polynomial Test of Order 1 (Linear)

Source	SS	df	MS	F	P
Time	3126.711	1	3126.711	61.421	0.000
Time*GROUP	1751.616	1	1751.616	34.409	0.000
ERROR	7992.239	157	50.906		

Table 4. Polynomial Test of Order 2 (Quadratic)

Source	SS	df	MS	F	P
Time	1921.549	1	1921.549	22.546	0.000
Time*GROUP	2333.046	1	2333.046	27.375	0.000
ERROR	13380.516	157	85.226		

Repeated measures analysis of variance indicated that there was a significant time by GROUP interaction for refusal skill ($F = 30.005$, $df = 2$, $P = 0.000$) at the $a = 0.01$ significance level.

Single degree of freedom polynomial contrasts supported that the time by treatment interaction was significant both linearly ($F = 34.409$, $df = 1$, $P = 0.000$) and quadratically ($F = 27.375$, $df = 1$, $P = 0.000$).

Treatment and control groups also differed greatly in the number of participants who improved their refusal skills posttest and follow-up scores. In the treatment group 88 percent scored higher on their posttest score than their pretest score, while in the control group 46 percent scored higher. In the treatment group 83 percent scored higher on their follow-up score than their pretest scores, while in the control group 56 percent scored higher.

DISCUSSION

This study has demonstrated that properly designed computer software can provide an economic, efficient, and effective means of improving student refusal skills. The *Refusal Challenges* program appears to have increased the ability of participants to use higher level refusal skills (asking questions, being assertive, providing alternative, using facts, predicting consequences) when challenged to do so in testing situations. The most exciting finding was that most of the improvement was maintained six months later. In light of the predictive validity of the measure used, there is a chance that this training could decrease the likelihood of some youth succumbing to negative peer pressure.

Table 5. Sample Pretest and Follow-Up Responses

Pretest Responses	Follow-Up Responses
I don't want to.	No. Look, that is bad for us. I dont want to have to do this all the time if I get addicted.
Not me	I'm your friend, but if you are my friend you will respect me and not force me. I just don't want to.
Not now. Maybe later.	No. With that you can get messed up.
It's wrong	There are other things that can be existing, like sports. We could play ball instead.
Not me.	Others may do it but not me. I am your friend, but I say no. I can be different.
I don't like it cause it's bad.	No. If you think about the future, can you see the consequences would be bad.

Table 5 shows how one student improved her responses to being asked to do something wrong.

Implications for Further Research

Further study could develop and apply software that focuses on different social skills in a wider range of treatment and educational applications. Additional computer programs could expand the use of interactive media in teaching, monitoring, and reinforcing other pro-social behaviors such as helping skills, conflict resolution skills, mediation skills, friendship initiation skills, self-control skills, etc. The structure of the software is best suited to skills that follow a predictable sequence of distinct steps.

This study looked at the effect of social skills software offered with no other social skills training. *Refusal Challenges,* or similar software, could be used in concert with other social skills training methods. Those conducting social skills training could use it as preparation for training, as in integral part of training, or as a way of providing booster sessions. Each of these applications could have different effects in terms of how well a skill is learned, how quickly it is learned, how efficiently the training is provided, how long skills are maintained, and how well skills transfer to real-world situations. One would be able to test the additive effect of social skills software on other treatment methods.

One could also manipulate variables within the software and test for differences in effect. Some software variables that could be manipulated include:

a) picture quality; b) sound; c) types of corrective feedback; d) types of reinforcement; e) user control; or f) additional instruction.

REFERENCES

1. C. U. Linquist, J. S. Lindsay, and G. D. White, Assessment of Assertiveness in Drug Abusers, *Journal of Clinical Psychology, 35*:3, 676–679, 1979.
2. S. J. Hover and L. R. Gaffney, Factors Associated with Smoking Behavior in Adolescent Girls, *Addictive Behaviors, 13*, pp. 139–145, 1988.
3. S. J. Hover and L. R. Gaffney, The Relationship between Social Skills and Adolescent Drinking, *Alcohol and Alcoholism, 26*:2, pp. 207–214, 1991.
4. S. P. Schinke, G. J. Botvin, and M. A. Orlandi, *Substance Abuse in Children and Adolescents,* Sage Publications, Newbury Park, 1991.
5. S. G. Millstein and C. E. Irwin, Accident-Related Behavior in Adolescents: A Biopsychosocial View, *Alcohol, Drugs, and Driving, 4*:1, pp. 21–29, 1988.
6. B. R. Flay, Psychosocial Approaches to Smoking Prevention: A Review of Findings, *Health Psychology, 4*:5, pp. 449–488, 1985.
7. P. L. Ellickson, R. M. Bell, and K. A. McGuigan, Preventing Adolescent Drug Use: Long-Term Results of a Junior High Program, *American Journal of Public Health, 83*:6 pp. 856–861, 1993.
8. L. Dusenbury, G. J. Botvin, and S. James-Ortiz, The Primary Prevention of Adolescent Substance Abuse through the Promotion of Personal and Social Competence, in *Protecting the Children: Strategies for Optimizing Emotional and Behavioral Development,* R. P. Lorion (ed.), The Haworth Press, Inc., New York, pp. 201–224, 1990.
9. S. G. Forman and J. A. Linney, School-Based Social and Personal Coping Skills Training, in *Persuasive Communication and Drug Abuse Prevention,* L. Donohew, H. E. Sypher, and W. J. Bukoski (eds.), Lawrence Erlbaum Associates, Hillsdale, New Jersey, 1991.
10. S. P. Schinke, G. J. Botvin, J. E. Trimble, M. A. Orlandi, L. D. Gilchrist, and V. S. Locklear, Preventing Substance Abuse among American-Indian Adolescents: A Bicultural Competence Skills Approach, *Journal of Counseling Psychology, 35*:1, pp. 87–90, 1988.
11. J. R. Davis and A. G. Glaros, Relapse Prevention and Smoking Cessation, *Addictive Behaviors, 11*, pp. 105–114, 1986.
12. S. Peele, What Works in Addiction Treatment and What Doesn't: Is the Best Therapy No Therapy? *The International Journal of the Addictions, 25*:12A, pp. 1409–1491, 1991.
13. W. R. Miller and R. K. Hester, The Effectiveness of Alcoholism Treatment: What Research Reveals, in *Treating Addictive Behaviors: Processes of Change,* W. R. Miller and N. K. Heather (eds.), Plenum, New York, pp. 121–173, 1986.
14. L. Eriksen, S. Björnstad, and G. Götestam, Social Skills Training in Groups for Alcoholics: One-Year Treatment Outcome for Groups and Individuals, *Addictive Behaviors, 11*, pp. 309–329, 1986.

15. N. S. Tobler, Meta-Analysis of 143 Adolescent Drug Prevention Programs: Quantitative Outcome Results of Program Participants Compared to a Control or Comparison Group, *Journal of Drug Issues, 16,* pp. 137–167, 1986.
16. N. Tobler, Updated Meta-Analysis of Adolescent Drug Prevention Programs, in *Evaluating School-Linked Prevention Strategies: Alcohol, Tobacco, and Other Drugs,* C. Montoya, C. Rigwalt, and R. Zimmerman (eds.), San Diego: University of California, San Diego Extension, pp. 71–86, 1993.
17. N. Tobler and H. Stratton, Effectiveness of School-Based Drug Prevention Programs: A Meta-Analysis of the Research, *Journal of Primary Prevention, 18*:1, pp. 71–128, 1996.
18. J. P. J. Sampson, An Integrated Approach to Computer Applications in Counseling Psychology, *The Counseling Psychologist, 11,* pp. 65–74, 1983.
19. M. Margalit and A. Weisel, Computer-Assisted Social Skills Learning for Adolescents with Mild Retardation and Social Difficulties, *Educational Psychology, 10*:4, pp. 343–354, 1990.
20. D. B. Malouf and MacArthur, S. Radin, Using Interactive Videotape-Based Instruction to Teach On-the-Job Social Skills to Handicapped Adolescents, *Journal of Computer-Based Instruction, 13*:4, pp. 130–133, 1984.
21. L. S. Appell, et al., *Using Simulation Technology to Promote Social Competence of Handicapped Students* (Report No. 300-85-0156). Macro Systems Inc. Silver Spring, MD: ERIC Document Reproduction Service No. ED 324 839, 1990.
22. P. Browning, W. A. T. White, G. Nave, and P. Z. Barkin, Interactive Video in the Classroom, *Education and Training of the Mentally Retarded,* pp. 85–92, 1986.
23. P. Browning and W. A. T. White, Teaching Life Enhancement Skills with Interactive Video-Based Curricula, *Educational and Training of the Mentally Retarded,* pp. 236–244, 1986.
24. R. Thorkildsen, Using an Interactive Videodisc Program to Teach Social Skills to Handicapped Children, *American Annals of the Deaf, 130*:5, pp. 383–385, 1985.
25. J. G. Barber, Computer Assisted Drug Prevention, *Journal of Substance Abuse Treatment, 7*:2, pp. 125–131, 1990.
26. J. G. Barber, An Application of Microcomputer Technology to the Drug Education of Prisoners, *Journal of Alcohol and Drug Education, 38*:2, pp. 14–22, 1993.
27. A. Eltringham and J. G. Barber, Can Microcomputers Help the Problem Drinker, *Australian Alcohol and Drug Review, 9,* pp. 169–176, 1990.
28. D. Weaver, *Technology Products for Substance Abuse Education,* Northwest Regional Educational Laboratory, Portland, 1992.
29. L. D. Gilchrist, W. H. Snow, D. Lodish, and S. P. Schinke, The Relationship of Cognitive and Behavioral Skills to Adolescent Tobacco Smoking, *Journal of School Health, 55,* pp. 132–134, 1985.
30. B. H. Schneider, *Children's Social Skills Training: What Works Best?* Paper presented at the meeting of the Annual Meeting, American Educational Research Association, New Orleans, Louisiana, 1988.
31. L. J. Kolbe and D. C. Iverson, Implementing Comprehensive Health Education: Educational Innovations and Social Change, *Health Education Quarterly, 8*:1, pp. 57–80, 1981.

32. S. N. Elliott and F. M. Gresham, *Social Skills Intervention Guide,* American Guidance Services, Circle Pines, Minnesota, 1991.

Direct reprint request to:

Ray Bryson, Ph.D.
54733 Avenida Diaz
La Quinta, CA 92253

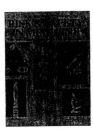

The International Journal of

Risk & Safety in Medicine

Side Effects of Drugs – Devices – Surgery – Prevention – Liability

Aims and Scope

The International Journal of Risk and Safety in Medicine is concerned with rendering the practice of medicine as safe as it can be; that involves promoting the highest possible quality of care, but also examining how those risks which are inevitable can be contained and managed. Particular attention is given to a number of major fields, including drugs and vaccines, surgery and anesthesia, gynecology and obstetrics, medical equipment and materials, and alternative medicine. The medical, ethical and legal aspects of risk in all these fields are examined.

Editor

M.N.G. Dukes
Trosterudveien 19
0778 Oslo, Norway
Tel.: +47 22 49 40 58
Fax: +47 22 92 11 35
E-mail: mngdukes@online.no

Editorial Board

D. Brahams (Law), P.R. Breggin (Psychiatry), E. Ernst (Complementary Medicine), L.M.C. Faro (Medical Technology), F.M. Haaijer-Ruskamp, (Medical Sociology), E. Helsing (International Health), W.J.A. van den Heuvel (General Practice), C. Hodgkin (Women's Health), J. Jagwe (Developmental Health), P.E. de Jong (Internal Medicine, Nephrology), L.T.W. de Jong-van den Berg (Pharmacy), M.B. Kapp (Legal Medicine), C. Laske (Medical Ethics), M. Mildred (Liability Law), B.A.J.M. de Mol (Safety Science), P. Peters (Pregnancy), M.V. Semenchenko (Drug Utilization), D.W. Sigelman (Public Health Law), T. Tijmstra (Health Sciences), D. Trichopoulos (Epidemiology), J. Turner (Health Services), G. van der Wal (Social Medicine), H. Wesseling (Clinical Pharmacology), B. Westerholm (Internal Medicine, Public Policy).

Call for Papers

Basic research, reports of clinical experience, and overviews will all be considered for publication, but since major reviews of the literature are generally written at the invitation of the Editorial Board it is generally advisable to consult with the Editor before embarking on papers of this type. News items will gladly be considered for publication, as will letters on topics which have been dealt with in the journal.

Subscription Information

The International Journal of Risk and Safety in Medicine (ISSN 0924-6479) will be published in one volume of 4 issues in 2000 (Volume 13). Regular subscription price: NLG 744/US$ 372 (including postage and handling). Individual subscription price: NLG 260/US$ 130.

Abstracted / Indexed in

Chemical Abstracts, Current Contents, Elsevier BIOBASE/Current Awareness in Biological Sciences, EMBASE/Excerpta Medica, Materials Science Citation Index, Research Alert, Risk Abstracts, SciSearch.

J. DRUG EDUCATION, Vol. 29(4) 373–386, 1999

PREVENTION TRAINING OF PARAPROFESSIONALS IN THE SCHOOLS: AN EXAMINATION OF RELEVANCY AND EFFECTIVENESS*

JOHN L. ROMANO
University of Minnesota

ABSTRACT

Prevention training programs for paraprofessional school personnel are examined in this article. Prevention training for the reduction of student alcohol and other drug use, incorporating a student well-being model, is described and evaluated. The prevention training, entitled "Enhancing Student Well-Being," took place in two urban school districts with over 200 paraprofessional school personnel participating. The training was evaluated using measures of knowledge gained, self-efficacy, and participant satisfaction. Pre- and post-training differences showed consistent gains in participant efficacy expectations but less consistent gains in outcome expectations and knowledge. Participant satisfaction and self-reports of knowledge enhanced and skill improvement were uniformly high across all training programs. Implications for inservice prevention training of paraprofessionals are discussed.

Recent studies show that alcohol and other drug (AOD) use among school-aged youth continues to be a concern. A 1997 U.S. government statistical summary of the well-being of U.S. youth reported regular alcohol use (defined as having an alcoholic beverage on two or more occasions in the previous 30 days) by 31 percent of twelfth graders, 20 percent of tenth graders, and 11 percent of eighth graders. In each grade level, males used more alcohol compared to females, with the largest difference being in grade twelve (36% vs. 25%) [1]. This same report showed substantial increases in illicit drug use for all three grades from 1991 to 1996 (e.g., increasing from 6% to 15% among 8th graders). Daily use

*Partially funded by the U.S. Department of Education, Safe and Drug Free Schools and Communities—School Personnel Training Grant.

of cigarettes also increased for all grades during these years but not as dramatically as illicit drugs. The 1996 Monitoring the Future study sponsored by The National Institute on Drug Abuse also reported student use increases in several illicit drug categories, including marijuana/hashish and cocaine, between 1994 and 1996 [2]. School and community based strategies have focused on direct curriculum and classroom interventions with youth [3-7], as well as the training of certified school personnel [8]. The focus of the research reported in this study is the AOD prevention training of a special group of school personnel: paraprofessionals—those who are employed by a school district to perform supportive activities within the school but who are not licensed or certified as a teacher or school specialist.

The inservice training of school personnel to promote the prevention of alcohol and other drug use is a priority for school districts. Districts, however, may allocate professional development funds for AOD training primarily to licensed or certified personnel in the district. These personnel can include those in positions of classroom teacher, school counselor, and principal. Too often, nonlicensed or noncertified personnel (i.e., paraprofessional) in the district are not given the same opportunities for professional development experiences as their licensed and certified colleagues. This discrepancy is unfortunate given that paraprofessional personnel often have less formalized training in education and child development, even though their positions require regular and important contact with students. Paraprofessional school personnel may hold positions in a school such as teacher aides or chemical health assistants. Their tasks can include student tutoring, monitoring student behavior during recess, and assisting with components of the educational and support programs of the school. Therefore, by not providing more inservice professional opportunities for this group of school personnel, districts are missing an opportunity to further the professional skills and knowledge of a large, important segment of the district's educational staff. Others have also strongly endorsed the value and importance of paraprofessionals or paraeducators in the educational enterprise [9, 10]. As Johnson, Lasater, and Fitzgerald state, "Aides have become a vital part of instruction for a growing number of students" [9, p. 6]. Although the numbers of school paraprofessionals have increased, their professional development experiences have not kept pace with their changing roles and responsibilities [10].

Four AOD training experiences of paraprofessional school personnel from two large urban school districts are described and evaluated in this study. Although each training experience was somewhat different because it was developed based on the needs of the district, there is sufficient commonality in types of school personnel trained, training protocols, and the evaluation of the training programs to make comparisons across the four training experiences.

BASIC TRAINING PROTOCOL
AND PHILOSOPHY

The training model implemented is based on a theoretical concept called "student well-being" (SWB). Romano defined student well-being as the "development of knowledge, attitudes, skills, and behaviors that maximize students' functioning (i.e., academic, inter- and intrapersonal, and physical and emotional health) in environments where they live and work (i.e., school, home, and community)" [8, p. 246]. This model is holistic, focusing on the whole student. The model argues that the promotion of student well-being within schools is a strong deterrent to students engaging in dysfunctional behaviors. Hill, Piper, and King support this concept by arguing that, in order to prevent student problem behaviors, school prevention programs must include "components that fundamentally challenge the way teachers are trained, the way schools are structured, the way students are organized for instruction, and the way 'learning' is defined" [11, p. S-15]. One of their study's major conclusions based on elementary and middle school personnel was that prevention must be an integral component of a school's basic structure and environment. O'Connor and Saunders [12] echoed this perspective by indicating that drug education and prevention must be addressed systematically at all levels of society to be effective. They criticize many school-based drug prevention programs for being too narrowly focused and not considering the influences of alcohol and drug use in families and communities.

Taking a different perspective, Benard's research review concluded "evidence demonstrates that a nurturing school climate has the power to overcome incredible risk factors in the lives of children" [13, p. 48]. Others have suggested similarly the importance of focusing on the school environment to reduce problem student behavior, such as school dropout [14]. The SWB model, utilizing a comprehensive approach, suggests that the prevention of alcohol and other drug use among students is best accomplished through prevention programs that involve the entire school community and include involvement of parents, family, and the broader social community in which the student lives. The importance of comprehensive AOD prevention programs has been supported by several authorities [15, 16]. Taking a systematic approach, the model recognizes social influences that promote student AOD use (e.g., media advertising of alcohol), as well as those that act as deterrents to AOD use (e.g., enforcement of laws regulating the sale of alcohol to minors). The need to broaden school-based prevention programs to give attention to community and societal norms and influences has received strong support in the literature [17, 18]. Finally, the SWB model appreciates the interrelationships between problem behaviors of youth [14], such as the relationships between poor school achievement, student aggressive behaviors, and AOD use [19, 20].

In addition to roots in the prevention literature, the SWB model evolved from more recent initiatives and conceptualizations to promote youth development [21]. Conceptualizations of youth development require paradigm shifts from focusing on youth problems and preventing them to focusing on initiatives and services that enhance youth development [22]. Pittman discusses youth development in terms of our goals for youth, their competencies and connections to the larger society, and their development into responsible and contributing adults [22]. Others have articulated similar dimensions of youth development [23-25].

Therefore, based on the SWB model, the training programs for paraprofessional school personnel evaluated in this article had four major objectives:

1. To articulate the SWB framework and discuss its conceptual use as a prevention model;
2. To give information related to several content areas requested by school personnel and important to the promotion of student well-being;
3. To give skills and strategies that school personnel can use in their work with students to promote student well-being;
4. To enhance the educators' self-efficacy related to their school positions.

TRAINING RESULTS

Four separate training programs were held for the paraprofessional school personnel. Each training program and its results are described separately below.

First Training

The training was held on four consecutive days, four hours each day, for a total of sixteen hours, prior to the start of the new school year. Paraprofessionals who were employed in positions such as educational assistant, health service assistant, and child development technician applied to attend the training. A total of 289 applications were received, but participation was limited to seventy-five employees. Applicants who had not received prior prevention training offered through the district were given priority. The large number of applications demonstrated the need for the training. Of the seventy-five applicants accepted for the training, sixty actually participated, and 78 percent attended all training sessions. Participants received continuing education unit credits and a stipend for their participation. These incentives were prorated for those who did not attend all of the sessions. Of the fifty-eight participants who completed the demographic survey, 90 percent were female and 64 percent were Caucasian. Other participant ethnic groups included 23 percent African-American and 4 percent each of Asian American, Hispanic, and Native

American. Most participants had at least some college coursework (84%), but the majority (81%) did not have a college degree. Over two-thirds of the group had "some," "little," or "none" previous training in prevention. Participants had been employed in the school district for an average of eight years, with 43 percent being employed for five years or less.

The training sessions included topics on student well-being and prevention, resiliency, cultural diversity, prenatal alcohol and drug effects on youth, inhalants, student behavior management strategies, communication skills training, and personal empowerment. All of the presentations were led by individuals familiar with the culture of schools and major issues facing contemporary youth. Presenters were selected to include representation from the community and school district and to represent ethnic and gender diversity. The presentation formats were designed to encourage participant dialogue and interaction with each other and the presenter.

In an effort to sustain the training effects, approximately two months after the initial training, participants were invited back for a follow-up training session to discuss how knowledge and skills gained in the initial training sessions were being applied to school problems that they were now facing. The three hour follow-up session was attended by twenty-four of the sixty trainees (40%). Continuing education units and a stipend were offered for this follow-up training, which occurred after school hours.

The training was evaluated in three ways. First, a participant satisfaction questionnaire was completed immediately after the training. This questionnaire revealed that participants were satisfied with the training (98% indicated at least "satisfied" on the Likert scale), 90 percent indicated gaining "much" or "very much" knowledge as a result of the training and 77 percent indicated that they increased their skills "much" or "very much" as a result of the training. Participant qualitative responses elicited by the questionnaire were generally positive, supporting the Likert item data.

The second evaluation measure was a Knowledge Questionnaire (KQ) to assess the amount of new knowledge that participants acquired as a result of the training. The 20-item true and false KQ was administered on the first day of training (pretest) and also at a two month follow-up (posttest). The follow-up KQ was sent to participants by U.S. mail. Approximately two weeks after the follow-up posttest was mailed, a reminder postcard was sent to nonrespondents. These procedures yielded a 62 percent return rate, as thirty-six usable pre- and post-questionnaires were available. These participants had an average score of 14.9 at pretest (score of 1 for each correct answer) and a standard deviation (SD) of 1.7. At posttest, the average score of respondents was 14.1, with SD at 2.5. Pre and posttest differences were not significant ($p > .05$).

The third evaluation measure was a Self-Efficacy Questionnaire (SE) completed by participants before and after training under similar conditions as the KQ (i.e., pretest on the first day of training and follow-up posttest approximately two months after the training). The SE has been utilized as an outcome assessment in previous school personnel prevention training [26]. A slightly modified version was used in this project. The SE consists of two parts: Efficacy Expectations (EE) and Outcome Expectations (OE); EE and OE emanate from Bandura's [27] self-efficacy theory. The EE relate to one's belief about his/her abilities to execute a particular behavior, whereas OE refer to one's belief about whether the behavior, if executed, will lead to desired outcomes. EE consists of twenty-two questions on a 7-point Likert scale, from "strongly disagree" (1) to "strongly agree" (7). The neutral response is 4. The questions focus on the respondent's beliefs about behaviors related to student well-being, starting with the phrase "I am able to . . . ." For example, Item 20 says, "I am able to identify students who are at high risk for using illegal substances." The OE scale consists of fourteen Likert items related to student well-being. However, respondents are instructed to answer each item as to how much each will "enhance student well-being in your school." For example, one item states: "Addressing media messages about tobacco, alcohol, and other drugs." The Likert scale ranges from "none" (1) to "very, very much" (7), with the neutral response being 4. A total of fifty-eight participants completed the SE at pretest, and thirty-seven questionnaires were available at posttest (64% return rate). Pre and posttest differences were significant for EE ($p < .05$) but not for OE ($p > .05$). Table 1 gives pre and posttest means and standard deviations for the KQ, EE, and OE.

Second Training

The second training sessions were similar in several ways to the first training but also different in some ways. As in the first training, the second training was sixteen hours in length and was based on the student well-being model. The recipients of the training were paraprofessional school personnel from the same urban district as in the first training. Participants received continuing education units (CEU) and a stipend to attend the training, which occurred over a three week period in four hours blocks of time.

Table 1. First Training Program: Pre and Post Self-Efficacy and Knowledge Questionnaire Measures Means and Standard Deviations

	N	Pre		Post		t	P<
		$\overline{X}$	SD	$\overline{X}$	SD		
EE	37	4.71	.66	5.02	.75	– 2.52	.05
OE	37	5.85	.16	6.01	.15	– 1.03	ns
KQ[a]	36	14.86	1.71	14.11	2.49	1.87	ns

[a]20-item questionnaire.

Paraprofessional school personnel were notified of the training opportunity, and sixty-seven were invited to participate. A total of fifty-five school personnel actually attended the three Saturday morning and one evening training sessions. CEUs and stipends were prorated for participants who missed training sessions. Of the forty-nine participants who completed the demographic questionnaire, 78 percent were female and 22 percent were male. Approximately 52 percent were Caucasian, 44 percent African-American, and 2 percent Asian-American. About 24 percent had completed a bachelor's degree or beyond, 49 percent some college, and 20 percent high school or GED diploma. The participants had been employed by the school district for an average of five years, with 77 percent having been employed by the district for five years or less. Most of the participants (84%) indicated either "some," "little," or "none" previous prevention training. Compared to the participants in the first training, this groups of trainees was more diverse with respect to sex and ethnicity. The two groups were comparable in educational levels, but the second training group had fewer years of employment in the district, and they had less previous prevention training.

As in the first training, the second training was entitled "Enhancing Student Well-Being" (ESW), emphasizing educator skills important to the development of student well-being. Content of the sessions included principles of prevention and their relationship to the prevention of student alcohol and other drug use, antisocial behaviors, and precocious and risky sexual behaviors; communication skills; resiliency and student asset building; and behavior management strategies. In addition to these sessions, teams of educators from two of the district's schools that had received ESW training and were implementing ESW projects in their schools were invited to share their experiences and the results of their projects with the participants.

The second training was evaluated in similar ways to the first training, i.e., measures of satisfaction, self-efficacy (SE), and knowledge (KQ) were administered. However, there were differences. The second training used a shorter KQ composed of ten true and false items taken from the first training KQ of twenty items. The KQ and SE were given on the first and last day of training. This was a departure from the first training when these questionnaires were given on the first day of training and at two-month follow-up. Since the second training occurred over several weeks, and to improve completion rates of the measures, it was decided to give them on the last day of training rather than rely on participants sending them back at follow-up. As in the first training, the satisfaction questionnaire was completed on the last day of training.

Of the fifty-five trainees, forty-two completed pre and post measures of EE and OE, a 76 percent completion rate, while thirty-nine completed the KQ both times (71% completion). These completion rates were higher than those obtained for the first training. The results, however, were comparable on the SE measure. The EE scale showed significant differences from pre to posttest

Table 2. Second Training Program: Pre and Post Self-Efficacy and Knowledge Questionnaire Measures Means and Standard Deviations

	N	Pre X	Pre SD	Post X	Post SD	t	p<
EE	42	4.78	.98	5.44	.77	−4.90	.001
OE	42	5.94	.84	5.90	.81	0.30	ns
KQ[a]	39	8.03	1.66	8.41	1.46	−2.15	.05

[a]10-item questionnaire.

($p < .001$), whereas the OE scale did not show significant differences ($p > .05$). The KQ showed differences from pre to posttest ($p < .05$), unlike the first training when no differences were found. The differences on the KQ between the first and second training groups is likely related to the second group having less previous prevention training. Table 2 summarizes these results.

Participants were "satisfied" or "very satisfied" (96%) with the training that they received. They also believed that the training increased their skills in working with youth either "much" or "very much" (80%), and they learned "much" or "very much" (89%) new knowledge as a result of the training. These percentages were similar to the first training where the percentages were 98 percent, 77 percent, and 90 percent respectively.

Third Training

The third and fourth training sessions were conducted in a large, urban school district, but a different one from the district of the first and second training sessions. The ESW training model was utilized in the third and fourth training sessions, although the content differed somewhat from the first two training sessions. The target population for these training sessions was again paraprofessional school personnel in the district. The number of training hours in this third training was sixteen hours, over four sessions, spread out over a forty-five day period. Participants were offered incentives of CEUs and a stipend if they attended all four sessions.

A total of ninety-five school personnel attended at least one training session; 85 percent of these attended all four sessions. The majority of participants were female (77%). Various ethnic groups were represented among the participants, with 51 percent Caucasian, 21 percent African-American, 10 percent Hispanic, 7 percent Asian-American, and 3 percent Native American. The educational background of the participants included 13 percent with a bachelor's degree, 46 percent with at least some college education, and 37 percent with a high school or GED diploma. The participants were employed by the school district for an average of six years, with 48 percent being employed by the district for three years or less. Although 63 percent of the trainees had "some," "little," or "none" previous prevention training, 37 percent had "much" or "very much."

The ESW training was interactive, combining presentations on several content areas with participant discussion. Content sessions included discussion of fetal alcohol effects, resiliency, home and school collaborations, and classroom management.

Again, measures of participant satisfaction, knowledge, and self-efficacy were used to assess the effectiveness of the training. The satisfaction questionnaire was administered on the last day of the training, and seventy-three participants (77% response) completed the questionnaire. The results showed that 56 percent gained "much" or "very much" knowledge as a result of the training, 52 percent increased their skills working with youth by "much" or "very much," and 82 percent were "satisfied" or "very satisfied" with the ESW training. The KQ and SE were the same as those given during the second training. However, the pretests were completed by participants prior to attending the first training session, and the posttests were completed on the last day of training. The KQ did not yield significant differences between the pre and posttests ($p > .05$). However, both scales of the self-efficacy measure showed significant differences between pre and posttests. The EE scale was significant at the .001 level and OE at the .05 level.

Fourth Training

The structure of this training differed from the previous three, as the training sessions were delivered on two consecutive Saturdays for a total of sixteen hours. The ESW conceptual model was again used as the training model, and content topics included student alcohol and drug use, fetal alcohol effects, resiliency, classroom management, sexual issues, and gangs and threat groups.

A total of thirty-three participants employed as paraprofessionals in the district attended at least one day, and twenty-seven attended both sessions. Those who attended both sessions received CEUs and a stipend. Demographic data showed that about 66 percent of the participants were female, most had at

Table 3. Third Training Program: Pre and Post Self-Efficacy and Knowledge Questionnaire Measures Means and Standard Deviations

	N	Pre X	Pre SD	Post X	Post SD	t	p<
EE	74	4.64	1.06	5.33	.76	−6.70	.001
OE	74	5.30	1.10	5.56	1.03	−2.12	.05
KQ[a]	71	7.99	1.41	7.94	1.42	.23	ns

[a]10-item questionnaire.

least some college education (83%), and 66 percent had either "some," "little," or "none" prior prevention training. About 65 percent of the participants have been employed by the school district for less than eight years. However, 35 percent have been employed by the district for more than ten years. Although the majority of participants were Caucasian (66%), African-American (17%) and American-Indian (4%) ethnic groups were also represented. Some individuals left the ethnicity question blank or indicated "other."

Evaluation was conducted through a satisfaction questionnaire given at the end of the last day of training and a shorter version of the SE measure given prior to the start of training and approximately six weeks after the training ended. Given the shortness of the fourth training (over two consecutive Saturdays) and the fact that the previous KQ did not discriminate well among trainees, it was decided not to include it as an evaluation measure. Further, it was hoped that a shorter questionnaire, measuring only self-efficacy, would increase the response rate of participants. The satisfaction questionnaire was completed by twenty-six trainees. It showed that 85 percent of the participants gained "much" or "very much" knowledge as a result of the ESW training. They also increased their skills in working with youth "much" (50%) or "very much" (31%), and they were either "satisfied" (58%) or "very satisfied" (39%) with the training. The SE measure was completed pre and post training by nineteen participants. Neither the EE (15 items) nor the OE (10 items) scales yielded significant differences ($p > .05$).

Discussion

Several observations can be made from these training sessions. First, schools must consider the training needs and professional development of paraprofessional school personnel. As these separate training programs showed, these school personnel usually come to their school position without a bachelor's degree and with relatively little training on prevention concepts and skills. Only 18 percent of the 221 paraprofessionals completing demographic questionnaires in the ESW training sessions had at least a bachelor's degree. Further, 32 percent indicated having "little" or "none" prior training in

Table 4. Fourth Training Program: Pre and Post Self-Efficacy Measures Means and Standard Deviations

| | N | Pre | | Post | | t | p< |
		$\overline{X}$	SD	$\overline{X}$	SD		
EE[a]	19	5.40	.77	5.37	.73	.23	ns
OE[b]	19	5.88	.83	5.99	.90	-.41	ns

[a]15-item questionnaire.
[b]10-item questionnaire.

prevention, whereas only 31 percent had "much" or "very much" prior prevention training.

Although the four training programs occurred in different school districts with slightly different training content and very different training structures, some interesting results were obtained. First, the efficacy expectations (EE) scale yielded significant pre/post training differences in three of the four training programs. Only the fourth training, occurring over two full days in consecutive weeks, did not show EE differences. The outcome expectations (OE) scale yielded significant results in only one of the training programs. The difference in results between EE and OE suggests an inability of paraprofessionals to exert influence in their schools. EE refer to the person's belief in his/her ability to execute a particular behavior, whereas OE refer to the individual's belief that executing the behavior will bring about change in the person's school. Paraprofessional school personnel may feel confident in their own abilities to enhance student well-being as a result of the training they received, but given their position as noncertified personnel in the school, they are less likely to believe that their behaviors will bring about change in their school. Therefore, they recognize their own improved skills to enhance student well-being but are less confident that engaging in these behaviors will bring about school change to enhance student well-being. Perhaps the paraprofessionals are reflecting on their inability to bring about school change due to their lack of influence in the school.

The KQ was significantly different from pre to post training in only one of the three training sessions. The school personnel in these training sessions scored high on the pretest, suggesting a ceiling effect on the KQ, that was likely contributed to by the "true" and "false" test item format. Further, the comprehensive and integrative ESW training model makes content-based knowledge questionnaires difficult to construct. In previous studies of school personnel training which have been more specifically focused on alcohol and drug content information, training differences in knowledge gained and retained were found [28, 29]. However, it is also recognized that increasing knowledge does not necessarily change behavior (12, 16).

In contrast to the more objective pre- and post-training measures, the end-of-training satisfaction questionnaires were generally very favorable in all four training sessions across all three Likert-type questions. Each Likert item had two favorable choices, two unfavorable, and one neutral choice. Taking the 194 participants collectively, 76 percent indicated gaining "much" or "very much" knowledge as a result of the ESW training, compared to 5 percent indicating "some" or "almost none." Further, 69 percent increased their skills working with youth "very much" or "much," whereas 11 percent answered "some" or "almost none" to this question. Finally, 91 percent were either "very satisfied" or "satisfied" with the ESW training, and only 2 percent were "dissatisfied" or "very dissatisfied."

The summary of the results of the four training sessions indicates that participants were very satisfied with the ESW training, and they believed that they learned new knowledge and increased their skills. They also improved their beliefs about their abilities and skills related to enhancing student well-being. However, they were less likely to believe that their improved skills would bring about changes in their school to enhance student well-being. A questionnaire designed to assess knowledge change as a result of the training did not yield consistently favorable results.

IMPLICATIONS

School districts employ paraprofessional staff to make important contributions to the educational mission of their districts. These employees often come to their positions with relatively little formal training and have limited professional, inservice opportunities once they are in their positions. Further, the nature of their positions often puts them in close and regular contact with students. This proximity to students gives paraprofessionals ample opportunities to apply prevention principles and skills with students, and support youth development strategies [25]. Their positions in the school may be seen by students as separate from the regular school establishment and power structure, and they may interact with paraprofessionals in more informal settings. Paraprofessionals have opportunities to observe students in less structured environments (e.g., the playground) or work with them individually or in small groups. The demographic data of the paraprofessionals participating in the training programs reported suggest that paraprofessional employees more closely represent the ethnic composition of the urban student body compared to licensed school staff. For these reasons, paraprofessionals are well situated to observe students and assist them before problems become major issues. Students may be more willing to discuss with the paraprofessional academic, social, and emotional concerns that the students are facing at school or at home. Paraprofessionals can act as a source of referrals to trained specialists who can assist the student (e.g., school counselor). They can also be a source of support for students who feel unsupported by the school community. Finally, paraprofessionals can work closely with the classroom teachers to design and implement educational interventions to meet student learning objectives.

Therefore, it behooves districts to consider the staff development needs of paraprofessionals and to include them in training opportunities [30]. The four training programs, based on the student well-being (SWB) conceptual model, that are described and evaluated in this article offer a training model and content, as well as structure and evaluation options for schools and districts. The SWB model offers a comprehensive, integrated approach to training that utilizes concepts from prevention science and the youth development literature. The evaluation of the SWB trainings showed that paraprofessionals were very satisfied with the training and that they increased their self-effacacy. The SWB training provides one vehicle through which paraprofessionals can increase their skills in enhancing youth development and feel appreciated as valued members of the educational enterprise through a greater sense of self-efficacy.

ACKNOWLEDGMENT

Jordan Orzoff provided assistance with the statistical analysis.

REFERENCES

1. K. K. Wallman, *America's Children: Key National Indicators of Well-Being. Federal Interagency Forum on Child and Family Statistics, 1997,* Office of Management and Budget, U.S. Federal Government, Washington, D.C., 1997.
2. R. Mathias, Marijuana and Tobacco Use Up Again Among 8th and 10th Graders, *NIDA Notes* (Publication No. 97-3478), National Institutes of Health and National Institute on Drug Abuse, Rockville, Maryland, pp. 12–13, March/April 1997.
3. G. J. Botvin, E. Baker, L. Dusenbury, E. M. Botvin, and T. Diaz, Long-Term Follow-Up Results of a Randomized Drug Abuse Prevention Trial in a White Middle-Class Population, *Journal of the American Medical Association, 273,* pp. 1106–1112, 1995.
4. J. A. Durlak, *School-Based Prevention Programs for Children and Adolescents,* Sage Publications, Thousand Oaks, California, 1995.
5. K. A. Komro, C. L. Perry, S. Veblen-Mortenson, and C. L. Williams, Peer Participation in Project Northland: A Community-Wide Alcohol Use Prevention Project, *Journal of School Health, 64,* pp. 318–322, 1994.
6. J. T. Shope, T. E. Dielman, A. T. Butchart, P. C. Campanelli, D. D. Kloska, An Elementary School-Based Alcohol Misuse Prevention Program: A Follow-up Evaluation, *Journal of Studies on Alcohol, 53,* pp. 106–121, 1992.
7. W. B. Hansen, School-Based Substance Abuse Prevention: A Review of the State of the Art in Curriculum, 1980-1990, *Health Education Research, 7,* pp. 403–430, 1992.
8. J. L. Romano, School Personnel Training for the Prevention of Tobacco, Alcohol, and Other Drug Use: Issues and Outcomes, *Journal of Drug Education, 27,* pp. 245–258, 1997.
9. M. M. Johnson, M. W. Lasater, and M. M. Fitzgerald, Paraeducator: Not Just an Aide, *Journal of Staff Development, 18,* pp. 6–11, 1997.
10. F. C. Welch and C. Daniel, Staff Development for Classified Staff: One School District's Approach, *Journal of Staff Development, 18,* pp. 12–15, 1997.
11. H. Hill, D. Piper, and M. King, The Nature of School-Based Prevention Experiences for Middle School Students, *Journal of Health Education,* pp. 15–23, November/December 1993 Supplement.
12. J. O'Connor and B. Saunders, Drug Education: An Appraisal of a Popular Preventive, *The International Journal of the Addictions, 27,* pp. 165–185, 1992.
13. B. Benard, Fostering Resiliency in Kids, *Educational Leadership,* pp. 44–48, November 1993.
14. D. S. Strebnik and M. J. Elias, An Ecological, Interpersonal Skills Approach to Drop-Out Prevention, *American Journal of Orthopsychiatry, 63,* pp. 526–535, 1993.

15. C. L. Fox and S. E. Forbing, *Creating Drug-Free Schools and Communities,* Harper Collins, New York, 1992.
16. M. Falco, *The Making of a Drug-Free America,* Times Books, New York, 1992.
17. J. M. Moskowitz, The Primary Prevention of Alcohol Problems: A Critical Review of the Research Literature, *Journal of Studies on Alcohol, 50,* pp. 54–88, 1989.
18. N. S. Tobler, Drug Prevention Programs Can Work: Research Findings, *Journal of Addictive Diseases, 11,* pp. 1–28, 1992.
19. D. Sztainer-Neumark, M. Storey, S. A. French, and M. D. Resnick, Psychosocial Correlates of Health Compromising Behaviors Among Adolescents, *Health Education Research, 12,* pp. 37–52, 1997.
20. P. Benson, *The Troubled Journey: A Portrait of 6th-12th Grade Youth,* Search Institute, Lutheran Brotherhood, Minneapolis, Minnesota, 1990.
21. *Contract with America's Youth: Toward a National Youth Development Agenda,* American Youth Policy Forum and the Center for Work Force Development (ERIC Document #ED395220), American Youth Policy Forum, 1001 Connecticut Ave. NW, Suite 719, Washington, D.C. 20036–5541, 1995.
22. K. Johnson Pittman, *A New Vision: Promoting Youth Development* [Testimony Before the House Select Committee on Children, Youth and Families], Academy for Educational Development, September 30, 1991.
23. K. A. Moore and D. Glei, Taking the Plunge: An Examination of Positive Youth Development, *Journal of Adolescent Research, 10,* pp. 15–40, 1995.
24. A. Meyer, S. Miller, and M. Herman, Balancing the Priorities of Evaluation with the Priorities of the Setting: A Focus on Positive Youth Development Programs in School Settings, *The Journal of Primary Prevention, 14,* pp. 95–113, 1993.
25. R. M. Robertson, Walking the Talk: Organizational Modeling and Commitment to Youth and Staff Development, *Child Welfare, 76,* pp. 577–589, 1997.
26. J. L. Romano, Evaluation of School Personnel Prevention Training: A Measure of Self-Efficacy, *Journal of Educational Research, 90,* pp. 57–63, 1996.
27. A. Bandura, Self-Efficacy: Toward a Unifying Theory of Behavioral Change, *Psychological Review, 84,* pp. 191–215, 1977.
28. R. E. Sherman, S. Lojkutz, and E. Rusch, An Evaluation of the ADE Program: A Teacher Training Strategy in Alcohol and Drug Education, *Journal of Alcohol and Drug Education, 30,* pp. 66–76, 1984.
29. L. DiCicco, R. Biron, J. Carifio, C. Deutsch, D. J. Mills, R. E. White, and A. Orenstein, Teacher Training in Alcohol Education: Changes Over Three Years, *Journal of Alcohol and Drug Education, 29,* pp. 12–26, 1983.
30. K. M. Anderson and O. Durant, Classified Staff Developers Unite! *Journal of Staff Development, 18,* pp. 18–21, 1997.

Direct reprint requests to:

Dr. John L. Romano
Department of Educational Psychology
University of Minnesota
130 Burton Hall
178 Pillsbury Drive S.E.
Minneapolis, MN 55455

J. DRUG EDUCATION, Vol. 29(4) 387-389, 1999

JOURNAL OF DRUG EDUCATION
Index—Contents of Volume 29, 1999

SUBSTANCE ABUSE PREVENTION:
A Multicultural Perspective
Edited by Snehendu B. Kar

Alcohol, tobacco, and other drugs (ATOD) abuse is a major threat to our health and quality of life. In this volume, nationally recognized substance abuse specialists, public health researchers, and community-based practitioners undertake an in-depth state-of-the-art review of substance abuse prevention intervention from a multicultural perspective.

Special emphasis is on the application of the lessons learned from fields of substance abuse and the new public health paradigm as a modus operandi for ATOD prevention in multicultural communities. The book further makes specific recommendations for prevention policy, research, professional preparation, and effective intervention strategies.

In thirteen chapters, twenty-four authors share their analyses, concerns, and conclusions in several domains including the: meaning and dynamics of multiculturalism affecting prevention intervention, relative risks and knowledge gaps across ethnic groups, social trends affecting health risks and substance abuse, lessons learned from substance abuse research and prevention, role of the media, promises and limits of the new public health paradigm for assessment, policy development, assurance of preventive services, and social action and empowerment for prevention in partnership with the public.

This pioneering volume will serve as a valuable resource to researchers, policy makers, educators, professionals and organizations interested in the health and quality of life of our communities as we approach the 21st century.

Format Information: 6" x 9", 336 pages, ISBN: 0-89503-194-9, $42.00 plus $4.00 postage and handling

Baywood Publishing Company, Inc. 26 Austin Avenue, Amityville, NY 11701
Call (516) 691-1270 Fax (516) 691-1770 **Orderline** (800) 638-7819
e-mail: baywood@baywood.com • **web site:** http://baywood.com

FOCUS ON ALCOHOL

Edited by SEYMOUR EISEMAN

PRIMARY ORIENTATION: prevention of drug misuse
A must for the drug educator

To adequately address and deal with the detrimental effects of alcohol, attempts must be made to learn and understand the motivations and attitudes which contribute to its use and misuse.

This essential collection represents a psychosocial perspective of the effects of alcohol while providing relatively unknown—but central research needed for a comprehensive understanding of the behaviors associated with alcohol use.

Table of Contents
Part I — Theory • Behavioral Intention as an Indicator of Drug and Alcohol Use • Pre-Service Teachers Use of and Attitudes Toward Alcohol and Other Drugs • Relationship Between Alcohol Consumption and Alcohol Problems in Young Adults • The Private Sector: Taking a Role in the Prevention of Drug and Alcohol Abuse for Young People **Part 2 — Research** • Early Onset of Drinking as a Predictor of Alcohol Consumption and Alcohol Related Problems in College • A Short- and Long-Term Evaluation of Here's Looking at You Alcohol Education Program • Evaluating the Effectiveness of a School Drug and Alcohol Prevention Curriculum: A New Look at "Here's Looking at You, Two" • Alcohol Education Research and Practice: A Logical Analysis of the Two Realities Long-Term • Evaluation of a Life Skills Approach for Alcohol and Drug Abuse Prevention • Does Drug and Alcohol Use Lead to Failure to Graduate from High School? Children's • Changing Attitudes Regarding Alcohol: A Cross-Sectional Study • Increased Exposure to Alcohol and Cannabis Education and Changes in Use Patterns **Part 3 — Practice** • Are Drinkers Interested in Inexpensive Approaches to Reduce their Alcohol Use? • Alcohol and Soap Operas: Drinking in the Light of Day • Effects of a Preventive Alcohol Education Program after Three Years • Public Attitudes to and Awareness of Fetal Alcohol Syndrome in Young Adults • College Students' Definitions of Social and Problem Drinking • Teaching Adolescents about Alcohol and Driving: A Two Year Follow-up • Alcohol and Drug Education Programs

Format: 6' x 9", 272 pages, Paper, ISBN: 0-89503-083-7

Price: $35.95 + $4.00 postage and handling

Baywood Publishing Company, Inc.
26 Austin Avenue, Amityville, NY 11701
call (516) 691-1270 **fax** (516) 691-1770 **orderline** (800) 638-7819
e-mail: baywood@baywood.com • **web site:** http://baywood.com

Journal of DRUG EDUCATION

INSTRUCTIONS TO AUTHORS

Submit manuscript to: Dr. Seymour Eiseman, Editor
Department of Health Science
California State University, Northridge
Northridge, CA 91330

Manuscripts are to be submitted in triplicate. Retain one copy, as manuscript will not be returned. Manuscript must be typewritten on 8-1/2" × 11" white paper, one side only, double-spaced, with wide margins. Paginate consecutively starting with the title page. The organization of the paper should be indicated by appropriate headings and subheadings.

Originality Authors should note that only original articles are accepted for publication. Submission of a manuscript represents certification on the part of the author(s) that neither the article submitted, nor a version of it has been published, or is being considered for publication elsewhere.

Abstracts of 100 to 150 words are required to introduce each article.

References should relate only to material cited within text and be listed in numerical order according to their appearance within text. State author's name, title of referenced work, editor's name, title of book or periodical, volume, issue, pages cited, and year of publication. Do not abbreviate titles. Please do not use ibid., op. cit., loc. cit., etc. In case of multiple citations, simply repeat the original numeral. Detailed specifications available from the editor upon request.

Footnotes are placed at the bottom of page where referenced. They should be numbered with superior arabic numbers without parentheses or brackets. Footnotes should be brief with an average length of three lines.

Figures should be referenced in text and appear in numerical sequence starting with Figure 1. Line art must be original drawings in black ink proportionate to our page size, and suitable for photographing. Indicate top and bottom of figure where confusion may exist. Labeling should be 8 point type. Clearly identify all figures. Figures should be drawn on separate pages and their placement within the text indicated by inserting: —Insert Figure 1 here—.

Tables must be cited in text in numerical sequence starting with Table 1. Each table must have a descriptive title. Any footnotes to tables are indicated by superior lower case letters. Tables should be typed on separate pages and their approximate placement indicated within text by inserting: —Insert Table 1 here—.

Authors will receive twenty complimentary reprints of their published article. Additional reprints may be ordered.

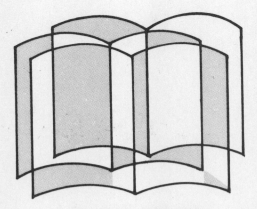